D0437711

1300

Health Care Delivery
in the United States

Steven Jonas

received his M.D. from Harvard and his M.P.H. from Yale. He is an associate professor in the Department of Community Medicine, School of Medicine, State University of New York at Stony Brook.

David Banta

received his M.D. from Duke and his M.P.H. and M.S.Hyg. from Harvard. He is a professional staff member with the Office of Technology Assessment of the U.S. Congress.

Carol McCarthy

received her M.S.H.S.A. from the State University of New York at Stony Brook. She is executive vice president of the Nassau-Suffolk Hospital Council.

Nancy R. Barhydt

received her M.S. from Albany Medical College. She is assistant professor in the Department of Preventive and Community Medicine, and director of the Primary Care Nurse Practitioner Program at Albany Medical College.

Ruth S. Hanft

received her M.A. from Hunter College. She is a visiting professor in the Department of Community Medicine, School of Medicine, Dartmouth College.

Lorrin M. Koran

received his M.D. from Harvard. He is an associate professor in the Department of Psychiatry and Behavioral Science, School of Medicine, State University of New York at Stony Brook.

Michael Enright

received his M.B.A. in Health Care Administration from George Washington University. He is a researcher in the Division of Intramural Research, National Center for Health Services Research, Health Resources Administration, USDHEW. He is also an associate professor in the Graduate Program in Health Service Administration, School of Allied Health Professions, State University of New York at Stony Brook.

Barbara Rimer

received her M.P.H. from the University of Michigan. She is program director for community resources in the Division of Cancer Control and Rehabilitation of the National Cancer Institute.

Health Care Delivery
in the United States

Steven Jonas
and contributors

with a Foreword by
Kurt W. Deuschle

Springer Publishing Company
New York

Copyright © 1977 by Springer Publishing Company, Inc.

All rights reserved

No part of this publication may be reproduced,
stored in a retrieval system, or transmitted, in any form
or by any means, electronic, mechanical, photocopying,
recording, or otherwise, without the prior permission of

Springer Publishing Company, Inc.
200 Park Avenue South
New York, N.Y. 10003

    78 79 80 81 / 10 9 8 7 6 5 4 3 2

For purposes of citation of copyrighted sources,
the credits on pp. xvii–xviii constitute an extension
of this copyright page.

Library of Congress Cataloging in Publication Data
Jonas, Steven.
   Health care delivery in the United States.

   Bibliography: p.
   Includes indexes.
   1. Medical care—United States. I. Title.
[DNLM: 1. Delivery of health care—United States.
2. Health services—United States. W84 AA1 J7h]
RA395.A3J65   362.1′0973   77–3253
ISBN 0–8261–2070–9
ISBN 0–8261–2071–7 pbk.

Printed in the United States of America

To Linda F. Jonas, Sandra S. Banta, Michael P. McCarthy,
Ruth L. Barhydt, Julius Richmond, Stephanie Koran,
Jerry R. Enright, Bernard Glassman,
and to the memory of E. Richard Weinerman

Contents

Foreword

Since World War I our health care delivery system has evolved from one featuring the general physician and the community hospital to one having an incredibly complicated and bewildering array of providers and institutions. The change from a physician-dominated to a systems-oriented model has brought into being a whole new language of health care, and has made health care a focus of nationwide attention and sometimes indignation.

This evolution away from the "family doctor" began slowly in the 1920s, when the technological revolution in medicine was in its early stages. Technological change—which was stimulated by World War II and has grown in quantum leaps ever since—begat specialization, because the vast armamentarium of new drugs and technical procedures made care-giving much more complex than ever before. No longer could the general practitioner handle all health problems, including surgery, and keep up to date on all new knowledge. Thus the superspecialist has come to outstrip the nonspecialist in status and in access to academic and financial rewards. Attention to organ systems, or even one part of an organ, has become the acceptable M.D.-university model.

Not only has the physician become specialized; he has been subsumed into (while remaining dominant over) a complex health team, and the system he works in has become organized into a regionalized referral network of institutions providing varying levels of specialized patient care. The specialist imperative extends to other workers in the system, including those involved in the highly sophisticated technology of, for example, intensive-care units, renal dialysis, and organ transplant centers.

Inevitably this specialization has created an increasing gap in general continuing health care at the community level. There is a serious contradiction between the need to provide basic

health services to the entire population and the specialist imperative resulting from the ever-increasing growth of scientific and
technological knowledge.

As a result, a whole field of community medicine has emerged
to redirect medical attention to general care. In July 1955, Cornell Medical College in New York City and the Navajo Tribal
Council, which governs the 100,000 American Indian Navajo
people, conducted an early experiment in this domain. The project was located in a remote area of the Navajo reservation in
northern Arizona, 90 miles north of the general hospital at Fort
Defiance, Arizona. The experiment was designed to find the most
effective way to provide modern medicine to a culturally different, indigenous population; it was hoped that the lessons learned
could help the U.S. Public Health Service improve the delivery
of general rural health services to Indian people throughout the
nation.

In that period of innocence, our language was informal; we
had little of today's ubiquitous terminology. Thus, although our
program involved "community participation," centered in a
"neighborhood health center," and employed "primary care doctors," "nurse-clinicians," and "community health workers," we
knew none of these terms. We did not speak of ourselves as
"health teams" practicing "community medicine," although, in
current parlance, that is what we were doing.

I use this example to show the rapid development of health
care–systems language and concepts during a 20-year period. In
public health as well as in specialized technology, whole new
principles have been formulated and a whole new vocabulary
invented to describe them.

Because these enormous changes have occurred, both providers
and consumers often have a confused picture of the current health
care delivery system. It is essential that health care education
keep pace with changes in the system, but it has not always
done so.

In this book Dr. Steven Jonas and his coauthors do much to
remedy the lack of basic texts conveying the knowledge required
by present and future decision makers in the health care system.
The book is basically descriptive in nature, examining the various
elements in the delivery system and elucidating their interactions; it succeeds in describing this labyrinthine system lucidly
and comprehensively. It does not neglect the economic ramifica-
tions of an industry that is now second only to defense in the

Gross National Product, nor the political controversies raging over accountability and the right to health care. Importantly, the book is up to date in terminology, and thus will help meet the urgent need of health workers to communicate with one another and with the public at large.

KURT W. DEUSCHLE, M.D.
Professor and Chairman
Department of Community Medicine
Mount Sinai School of Medicine

Preface

Health services, affecting as they do the lives of all of us, have become a major social issue. The rapidly rising costs of health services make them a major economic issue too. There are frequent political debates and innumerable statements of policy. Thus, the main topic of this book—how personal health services are organized and delivered—has come to interest a wide array of professionals, as well as many laypersons.

For these reasons, in describing the health care delivery system in the United States, we do not address ourselves to one specialized audience. The book is designed primarily as a text for introductory courses in health care delivery offered in medical schools, schools of public health, health services administration programs, nursing schools, schools of allied health professions and of social welfare; but it can also be used in such non-health-oriented academic programs as law, architecture, engineering, economics, political science, history, sociology, community planning, and the like.

Moreover, we have attempted to produce an integrated work that can be read by interested persons who are not students, but want to locate in one place the basic, essential information about health care delivery in the United States. We hope that health professionals, lay members of health-related boards, policy makers, observers from abroad, and the concerned general public will find this book useful and enlightening.

We attempt to be reasonably objective in our description of the health care delivery system; this is not intended to be another "health care crisis" book. As we point out in the Introduction, over the years there has been a plethora of such books, many serving a useful purpose. However, we do not believe that there is actually a health care "crisis," as the word is customarily defined; rather, we think that our complex health care delivery system has a number of serious problems, most of which have a long history. In our analysis of the system, we recognize both its good points and its failings. Its outstanding strengths include a large and dedicated manpower pool, a strong institutional base, fine education and research establishments, and a supporting industry that has produced many significant technological advances over the years. Our society now faces the task of attempting to build creatively on the strengths in order to deal with the shortcomings.

The authors do, of course, hold individual opinions and, to a certain extent, a collective point of view. We represent a variety of health care professions, but in our work we are all involved in continuing analysis, evaluation, and program development in one or more parts of the system. In work of this type, one naturally tends more toward involvement with change and reform than toward defense of the status quo: we are aware of the system's strengths, but we are likely to be more directly concerned in our day-to-day work with its weaknesses. Thus, we have allowed ourselves the privilege of "editorializing" from time to time, often critically, without, however, succumbing to the natural temptation to offer our own sweeping prescriptions for change. Based on the facts as they are presented, we feel that readers who are so inclined should be able to develop their own proposals for reform.

We do feel that without some comments from us, however, this book would be very dry indeed. Some readers will undoubtedly feel that we have been too factual, whereas others will think that we have overeditorialized. Nevertheless, we hope that our descriptions are clear enough for the reader to be able to judge for him or herself which of our subjective evaluations are closest to reality.

The reader should note several important technical features in the book. Most tables are from public sources, published on a regular, periodic basis. Part A of Appendix I ("Guide to Sources") briefly describes all of the important sources of health and health care data in the United States, and numbers each source. Each table in the text taken from a source listed in Appendix I is keyed to the Appendix. By using Appendix I, the interested reader can thus find the most recent versions of all tables from public, recurring sources. We hope that this feature will allow the book to remain up to date longer than most textbooks.

Part B of Appendix I lists the important categories of data (population, mortality, health manpower, and so on) ; the reader is told in which sources the data may be found. For example, in Appendix I, Part B, under "Institutions," there is a list of the principal recurring sources of data on health care institutions in the United States, keyed to the source descriptions in Part A.

Even in a book of this size, it is not possible to cover every important topic. In Appendix II, "Additional Topics," the reader will find a few selected references on a number of matters not considered elsewhere.

Most of the chapters have fairly lengthy reference lists. This was done in order to document our material satisfactorily and to provide instructors with an ample selection of supplementary readings, if they wish to use the bibliographies for that purpose.

Please note that in general the male pronouns are used, only because that is the customary mode at this time and because the alternatives—using he/she or changing from male to female pronouns in alternate chapters—are artificial and linguistically cumbersome. We trust that readers will not invest this point of usage with political implications.

Acknowledgments

In part, the genesis of our book is to be found in "The Delivery of Health Care," by Steven Jonas and Victor W. Sidel, Chapter 21 in *Practice of Medicine* (New York: Harper and Row, 1973). Portions of that work appear in this book, particularly in Chapters 2 and 6, and are used with the special permission of Harper and Row. Dr. Sidel's contributions to the earlier chapter are gratefully acknowledged, and the material is used with his permission as well.

Parts of two other chapters have also appeared elsewhere. A portion of Chapter 14 is drawn from "Health Services Research and Health Policy," by David Banta and Patricia Bauman (*Journal of Community Health, 2,* 1976). It appears with permission of the publisher. An excerpt from Chapter 15 appeared in *Medical World* (England) in May 1976.

The material in Chapter 7 attributed to *The American Health Care System,* by John Gordon Freymann, is used with the kind permission of Dr. Freymann and the publisher, Williams & Wilkins, Baltimore (© 1974).

The sections on the Veterans' Administration and the Department of Defense in Chapter 10 are based on material written by James Korjus. We acknowledge his contribution with thanks.

Figure 2.1 is reprinted, with permission, from Kerr White's "Life and Death in Medicine," Copyright © September 1973 by Scientific American, Inc. All rights reserved.

Figure 2.2 is reprinted, with permission, from the *Medical Care Chart Book*, 5th edition, 1972, Department of Medical Care Organization, School of Public Health, University of Michigan, Ann Arbor.

This book could not have been produced without the help of many people. For reading, commenting on, and helping with the preparation of various chapters, we would like to thank

Patricia Bauman, Martha Blaxall, James Brindle, Helen Burnside, Robert Carroll, Tom Christoffel, Barbara Cohen, Kathleen Dolan, H. Jack Geiger, Bernard Glassman, Frederick Jerome, Howard Kelman, Marvin Leeds, Raymond Lerner, Thomas Mann, Joyce Page, Ian Porter, Wanda Robinson, Ruth Roemer, Joshua Sanes, Richard Seggel, Milton Terris, John Thompson, and Andre Varma. We received valuable help from student assistants. Among them are Charles Andrews, Daniel Ricciardi, Harold Rosenthal, and Zakhar Spektor.

Many people participated in the typing and we are grateful to them all. The heroic dedication of Eleanor Lindwall and Eugenia DiGirolamo in the editor's office deserves special mention. They typed, and retyped, not only the editor's own chapters but also the entire manuscript. Their participation proved invaluable.

Our editors at Springer Publishing Co., Ellen Tumposky and Isabel Stein, were able, despite little direct knowledge of this rather technical field, to find that fine line between doing too much and too little. In their hands, on many occasions, ponderousness gave way to brevity and grace.

Our publisher, Ursula Springer, reviewed every chapter in detail. Her suggestions were very helpful. More important, however, in accepting our book for publication in the first place, Dr. Springer demonstrated her faith that a group of generally young, generally unknown authors could produce something of value. We hope that with this work we have justified her faith.

Finally, we gratefully acknowledge that the publication of this manuscript was assisted by a grant from the Josiah Macy, Jr., Foundation.

Health Care Delivery
in the United States

1

Introduction

Steven Jonas

The State of Health Care Delivery in the U.S.

Over 40 years ago, a study of health care delivery in the United States summarized its findings in these terms:

> The problem of providing satisfactory medical service to all the people of the United States at costs which they can meet is a pressing one. At the present time, many persons do not receive service which is adequate either in quantity or quality, and the costs of service are inequably distributed. The result is a tremendous amount of preventable physical pain and mental anguish, needless deaths, economic inefficiency, and social waste. Furthermore, these conditions are, as the following pages will show, largely unnecessary. The United States has the economic resources, the organizing ability, and the technical experience to solve this problem. (Committee on the Costs of Medical Care, p. 2)

So commenced the final report of the Committee on the Costs of Medical Care, published in 1932. The committee, chaired by Ray Lyman Wilbur, a past president of the American Medical Association (AMA), had been appointed in 1928 by President Herbert Hoover to look into problems of health care delivery. Strikingly, the statement is entirely applicable to our current health care system.

Observers of the U.S. health care system in the 1960s and 1970s often spoke in terms of "crisis." For example, in 1970 the editors of *Fortune* said:

> American medicine, the pride of the nation for many years, stands now on the brink of chaos. To be sure, our medical practitioners have their great moments of drama and triumph. But much of U.S. medical care, particularly the everyday business of

1

preventing and treating routine illnesses, is inferior in quality, wastefully dispensed, and inequitably financed. Medical manpower and facilities are so maldistributed that large segments of the population, especially the urban poor and those in rural areas, get virtually no care at all—even though their illnesses are most numerous and, in a medical sense, often easy to cure. (1970, p. 9)

In a similar vein, Senator Edward M. Kennedy, speaking to an audience of doctors in New York City in 1971, said: "America is beginning to realize that we have a health care crisis on our hands, and that the magnitude of the crisis is enormous. . . . I challenge even the most reactionary pillars of organized medicine, even the most affluent physicians in the most affluent suburbs of this rich city, to deny that a crisis exists, or that it exists for all Americans—not just the poor, not just the black, but each and every one of us" (Klaw, p. xi).

In 1968, an article called "Crisis in American Medicine" in the British journal *The Lancet* began:

In terms of gross national product the U.S.A. spends more on health than does any other country. But costs are rising at such a rate that more and more people will find it difficult to get complete health care. This particularly applies to the poor, the old, the Negroes, and other disadvantaged groups. Doctors and hospital beds are distributed most unevenly both in broad geographic regions and between States. There are indications, too, that the quality of care has been inferior, especially in terms of antenatal and infant mortality. The whole organization of medical care in the U.S.A. has failed to respond to changing disease patterns, the move from country to cities, industrialization, and the increasing proportion of old people in the population. (Battistella and Southby)

There have been many other reports in recent years (*Fortune;* Moskin; National Commission on Community Health Services; Report of the Health Citizens' Board of Inquiry; Kennedy; Ribicoff; Ehrenreich and Ehrenreich; Schorr; Klaw). Milton Roemer has cited a series of critical studies going back many years.*

* Roemer listed these studies as follows:

"Every few years, more recently in the last decade, there appears a book analyzing the serious defects of health care in America. In 1927, Harry H. Moore produced *American Medicine and the*

Social critics are not alone in holding negative views. Eliot Richardson, one of the Secretaries of the United States Department of Health, Education and Welfare (USDHEW) in the Nixon Administration, said in Senate testimony:

> In general our critical health problems today do not arise because the health of our people is worsening, or because expenditures on health care have been niggardly, or because we have been negligent as a Nation in developing health care resources, or because we have been unconcerned about providing financial protection against ill-health. We must look elsewhere. I should like to suggest that our present concern is a function of two broad problems. The first is the inequality in health status and care, and in access to financing. The other is the pervasive problem of rising medical costs. . . . The impressive growth in the number of people covered by health insurance conceals the fact that only 29 percent of all personal health expenditures were paid by insurance in 1968. The indices of general improvement in health pale in importance when we look behind them and see that the poor and non-Whites are doing far worse than whites and those with decent incomes. . . . When we look beyond our borders and compare ourselves with other nations, any sense of accomplishment over our long-run gains in health status is mitigated by the fact that other advanced nations are doing better than we are. . . . These disparities point to a gap between what we have accomplished and what remains to be accomplished, between our achievements and our expectations, between what is and our impatience for what might be. . . .

On the other hand, some observers—the American Medical Association for example—vehemently deny that a crisis exists:

> The constantly improving American health system is the best in

---

People's Health, in the 1930's were the magnificent 27 volumes of the Committee on the Costs of Medical Care, in 1939 there was James Rorty's *American Medicine Mobilizes,* and in 1940 Hugh Cabot's *The Patient Dilemma*. After World War II Carl Malmberg wrote *140 Million Patients* in 1947, Michael Davis wrote *Medical Care for Tomorrow* in 1955, and Richard Carter wrote *The Doctor Business* in 1958. In 1965 there was Selig Greenberg's excellent *The Troubled Calling: Crisis in the Medical Establishment.* The year after Medicare, 1966, saw two critical outputs: *The American Health Scandal* by Raul Tunley and *The Doctors* by Martin L. Gross. In 1967 there was Fred J. Cook's *Plot Against the Patient* and in 1970 Ed Cray's *In Failing Health.*" (1972)

the world and must not be stifled by adopting a government-
controlled national health insurance program, the American
Medical Association told Congress.

AMA President Max H. Parrott, testifying before Congress,
said: "When considering a national plan for this country, it is
necessary to take cognizance of the strengths of our own method
of health care delivery . . . this will assure that our excellent
system will continue to improve and will not suffer the stifling
effects experienced in other countries." He further stated, "American medical service and technology have developed at an unparal-
leled rate . . . presently there is more and better medical technology here than anywhere else in the world." (*American Medical
News*, November 17, 1975)

And in 1972, in his book *The Case for American Medicine*,
journalist Harry Schwartz wrote that cries of "crisis" were just
so much hyperbole; United States medicine has been doing an
outstanding job, and new research and sociological change is
needed to improve the nation's health further.

The debate, then, has centered on the soundness of the system,
whether it is moribund or dynamic, whether it is "in crisis" or
whether it is on the contrary smoothly functioning and effective.
In our opinion, available statistical data, data from quantitative
research, and descriptive analysis confirm that major problems
confront the health care system: rising costs; financial and other
barriers to care; geographic maldistribution of manpower and
facilities; overspecialization of providers; overutilization of hospitals; deficiencies in quality and quality control; a tendency,
particularly among physicians, to stress the unusual at the
expense of the commonplace; barriers to provider-patient communication; training and educational programs and research
undertakings that are not always directly relevant to patient
needs; an emphasis on treatment rather than prevention; and an
orientation toward patients with acute, physical problems at the
expense of patients who are chronically ill or have mental problems.

However, few if any of these problems are new; over time they
have simply undergone gradual changes in magnitude. Indeed,
many of the major problems considered by the Committee on the
Costs of Medical Care and still pressing today originated in our
country and those of our European forebears in the seventeenth,
eighteenth, and nineteenth centuries (Freymann, 1974, Sections
I, II). Thus it is not quite accurate to say we face a "crisis" in

health care. Our health care delivery system has serious problems with deep historical roots embedded in the whole fabric of American society. This fact should not be a cause for complacency, however. As modern medical practice itself illustrates, it is often easier to deal with a crisis, even a major one, than with long-standing, chronic problems. Nevertheless, with its enormous resources, its dedicated health manpower pool, and its talent for problem-solving, the United States should be equal to the task.

In this book we undertake the difficult task of describing our health care delivery system. The United States presents a particular problem in this regard: in most industrialized countries there is a Ministry of Health that plays a central role in financing and operations and that often provides a framework for the various components of the system. The Ministry may not directly operate the system, but at least it creates the structure within which the system functions. In the United States, however, no such central organizational structure exists. There is of course a system; there are loci of power and control; but they are difficult to recognize and to describe.

In order to delineate the shape of this rather amorphous system, we will deal with the major components of any health care delivery system: the people for whom it provides care; the people who provide the care; the institutions and organizational structures within which they work; the financing mechanisms that allow the first three components to interact; and the government under which the system functions.

What Is Health Care and Who Is Served?

The United States has one of the largest populations in the world, approaching 215,000,000 in 1976. The population is aging: the proportion of persons 65 and over is approximately 10%. Many ethnic and national groups are represented. There is a broad range of social classes and large income differentials exist. Non-white persons are represented in the lower social class and income groups in a proportion greater than their representation in the total population. Unemployment, or the threat of it, substandard housing, and dysnutrition are major socioeconomic problems in rural as well as urban areas.

The crude death rate in 1976 approached 9 per 1,000 population and the infant mortality rate approached 15 per 1,000 live births. The major causes of death are heart disease, cancer, stroke, and accidents. The major causes of morbidity are upper respiratory infections, influenza, injuries, heart conditions, arthritis, impairments of the lower limbs, impairments of the back and spine, asthma and hay fever, and mild emotional disorders.

In Chapter 2 ("What Is Health Care?"), we discuss what constitutes health, disease, and illness, and consider the efficacy and utility of the several types of health services. In Chapter 3 ("Data for Health and Health Care"), we present the principal quantitative measures used to describe the population, its health and illness levels, how it uses the health care system, and how the health care system functions. Thus the reader is introduced to the first and most important component of any health care delivery system, the people whom it serves.

Inputs to the System

The more than 4,000,000 people who work in the health care delivery system may be divided into three major groups: independent practitioners, dependent practitioners, and supporting staff, although the lines between the groups are at times unclear. The largest manpower categories are the nurses, clerical staff, hospital manual workers, physicians, dentists, pharmacists, and technicians. The physicians, of whom over 300,000 are active, are the dominant group. Indeed, as shall be seen in later chapters, this dominance is guaranteed by law.

The principal mode of physician organization is private practice. Excluding hospital house staff in training, about 80% of all physicians in active practice are in private practice. This means that they are self-employed private entrepreneurs, administratively responsible to no one but themselves. Since physicians are in a controlling position in the delivery of care, this mode of physician organization is one of the major features of the U.S. health care delivery system.

Chapter 4 ("Health Manpower") provides basic information on supply, types, distribution, and education of health workers. There is not space in a book of this type to give due consideration to all of the categories of health worker. However, Chapter 5 ("Nursing") is entirely devoted to the single largest health care provider group; it discusses nursing roles and functions, current issues in nursing, and key aspects of the relationships between nurses and other categories of providers. It is an example of the kind of analysis that can be carried out for each and every health manpower type.

Since physicians are the dominant manpower group, they receive the most attention throughout the book. Aspects of their work are discussed in chapters that deal primarily with the organization/institutional and financing sectors. More detail on the distribution and functions of physicians can be found in Chapter 6 ("Ambulatory Care") and Chapter 7 ("Hospitals"). Certain special aspects of the work of health care personnel are presented in Chapter 8, "Mental Health Services." In Chapter 13 ("Measurement and Control of the Quality of Medical Care") the licensing system is discussed, along with the various modes of regulation and quality control that pertain to all health care personnel.

Various types of institutions provide health care services. The most frequently used type of care is ambulatory—care provided to patients other than in institutional beds. About 80% of ambulatory care is delivered in private doctors' offices; other sites include hospital ambulatory services, group practices, neighborhood health centers, and health department health centers. The most common loci for ambulatory care are described in Chapter 6.

Of the institutions housing and caring for patients in bed, hospitals are the most numerous. In the United States, there are more than 7,000, with more than 1.5 million beds. They are categorized in a variety of ways: by ownership, size, function, and average length of stay. There are three principal types of ownership: government (federal, state, and local), private not-for-profit (voluntary), and private for-profit (proprietary). There are four functional categories for hospitals in the United States: general, tuberculosis, mental, and other special. The American Hospital Association also defines the "community hospital": a nonfederal short-term general or other special hospital. It is the predominant type in the United States. The basic descriptive material on hospitals is presented in Chapter 7. Mental hospitals are discussed in Chapter 8 ("Mental Health Services"); other government hospitals are touched upon in Chapter 10, while certain aspects of regulation of hospitals are considered in Chapter 12 ("Planning for Health Care") and Chapter 13, on quality control.

The principal category of institution for inpatients other than hospitals is the nursing home, primarily long-term care facilities for the aged. There are more than 20,000 of these institutions with over 1.2 million beds. They are considered briefly in Chapter 7.

Institutions for education and research in the health sciences are also important. Issues in health sciences education are considered in Chapter 4 ("Health Manpower"), Chapter 5 ("Nursing"), and Chapter 13. Chapter 14 deals with policy issues in both biomedical and health services research.

American medical practice is organized primarily along the lines of the private entrepreneurial model. Medical care is mainly provided on the basis of a private, direct contract (usually unwritten), between physician and patient, even when the source of payment is not the patient. Since medical care—that is, the treatment of sick persons by physicians—is the focus of the United States health care delivery system, and since medical care is provided primarily on a private basis, the organizational framework of the health care system is rudimentary compared to that found in other countries. The care provided by health care institutions themselves is discussed in Chapters 6, 7, 8, and 10.

Financing

In the fiscal year 1975, the United States spent over 8% of its Gross National Product on health care services. Expenditures on health care surpass the total GNP of most other countries in the world. Health care costs rise more rapidly than most other categories of consumer spending in the United States. Ultimately, of course, all money paid for health services comes from the people. However, there are three major means by which money is transferred from the people to the providers: government (about 40% of total expenditures), insurance companies (about 25% of the total), and direct payment (about 35% of the total). Government expenditures are both for services that it operates directly and for services obtained by patients from independent providers, in which case government is a third-party payor. The two major factors in the insurance mode of financing are Blue Cross/Blue Shield (not-for-profit) and the commercial (for-profit) companies, which share almost equally over 90% of the premium flow.

The major recipients of funds are the hospitals (39%), physicians (19%), dentists (6%), nursing homes (8%), and the drug companies (9%). The vast majority of health care personnel are paid on salary, although the independent practitioners are usually paid on a fee-for-service basis. Institutions for the most part operate on a global budget, or a cost-reimbursement basis.

Chapter 9 ("Financing Health Care") considers these matters in depth, while Chapter 15, on national health insurance, looks at the implication of NHI for health care financing and of the present system of financing for NHI.

Government, Policy-Making, Quality, and the Future

Although the government operates no piece of the health care system in its entirety by itself, it is closely involved in one way or another in all of them: collecting and disseminating information, training personnel, operating institutions, providing services, participating in financing, supporting and carrying out research, planning, evaluating, and regulating. Some aspects of government activities in health care delivery are covered in the chapters on personnel, institutions, and financing. In Chapters 10 through 14 we look at some of the various functions of government not considered in earlier chapters.

In Chapter 10, we describe the major government activities in the delivery of personal health and medical services. Chapter 11 describes the process by which health and health care policies and legislation are developed in the United States Congress, as an example of the role of legislatures in the health care delivery system.

We then proceed to examine several important functions of the health care system in which government plays a critical, although not exclusive role: planning, quality control, and research. Chapter 12 considers the health care planning process and the major pieces of federal legislation that have appeared over time. Chapter 13 discusses the problems of quality assessment and regulation.

Biomedical and health services research constitute an essential component of the life-blood of the health care delivery system. We do not examine the vast fields of research per se, but in Chapter 14 we do describe the process by which research policy decisions are made, particularly at the federal government level.

National health insurance, by its very name, means government participation at one or more jurisdictional levels throughout the country in the health care financing system. Chapter 15 first traces the history of proposals for NHI in the United States, then examines the major policy issues in NHI in the mid-70s and the positions of the major interest groups on them. Finally, it considers the relationship between NHI and health.

In the course of our book we offer some suggestions for change but do not propose a single plan for reform (or for revolution). We hope that after assimilating the facts as we see them and present them, the reader will be able to develop his or her own conclusions about what is to be done.

References

American Medical News. "AMA Hits Federal NHI Plans." November 17, 1975, p. 1.
American Medical News. "The Case for American Medicine. Chapter II: What Health Crisis? From the New Book by Harry Schwartz." October 16, 1972.
Battistella, R., and Southby, R. McK. "Crisis in American Medicine." *The Lancet,* March 16, 1968, p. 581.
Business Week. "The $60-billion Crisis over Medical Care." January 17, 1970.
Committee on the Costs of Medical Care. *Medical Care for the American People.* Chicago, Ill.: University of Chicago Press, 1932. Reprinted, Washington, D.C.: USDHEW, 1970.
Ehrenreich, B., and Ehrenreich, J. *The American Health Empire: Power, Profits, and Politics.* New York: Vintage Books, 1971.
Fortune. Our Ailing Medical System: It's Time to Operate. New York: Harper and Row, Perennial Library, 1970.
Freymann, J. G. *The American Health Care System: Its Genesis and Trajectory.* New York: Medcom Press, 1974.
Harper's Magazine. "The Crisis in American Medicine." October, 1960, pp. 123–168.
Kennedy, E. M. *In Critical Condition.* New York: Simon and Schuster, 1972.
Klaw, S. *The Great American Medicine Show.* New York: The Viking Press, 1975.
Moskin, J. R. "The Challenge to Our Doctors." *Look,* November 3, 1964, p. 26.
National Commission on Community Health Services. *Health Is a Community Affair.* Cambridge, Mass.: Harvard University Press, 1966.
Report of the Citizens Board of Inquiry into Health Services for Americans. *Heal Yourself.* Washington, D.C., 1971.
Report on the Health Task Force of the Urban Coalition. *Rx for Action.* Washington, D.C., 1969.
Ribicoff, A., with Danaceau, P. *The American Medical Machine.* New York: Saturday Review Press, 1972.

What Are "Health" and "Disease"?

The philosophical distinction between health and disease goes back to antiquity. As Henry Sigerist (p. 57) points out, "the [ancient Greek] physicians had an explanation for health. Health, they believed, was a condition of perfect equilibrium. When the forces or humors or whatever constituted the human body were perfectly balanced, man was healthy. Disturbed balance resulted in disease. This is still the best general explanation we have." However, the cult of Asklepios concentrated on disease and miracle cures, and, with the rise of Christianity, the idea of disease was given a preferential place. The Greek ideal of health as a perfect balance had little meaning to the masses of that day, living as they did in poverty, sickness, and oppression. Later, scientific medicine began to develop, but the idea of miracle cures persisted, as it does in present-day medicine. It is a seductive dream: a cure that can compensate for the abuses the individual and society have perpetuated, correcting at a stroke the effects of smoking or of breathing polluted air or of eating saturated fats over a period of years.

Webster's Unabridged Dictionary reflects the conflict, defining health as "physical and mental well-being," but continuing, "freedom from defect, pain, or disease." Health statistics, of course, are actually disease statistics, and health care is often disease care. Jago lists 43 usages of "health" as an adjective, most of which add to the confusion. Examples include "health status," "health center," and "health worker."

The World Health Organization defines health as a "state of complete physical, mental, and social well-being, and not merely the absence of disease or infirmity" (World Health Organization). This definition has been criticized as being utopian (Dubos) and is certainly not measurable. Nonetheless, the concept of health as a positive rather than a neutral state is significant.

Disease is also frequently defined rather ambiguously. Webster's suggests "uneasiness or distress," and, more sweepingly, "any departure from health." Blakiston's *New Gould Medical Dictionary*, quoted by an authority in the field, terms disease "a failure of the adaptive mechanisms of an organism to counteract adequately the stimuli and stresses to which it is subject, resulting in a disturbance in function or structure of some part of the body" (Clark, p. 4).

More recent definitions of health have stressed life functioning, seeing health as the "state of optimum capacity for effective performance of valued tasks" (Parsons, 1958, p. 168) or as "personal fitness for survival and self-renewal, creative social adjustment, and self-fulfillment. The most exacting test of one's health is to stay alive and to retain the capacity for self-repair and self-renewal" (Hoyman, p. 189). This trend underlies the growing development of health status indices. Although the early health status indices focused on mortality and morbidity, Bush and Fanshel have developed a promising functional index. Such an index becomes particularly important as government funding of health care increases. Cost-consciousness, along with an emphasis on evaluation, will inevitably develop because of the need to justify the expenditures of tax monies. If health is the ultimate goal of health services, then evaluation of health care activities is dependent on valid and reliable indicators of health.

Biological Factors in Health

Health is generally conceived of as a biological state. It is obviously dependent upon biological factors. Genetic endowment of the individual is the starting point, but health is to a large extent the result of the complex interaction of this soma with the environment. The environment comprises physical surroundings, social factors (largely beyond the control of the individual), and personal life-style.

The environment is a crucial determinant of health. In 1857 the tuberculosis death rate in Massachusetts was 450 per 100,000; by 1890, the figure had fallen to 250; by 1920 to 114; and by 1938 to 35.6 (Sigerist, 1970, p. 46). Yet the first specific antituberculosis therapy was not in general use until after 1938 —convincing evidence that the prevalence of a disease can decline dramatically without effective medical care, probably owing to environmental factors.

An analysis of falling death rates and rising populations in England and Wales for the last 140 years has shown that the changes considerably preceded any direct medical intervention (McKeown, pp. 27–50). Improvements in water supplies and sewage disposal began about 1870, but there was a large reduction in infectious disease deaths, including deaths from tuberculosis, between 1840 and 1870. He concludes that a better food supply, with concomitant improved nutrition, was the prime factor. By the time specific therapeutic agents were available against microorganisms during the 1930s, death rates from several major infectious diseases had fallen to relatively low levels compared to Western European rates in the 1800s. Diseases caused by microorganisms have been the scourge of man throughout recorded history, and have been the largest biological determinant of death and disability. Now, although infectious diseases persist, they are of limited importance for most of the population of the United States. Figure 2.1 shows different categories of disease along with their impact on death, hospital admissions, and activity. Diseases of the circulatory system account for more than 50% of the deaths in the United States annually. But the most important cause of limitation of activity is apparently disease of the musculoskeletal system, including arthritis. Overall, chronic diseases have become the most prevalent and troublesome.

Chronic disease is largely dependent on biological factors as well, although no specific etiology such as a microorganism can be identified for most such conditions (Lalonde). The importance of genetic factors to the basic biological makeup of the individual is being recognized, and it is becoming increasingly apparent that congenital causes of sickness, disability, and death have been relatively unresponsive to changes in environment and in medical care. But the role of environmental factors is receiving the greatest attention. We now know beyond question that diet, air and water pollution, occupational hazards, and cigarette smoking are critical in the genesis of chronic disease. For example, epidemiological studies indicate that up to 90% of cancers may be environmentally induced by just such factors (Schneiderman; Higginson).

The essential point is that the interaction between genetic factors and the environment in producing individual disease is enormously complex, and much research is needed to elucidate the relationship.

Perceptual Factors in Health

It is crucial to recognize that there are different perceptions of what constitutes health and illness (R. White). The stimuli that affect behavior range from vague feelings of uneasiness to severe pain. Although health care providers react quickly to a patient's pain, they often tend to dismiss the vague anxieties of careseekers unless physiological evidence can be found. However, such vague feelings are often indicative of real disease: it has been shown that such self-perceptions and symptoms predicted mortal-

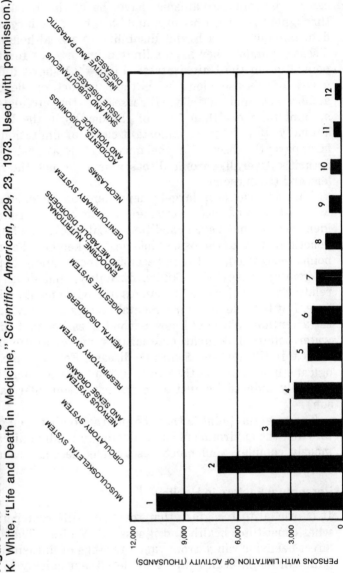

Figure 2.1. Disease categories: their impact on activity, hospital admissions, and death. (*Source:* K. White, "Life and Death in Medicine," *Scientific American*, 229, 23, 1973. Used with permission.)

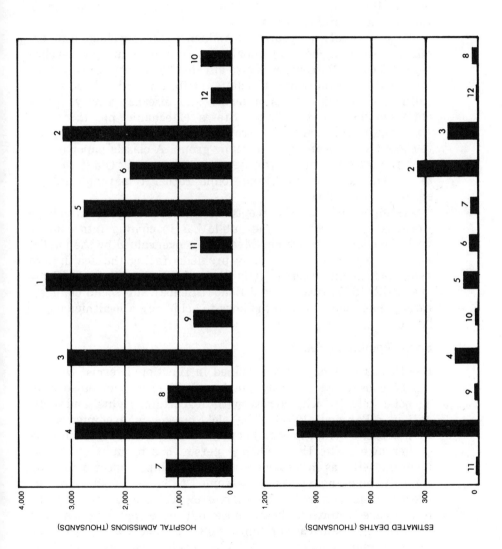

HOSPITAL ADMISSIONS (THOUSANDS)

ESTIMATED DEATHS (THOUSANDS)

17

ity over an 11-year period (Daly and Tyroler) and that symptomatic cancer patients do much worse than matched controls without such symptoms (Feinstein). This seems to indicate that self-
perceptions have more validity than the medical profession has
been willing to grant them, and points up one area in which medical practice is still ignorant.

An individual's perception is influenced by physiologic determinants such as chemical imbalances or hunger and by psychological factors. Perception is also affected by sociocultural factors
influencing the individual's beliefs, attitudes, and values. Other
cultures have conceptions of health and disease entirely different from those of the United States (Mechanic, pp. 129–130).
And even in this country, perception of disease varies according
to class (Koos; Kunitz) and ethnic group. A classic paper examined the meaning of pain in Jews, Italians, and "Old Yankees"
in an American hospital, and found rather remarkable differences (Zaborowski).

An important part of perceptual influences on health in today's
world is the expectation the public has in coming into contact
with the health care system. Medicine is overvalued by the public,
and this is at the root of many problems facing the health care
field, such as malpractice. It is likely that "right living" (Breslow, 1972, 1975; Breslow and Belloc; Belloc) and social changes,
rather than medicine, are the keys to achieving a healthier population.

Social Factors in Health

Health has previously been defined in functional terms. Disease
can be considered to be dysfunctional. Sickness can be seen as
a social role, which carries with it certain rights and obligations (Parsons, 1951). The sick person is exempted from
normal social obligations and is not considered responsible for his
or her own state. Even when a person has brought an illness
upon himself—as in a careless accident or lung cancer caused by
cigarette smoking—he is not assumed to be responsible for the
process of getting well. With increasing cost-consciousness in the
health care sector, one hears more and more that a person who
has brought his disease on himself should somehow pay a higher
price. A smoker might pay a higher health insurance premium,
for example, or even be denied coverage under a national health
insurance program. This proposal seems to be dangerous and
inhumane. First, knowledge is not perfect enough to enable us to

make such clear-cut causal determinations. But that point aside, the logical extreme of this position is to deny care to those responsible for their own disease state unless they can pay for it; such a policy would lead to a class-bound system of health care perhaps even more pernicious than the one we have now.

The sick role also entails responsibilities. The sick person is expected to cooperate in his treatment and to return to normal functioning as soon as possible (Parsons, 1951). The physician shares his society's disdain for hypochondriacs, who are felt to be using illness symptoms to gain special status.

The role of value systems and social structures is evident, as the example of other countries helps to make clear. People in developing countries may suffer from malaria or schistosomiasis without assuming the sick role or considering themselves sick (Susser). Every physician is familiar with patients who function well despite organic disease that should be incapacitating. A renowned physician described his long-standing competition with a famous faith-healer, some of whose patients go back to a functional status despite quite severe disease (Stead). The physician or other health care provider can also assume this healer's role of encouraging independence. In short, health is a relative, not an absolute, concept.

Society has increasingly viewed the medical profession as acting at the organic level in curing and preventing disease. But medicine must also function at the psychological level, giving reassurance to those who seek help, and at the social level, legitimizing the sick role. Further, society's categorization of health and disease changes over time. Within recent memory, social problems such as suicide and attempted suicide and drug addiction have been redefined, and are now considered to be illnesses (Mechanic, pp. 192–194). This broader conception of ill health carries dangers (Szasz; Illich) : for example, psychiatrists play an increasing role in the courts, where a person may be considered to be insane and locked up indefinitely. Psychiatry seems particulary prone to abuse in such ways (Mechanic, pp. 192–194).

Personal and Community Health Services

Given our broad definition of health, we may examine health services in a broad context as well. Health services have been defined as those services delivered by personnel engaged in medical occupations, such as physicians and nurses, plus other personnel working under their supervision; the physical capital involved, such as hospitals; and the other goods and services, such as drugs and bandages (Fuchs, 1966). Weinerman (1971) defines the health services system as "all of the activities of a society which are designed to protect or restore health, whether directed to the individual, the community, or the environment."

A critical distinction must be made between health care and medical care. Medical care is generally thought of as that care provided by a physician. It is generally restricted in scope, focusing on pathophysiological and social problems, and contains a strong element of "caring."

Health and health care services may generally be divided into two broad categories: personal and community. Personal health care services, familiar to everyone, deal directly with individuals for the maintenance of health or the control or cure of illness. Community health services are directed toward groups, not discrete individuals. The public today takes pure drinking water and sewage disposal for granted, but pure water has probably had a greater impact on health than any factor except nutrition. Other community health services include solid waste disposal; food, milk and drug control and inspection; fluoridation of water; and control of air and noise pollution.

A number of health services—which we call "combined" services—have aspects of both community and personal health services. Mass immunization programs, by protecting each immunized individual, protect the community as a whole. "Herd-immunity" makes epidemics impossible. This is especially true of diseases caused by obligatory human parasites, like the now-eradicated smallpox virus. Other such combined community and individual services include tuberculosis and venereal disease case-finding and treatment programs, which gradually reduce the total number of sources of infection to healthy persons, and thus contribute to community health.

A definition of health care must take into account its boundaries and its providers. If health is to have a functional definition, stressing the positive, health care must in some way affect outcomes, by having an active role in improving or assisting in social functioning. Rudolph Virchow, the great German pathologist, fought on the barricades against Bismarck's government as a youth, and described his profession with these well-known words: "Medicine is a social science and politics is nothing else but medicine on a large scale" (Sigerist, p. 93). Should the physician be a revolutionary? Drs. Che Guevara and Salvador

Allende thought so, but most physicians have seen their main task as helping people with their immediate ills. Yet in a day when cancer is the second greatest cause of death in the United States, and 40% of cancer could probably be controlled by changing the environment (Lilienfeld), can the physician stand by, merely providing personal care and ignoring a work place exposing his patients to carcinogens, or a refinery whose fumes may be causing cancer? There is no easy answer to such a question.

There is also the danger, alluded to in the previous section, of defining health care too broadly, so as to encompass all areas of life. The patient generally initiates contact, seeking skilled assistance, and must be assumed to be in control of his overall life. But increasingly medicine is fostering a dependency role (Mechanic, pp. 15, 169), a situation made more acute in an era of chronic disease, where patients need care at frequent intervals for a period of years. Illich (1974) is particularly concerned about the social iatrogenesis that develops, with an individual losing control over his own life. The public has already lost sight of the fact that its own health behavior has far more impact on its health than medical care. There is also a risk in the tendency to broaden the definition of mental illness, thus taking away an individual's autonomy and personhood by calling him or her sick (Szasz). Health care could become a tyranny. For this reason, a somewhat limited definition seems more desirable.

The question of who provides health care is closely related to its definition. There are more than 12 health workers for every physician in the United States, yet when most people think of health care, they think of physicians. If health care is to live up to a dynamic definition, the contributions of such providers as social workers and medical administrators will need to be recognized by both the public and the health workers themselves. Physicians have perhaps been slowest to acknowledge these contributions; yet they too are beginning to be aware of the importance of team work in health care, and of the need for special efforts to foster such team work. At least one project is under way to train health care providers to be effective team members (Wise).

Health Care as a Right

As early as 1787, Thomas Jefferson said: "Without health there is no happiness. An attention to health, then, should take the place of every other object" (R. White). With the growing

affluence of the United States, this seems to be an idea whose time
has come. Although high quality health care is certainly not
available at present to the entire population, it is generally
accepted that this country is in the process of putting the concept
into operation.

This idea of "health care as a right" is different from "health
as a right." Health is first and foremost the concern of the individual: he can strive for it, but the health care system cannot give it
to him. However, health *care* for all is a realizable goal.

The United States has been slow, however, to take the necessary steps. Up to the time of the enactment of Medicare in 1965,
no unit of government had taken general responsibility for
aiding nonindigent individuals when they were ill (R. White).
The roots of this inattention can be found in the American ethic
of freedom and equality. Harlow (R. White, p. 56) says it well:
"There has been a stubborn insistence on protecting the individual's freedom by making him responsible for his own tragedy."

A significant percentage of people in the United States can be
said to have a right to health care already. More than 150 million
people have work-related health insurance, including more than 5
million enrolled in prepaid comprehensive group practices
(Banta and Bosch). Of course, a time of high unemployment
points out the fallacy of using this mechanism to assure access to
health care. In addition, in 1975 about 20 million elderly people
had a right to care under the Medicare program, and about 25
million poor people had such a right through Medicaid. However,
the Social Security Administration estimated that in 1975 there
were 41 million people with no health insurance of any kind
(Mueller). Even those who have chosen not to buy health insurance must be covered by a compulsory program. In a just and
humane society, one does not turn a sick person away from a hospital for lack of health insurance.

Many who endorse the concept of health care for everyone are
unsure how to put it into effect. Dr. Hanlin's prescription, "The
best care—to everybody—now" (R. White, p. 66) is appealing,
but, as a later chapter will make clear, "best care" is difficult to
define. It is simply not feasible to make available everything any
individual could want at all times. Likewise, health care providers cannot have everything they want to do a good job. Limits
must be set to avoid falling into the "bottomless pit" of medical
expenditure.

The Value We Place on Health

It is commonly felt among health professonals that all possible services should be provided by a health system. But are people willing to support health services to that extent? Health is certainly an important value, but it is not the only value. Achilles recognized this in the *Iliad*: "Either, if I stay here and fight beside the city of the Trojans, my return home is gone, but my glory shall be everlasting; but if I return home to the beloved land of my fathers, the excellence of my glory is gone, but there will be a long life left for me, and my end in death will not come to me quickly" (*Iliad* of Homer, p. 209). Achilles chose to stay and die. The modern analogue might be the skydiver or skier who intentionally takes a risk for the sake of the thrill he derives from the sport. To the extent that the public is aware of risk factors, one could say that the person who smokes cigarettes, eats saturated fats, or refuses to wear seat belts is deciding that other values are more important than good health.

Society can invest more in justice, beauty, or knowledge, just as it invests in health (Fuchs, 1974). The yearly federal budget is to a large extent a reflection of the values and choices of society and its leaders. The aggregated requests of the health programs in the Department of Health, Education, and Welfare would far exceed the approximately $28 billion budget allocated for those health programs in 1975. Health economists deal with this problem of limited resources by speaking of marginal benefit and marginal cost. Is the added benefit—of a day in the hospital, for example—worth the added cost?

Every practicing physician confronts conflicting values every day in his practice. A person may be fully knowledgeable about the risks of smoking but continue to smoke. Overeating, drinking alcohol, or not exercising are other examples of behavior with profound health implications which may be impossible to alter because the values of a person make that behavior more important than theoretical future health consequences. Such problems can only be dealt with by active intervention in matters which the society generally considers personal.

However, this society already intervenes rather aggressively in human behavior, particularly through the economic system. Navarro criticizes the recent emphasis on individual behavior as a way of avoiding the more important questions of the changes

needed in society as a whole. As he says: "But a far better strategy than self-care, and changes in life-style to improve the health
of the individual would be to change the economic and social
structure that . . . conditioned and determined that unhealthy
individual behavior to start with." His example of unhealthy diet
is a convincing one. Specific corporate interests have economic
needs to determine consumption and stimulate certain kinds of
production. Navarro cites the well-known nutritionist, Dr. Jean
Mayer, who maintains that the food conglomerates have a primary responsibility for the poor diet of United States citizens.
One can readily recall seductive advertisements for snack food
and fast-food restaurants, as well as the difficulty one sometimes
faces in trying to find tasty fresh vegetables.

It may also not be necessary to intervene so actively in affecting values and behavior in all cases. It has been pointed out that
changing the definition of the "prime" designation for beef would
have great potential benefits to health, because the marbling that
allows the prime rating is made up of saturated fat. The National
Institutes of Health is trying to produce a safe cigarette that
preserves good taste—already the amount of tar and nicotine in
the average cigarette has been reduced approximately 25% over
the past 20 years. Air bags to replace seat belts is another example of engineering protection against risk factors. Some object
that these regulations infringe on personal freedom, but society
can no longer afford to be so passive in the face of mounting evidence of risk factors which could in many cases be controlled.
Society has already determined that some interventions are necessary to protect the public, as when it made vaccination against
smallpox compulsory, over the objections of a vocal minority.

Clearly, both personal and governmental action are needed.
The society needs a health policy similar to that being developed
in Canada, which will deal with four elements seen to affect
health: human biology, environment, life-style, and health care
organization (Lalonde). Sigerist said it well:

> . . . knowledge alone is not enough. In order to become effective it
> must be applied and this is only possible if it is shared by all the
> people. Education, therefore, is all-important. I must repeat that
> the people's health is the concern of the people themselves. They
> must be enlightened in matters of health. They must want it and
> take an active part in its administration. And since the protection
> of health is a task of great magnitude, the people will endeavor to

fulfill it collectively through the state and its organs. That is why health is a primary concern of the people *and* of government. (p. 102)

The Efficacy of Health Care

Work showing that mortality rates began to fall about 100 years before medical care had anything to offer other than warm personal support has previously been cited (McKeown). The decline continued into the period after World War II, although it has now leveled off (Table 2.1). Of course, the treatment for tuberculosis probably lowered the rates even further, and prevented new cases. It has also unquestionably aided many sick individuals. Other therapeutic procedures of apparently proven value are antibiotics and modern surgery; however, the examples are fewer than one might think. It has been estimated that only 10 to 20 of procedures employed by health professionals have objective, controlled clinical trials to support the view that they will be helpful (K. White). Clinical physicians will counter the evidence with "clinical experience," but in a scientific age that is not sufficient. The practitioner has unconscious reasons for wishing therapy to succeed, and he also sees a limited spectrum of the population and its problems (Mechanic, p. 11). The practitioner is unable to avoid bias or to compare therapies to a control, and these are two essential aspects of a controlled clinical trial. Clinical judgment must be supported by such studies. Cost-consciousness is likely to lead to more and more scrutiny of unproven procedures.

The British National Health Service has been moving in that direction. A director of a British Medical Research Council Epidemiology Unit in Cardiff, Wales, has stated that the problem of evaluation is the first priority of the National Health Service, and has reviewed the evidence concerning selected preventive, therapeutic, and diagnostic procedures (Cochrane). Perhaps the most interesting example is a study carried out in Britain (Mather et al.) comparing treatment of patients with acute myocardial infarctions randomly allocated to treatment at home or to specially equipped and staffed coronary-care units in hospitals. Those patients at home had a lower mortality. Practically every hospital in this country has a coronary-care unit, at enormous capital and staffing costs, yet this modality of care has not been proven to be better than home treatment. This case illustrates the fallacy of relying on logic and clinical judgment in medical care. Yet no study is under way in this country to prove the effectiveness of such units, because the profession is convinced of their efficacy and feels that a clinical trial would be unethical. The case could easily be made that it is instead unethical to subject a patient to the pain, inconvenience, and costs of procedures that have not been proven beneficial, and may even cause harm.

Personal health care has developed an unfortunate mechanical orientation, which can be traced back to the seventeenth-century philosopher René Descartes (McKeown). Descartes separated mind and body in his thinking, and held that the body was merely matter. As Freymann (p. 172) says, "Cartesian mechanism and dualism encourage the naive faith that, because the universe is composed of elemental particles, the total explanation of its complex systems can be found in information derived from these particles. There are many examples of this faith in medical literature." The resources of physical and chemical sciences have intensified this "engineering" approach during this century. Medical care is thus dominated by the acute hospital, where the technology of medicine is concentrated. Transplantation of organs is a logical outgrowth of this view of man, which de-emphasizes the possibilities of disease prevention. Although perhaps 40% of cancers could be prevented based on what is now known about them (Lilienfeld), the society will spend literally billions of dollars attempting to cure these cancers every year. Medicine is increasingly dominated by what Thomas has called halfway technology, which only deals with the symptoms of a condition already far advanced. Examples are renal dialysis, respirators, and cardiac monitors and pacemakers.

Taking all of these factors into account, we still find it difficult to determine whether or not health care "does any good." It is true that in the United States there have been some remarkable improvements in health levels since 1900. The use of various types of health and disease level statistical indicators can be of great help in understanding the reasons for these improvements. Among them are crude, age-adjusted, and disease-specific mortality rates, life expectancy, infant mortality rate, and average remaining lifetime in years at specified ages. Unfortunately, since these indices are all related to mortality, they are rather crude measures of health levels. However, data on morbidity are difficult to obtain and verify; thus, for long-term historical analysis of health levels, we are forced to rely upon mortality data.

Between 1900 and 1960 in the United States the crude and infant mortality rates fell, while the life expectancy from birth rose (Tables 2.1). However, while crude mortality declined by about 45% from 1900 to 1970, the infant mortality declined by more than 80% from 1915 to 1970. In fact, the major portion of the decline in the crude mortality rate is due to the remarkable drop in mortality that occurred generally in the younger age groups in the population. Table 2.2 shows the 1970 age-specific mortality rates as percentages of the 1900 age-specific mortality rates. The death rate for the one- to four-year age group in 1968 was only 4% of the rate in 1900, while for people over 65 in 1968 it was still almost two-thirds of the 1900 rate. Note too the large gap in percentage improvement between the 15 to 34 age-group and 45 to 65 age-group.

This evidence is corroborated if one looks at mortality data in yet another way. Table 2.3 shows the average number of years of life remaining at specific ages in 1900 and in 1970 and the percentage change in life expectancy at specified ages between those two years. The percentage increase in life expectancy from birth is almost double that seen at all other ages. Further, in 1970 one could expect to live 21.8 years longer from birth than one could in 1900. However, upon reaching age 65, one could expect to live

Table 2.1

Mortality Rate, Infant Mortality Rate, and Life Expectancy from Birth, U.S., 1900–1970

	Crude Mortality Rate per 1,000 Pop.	Infant Mortality Rate per 1,000 Live Births[a]	Life Expectancy from Birth (in years)
1900	17.2	(99.9)	47.3
1920	13.0	85.9	54.1
1940	10.8	47.0	62.9
1960	9.5	26.0	69.7
1970	9.4	19.8	71.0

Source: Data for 1900–1960 derived from R. D. Grove and A. M. Hetzel, Vital Statistics Rates in the United States, 1940–1960 (National Center for Health Statistics, U.S. Dept. of Health, Education, and Welfare, 1968), Tables 38, 51, and 53. Data for 1970 derived from Statistical Abstract of the United States, 1971 (Bureau of the Census, U.S. Dept. of Commerce, 1971), Tables 57 and 69, and Statistical Abstract, 1974, Table 82. (See Appendix I, A1 and A5.)
[a] Data available only from 1915.

only 3.2 years longer than one could have in 1900. Tables 2.2 and
2.3 thus indicate that the most important factor in the fall in the
crude mortality rate and the rise in life expectancy from birth is
the decrease in the infant mortality rate. If many more individu-

Table 2.2

Age-Specific Mortality Rates, U.S., 1900 and 1970

Age Group (years)	Age-Specific Mortality Rate (per 1,000 pop.)		1970 Rate as % of 1900 Rate
	1900	*1970*	
1–4	19.8	0.8	4.0
5–14	3.9	0.4	10.3
15–24	5.9	1.3	22.0
25–34	8.2	1.6	19.5
35–44	10.2	3.1	30.4
45–54	15.0	7.3	48.7
55–64	27.2	16.6	61.0
65–74	56.4	35.8	63.5
75–84	123.3	80.0	64.9
85 and over	260.9	163.4	62.6

Source: Statistical Abstract of the United States, 1974,
(Bureau of the Census, U.S. Dept. of Commerce, 1974), Table
83. (See Appendix I, A1.)

Table 2.3

Average Remaining Lifetime in Years at Specified Ages, U.S., 1900 and 1971, and Percent Change between 1900 and 1971

Age in Years	Life Expectancy		Years Difference	% Change
	1900	*1971*		
0	49.2	71.0	21.8	44.3
5	55.0	67.6	12.6	22.9
15	46.8	57.9	11.1	23.7
25	39.1	48.8	9.5	24.3
35	31.9	39.3	7.4	23.2
45	24.8	30.3	5.5	22.2
55	17.9	22.1	4.2	23.5
65	11.9	15.1	3.2	26.9
75	7.1	9.1[a]	2.0[a]	28.2[a]
85	4.0	4.8[a]	0.8[a]	20.0[a]

Source: Statistical Abstract of the United States, 1971 and 1974
(Bureau of the Census, U.S. Dept. of Commerce, 1971 and 1974.)
(See Appendix I, A1.)
[a] Figures for 1968.

als survive the first year of life to then live into their sixties or seventies, it is obvious that the overall life expectancy of any one group of such fortunate infants is going to rise.

Figure 2.2 indicates how the important causes of death changed between 1900 and 1967. In 1900, the 10 leading causes of death were influenza and pneumonia, tuberculosis, gastritis, diseases of the heart, vascular lesions affecting the central nervous system, accidents, chronic nephritis, malignant neoplasms, diseases of early infancy, and diphtheria. Six of these remain in the top ten causes of death, but their relative importance has changed. Diseases of the heart and blood vessels now account for more than half of all deaths, whereas they accounted for less than 20% in 1900. Diseases of early infancy remained in the top 10, but are much less important, as indicated by the 95% reduction in mortality in the age group under the age of four. More specifically, infant mortality fell from approximately 100 per 1,000 live births in 1900 to below 20 in 1970.

Since the improved life expectancy results primarily from the change in infant and child mortality, it is worthwhile to look specifically at that group. The major killers of infants and young children early in the century were the major infectious diseases, including infantile diarrhea, tuberculosis, typhoid fever, measles, diphtheria and influenza, and pneumonia. Most of the decline in infant mortality has resulted from the decline in infectious diseases. Some were probably most affected by nutrition—certainly that was the case with tuberculosis. Others, such as infantile diarrhea and typhoid fever, were probably more affected by provision of a pure water supply and sewage disposal. Diphtheria was on the decline prior to development of a vaccine, but it is reasonable to assume that the vaccine contributed greatly to its near disappearance. Public health case-finding contributed to the decline in tuberculosis rates by removing infected individuals from the community. Finally, pneumonia was probably affected by improved environments, including housing, but antibiotics must be given the credit for making a once-dread disease a fairly rare and almost benign one. It is worth noting that only the use of antibiotics falls into the area of purely personal health services.

Infant mortality is also a useful index to consult in considering other influences on health, such as social class. Maternal age and parity, birth weight of the infant, rapidity of childbearing, loss by the mother of a previous child, paternal social class, and the

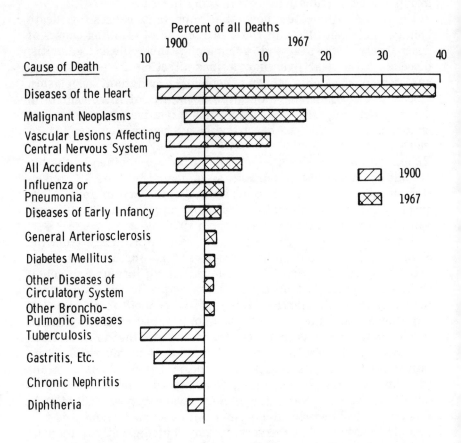

Percent of all Deaths

Figure 2.2. Percent of All Deaths, by Specified Causes of Death, U.S., 1900 and 1967. (*Sources:* For 1900: U.S. National Office of Vital Statistics, *Vital Statistics of the United States, 1950, Vol. 1* [Washington, D.C., 1950], Table 2.26, p. 170; Figures include death registration states only. For 1967: U.S. Department of HEW, Public Health Service, *Vital Statistics of the United States, 1967, Vol. II—Mortality, Part A* [Washington, D.C., 1969], Table 1–5, p. 1–6. Reprinted with permission from: University of Michigan, School of Public Health, *Medical Care Chart Book,* 1972 ed., Chart B-4.)

region of the country in which the child is born have all been shown to be related to infant mortality (Morris, pp. 56, 267). The infant mortality rate is sensitive to environmental conditions, such as housing, sanitation, and pure food and water (Rosen, 1958). The birth weight of the infant, one of the factors in infant mortality, has itself been related to a variety of factors, including smoking habits of the mother.

The infant mortality rate has been cited a great deal in the last few years as indicating that the United States has an inferior medical care system. Table 2.4 shows the relation of the United States rate to other countries' rates in 1973, with the United

Table 2.4

Infant Mortality Rates, Selected Countries, 1973

Rank	Country	Rate
1	Sweden	9.6
2	Finland	10.1[a]
3	Norway (1972)	11.3
4	Netherlands	11.6[a]
5	Japan (1972)	11.7
6	Switzerland	12.8[a]
7	Denmark (1971)	13.5
8	France (1972)	16.0[a]
9	German Democratic Republic	16.0
10	New Zealand	16.2
11	Australia (1972)	16.7[a]
12	Canada	16.8
13	Belgium	17.0[a]
14	United Kingdom (1972)	17.5
15	UNITED STATES	17.6[a]
16	Ireland	17.8[a]
17	Federal Republic of Germany (1972)	20.4[a]
17	Singapore	20.4[a]
19	Czechoslovakia	21.2[a]
20	Israel	22.1
21	Austria	23.7[a]
22	Spain (1971)	25.2[a]
23	Italy	25.7[a]
24	Bulgaria	25.9[a]
25	Jamaica	26.2
25	Trinidad and Tobago (1972)	26.2
27	USSR	26.3[a]
28	Greece (1972)	27.8[a]

Source: National Center for Health Statistics, Department of Health, Education, and Welfare, 1975.
Note: Rate represents deaths under one year of age per 1,000 live births
[a] Provisional.

States fifteenth on the list, despite a considerable reduction in the United States rate over the last few years. Most of the factors known to influence infant mortality can be changed for the better by enlightened social policy, but some of these, such as child spacing by birth control, can be approached through medical care itself. Thus, the standing of the United States indicates its investment in the welfare of infants, a part of which is in medical care.

Medical care certainly has a positive effect on infant mortality. In Denver, Colorado, the extension of comprehensive health services to low-income areas helped to reduce the infant mortality rate in those areas from 34.2 in 1964 to 23.5 in 1968, while the rate for the rest of Denver decreased only from 24.5 to 19.2 (Morris, pp. 56, 267). An analysis of infant death in New York City carried out by the Institute of Medicine found that adequacy of care was strongly associated with infant birth weight and survival, and estimated that adequate health services could reduce the overall 1968 rate of 21.9 per 1,000 live births as much as 33% to 14.7 per 1,000 (Kessner).

Further, even though it is not possible to show that personal health services substantially influenced the health of the population (as it can currently be measured), such services are certainly important to the health of individuals with various disease processes. And, aside from needs for personal health services which can be recognized by professionals, services to deal with other human needs are being demanded to an increasing extent by the consumers of care. It is clear that many persons, both providers and consumers, have overestimated the importance of medical care as a determinant of health. Human biology, environment, and life-style have important effects on health status. Furthermore, not a great deal of health care is of proven efficacy. Nonetheless, there is evidence that for certain conditions medical care positively affects the health of individuals, and sometimes of population groups. A major challenge for the future is to greatly expand the scientific basis of medical treatment.

The Caring Function

Health professionals sometimes become so involved in delivering services that they neglect medicine's traditional role, caring for people. As Sigerist says:

Disease, then, is a biological process. . . . But this process takes place in man, and thus always involves the mind. . . . Disease, a destructive process that threatens life, may destroy only a few cells that can easily be replaced, but it may destroy the entire organism and with it the individual. For this reason, man suffers and is afraid: disease reminds him that he is mortal, that he must die sooner or later, and, if the illness is serious, it may be very soon. . . . Elementary fears, age-old views, come from the depth of the unconscious, breaking through the thin crust of education. (p. 93)

Although care has a long history, it is little talked about in today's technological world of medicine. But the public is beginning to demand more than machines.

Studies have supported the importance of care. It has been shown that patients with acceptance—measured by a scale including trust in the surgeon, optimism about the outcome, and confidence in their ability to cope—healed faster in a trial involving eye surgery (Frank). Another study showed that when mothers were reassured and given an opportunity to ask questions, their children undergoing tonsillectomy adapted more easily to the hospital and recovered faster after surgery (Skipper and Leonard). Perhaps more important, it is known that disability from chronic disease is probably more dependent on the patient's attitudes than on his actual physical state (Mechanic, pp. 117–119, 133–134).

Studies of primary-care settings have indicated that a large majority of patients present either with psychological problems or with physical complaints which a physician is trained to regard as trivial (Mechanic, p. 119). Yet caring is really the essence of health care. The conclusions of the 1972 Sun Valley Forum on "Medical Cure and Medical Care" are germane: "Traditionally, medical care has served as much to relieve pain and anxiety and system function as it has to effect cures. Medical care is a highly personalized service with both physical and psychologic elements; these are highly related in the consumer's motivation to seek service and in the physician's ability to achieve cooperation by his advice and to change behavior to be conducive to health. There was widespread agreement that both the 'curing' and 'caring' functions are central to high-quality care, and that models for delivering health services must allow for the effective integration of both concerns" (Sun Valley Forum on National Health).

It seems clear that if the traditional system is unable or unwilling to provide practitioners to deal with problems in a warm and caring way, the public will either force it to change or will find other types of providers who can meet those needs. As McKeown notes, "Since most serious diseases and disabilities are likely to prove relatively intractable if they cannot be prevented, the role of therapeutic medicine should be modified to include as the major commitment the concept of care. Such a change would carry important implications for medical science and service and should affect the content and orientation of medical education."

The Future of Health Care

The engineering approach to man's diseases (Freymann, p. 172) is not going to be abandoned, nor should it be. The major criticism of this approach is that it has limited applicability, but research will surely produce new and valuable advances. Advances that have been predicted include genetic transfer, understanding the genetic origin of many diseases, regeneration of tissues, slowing of aging, and increased epidemiological knowledge resulting from databank records. Two recent advances of great potential importance are prenatal genetic analysis, with abortion to prevent birth defects, and behavior therapy and biofeedback, which already appear to be effective against stuttering, bed-wetting, obesity, anorexia, and high blood pressure, and may be useful in many other disorders (Platt).

In 1972, a panel of 102 "experts" were asked to predict future events in health care. The results are particularly interesting because they go beyond the technical advances mentioned above. In the section on organization and control, for example, the predictions include the following: the disappearance of solo practice (the entire population being served by strategically located neighborhood health centers); the extension of national health insurance to cover more than 95% of the population; and effective coordination of medical care disbursement and planning on a regional basis throughout the country. Most of the changes are predicted to occur before the end of the next 10 years (McLaughlin and Sheldon).

One can also predict that the importance of care will not decline. McKeown sees a group of intractable problems in technologically advanced countries made up of congenital, psychological, and geriatric conditions, as does Weinerman (1965). Congenital conditions could be possibly prevented by prenatal diagnosis and abortion, as noted. Practically the only information available about psychiatric illness indicates that social institutions and social behavior contribute to its occurrence, so further research and societal changes could eventually ameliorate the problem. But the many mild emotional, sexual and social problems of adjustment for which people seek care will surely not disappear. And geriatric illness, with death coming after a prolonged course of chronic disease, will remain.

The Future of Man

Earlier sections of this chapter have argued that the concept of health depends greatly on psychological, social, and cultural factors. Thus, the future of health and health care is intertwined with man's image of himself and the ways he acts on that image. The Stanford Research Institute has undertaken to study how "the structure and history of society are related to the dominant image(s) of man in that society, and in particular to examine our own technological-industrial society from this point of view" (Markley p. 1). The researchers have concluded as follows:

"1. There are increasingly evident signs of the imminent emergency of a new dominant image of man.

"2. The increasingly serious dilemmas of industrialized society appear to require for their ultimate resolution a drastically changed image of man-on-earth."

One's image of man depends on one's answers to such questions as whether man is good or evil, whether man has free will, whether man is essentially physical or spiritual in nature, whether men and women are essentially equal, and so on. An appraisal of industrialized society deals with such issues as whether human progress is synonymous with economic growth and increasing consumption, whether man's destiny is to conquer nature, and whether economic efficiency is the most trustworthy approach to the fulfillment of man's goals. Survey and poll data indicate changing attitudes toward spiritual and transcendental experience, questions as to the continuation of the growth-and-consumption ethic of business, and a changing attitude within science itself toward subjective experience, varied states of consciousness, psychic phenomena, and so forth (Harman).

Some of the implications for health care are described in a report from the Institute (Harman). These include a broadened definition of health, reduced status for professionals, recognition that the whole society is the environment that affects health, blurring of the distinction between mental and physical illness, changing attitudes toward death, and control over medical technology.

One may hope that the optimism of the Institute is justified.

Summary and Conclusions

This chapter has argued for a broadened conception of health and health care, and has supported the idea of health care as a right. Evidence has been cited that curative medicine is less efficacious than the public, or even the professions, believes. This and other considerations lead to the conclusion that "caring" in medicine and health care must and will increase. However, it is recognized that within limits the individual can still determine his or her own destiny, although many factors in society act to produce unhealthy behavior. Unquestionably, great possible health benefits could result from controlling the physical and social environment.

However, it is important to emphasize that treating disease is not the same as creating health. Dubos sees health as a mirage that will continue to recede just beyond reach; he believes that this is all to the good. "Human life implies adventure, and there is no adventure without struggles and dangers. . . . Attempts at adaptation will demand efforts, and these efforts will often result in failure . . . . Disease will remain an inescapable manifestation of his struggles. While it may be comforting to imagine a life free of stresses and strains in a carefree world, this will remain an idle dream. Man cannot hope to find another Paradise on earth, because Paradise is a static concept while human life is a dynamic process" (Dubos, p. 278).

References

Balinsky, W., and Berger, R. "A Review of the Research on General Health Status Indexes." *Medical Care, 13*, 283, 1975.

Banta, D., and Bosch, S. "Organized Labor and the Prepaid Group Practice Movement." *Archives of Environmental Health, 29,* 43, 1974.

Banta, D., and Fox, R. "Role Strains of a Health Care Team in a Poverty Community." *Social Science and Medicine, 6,* 697, 1972.

Belloc, N. B. "Relationship of Health Practices and Mortality." *Preventive Medicine, 2,* 67, 1973.

Belloc, N. B., and Breslow, L. "Relationship of Physical Health Status and Health Practices." *Preventive Medicine, 1* 409, 1972.

Breslow, L. "A Quantitative Approach to the World Health Organization Definition of Health: Physical, Mental and Social Well-Being." *International Journal of Epidemiology, 1*, 347, 1972.

Breslow, L., Chairman. "Theory, Practice and Application of Preventive Medicine in Personal Health Services." Task Force III Report, The National Conference on Preventive Medicine, *Summaries and Recommendations.* Fogarty International Center, Bethesda, Md., November, 1975.

Bush, J., and Fanshel, S. "A Health Status Index and Its Application to Health Services Outcomes." *Operations Research, 18*, 1021, 1970.

Clark, D. "A Vocabulary for Preventive Medicine." In Clark, D., and MacMahon, B., Eds., *Preventive Medicine*, Ch. 1. Boston, Mass.: Little, Brown and Co., 1967.

Cochrane, A. *Effectiveness and Efficiency.* London: The Nuffield Provincial Hospitals Trust, 1971.

Daly, M., and Tyroler, H. "Cornell Medical Index Response as Predictor of Mortality." *British Journal of Preventive & Social Medicine, 26*, 159, 1972.

Dubos, R. *Mirage of Health.* New York: Harper & Row, Perennial Library, 1971.

Feinstein, A. "Symptoms as an Index of Biological Behaviour and Prognosis in Human Cancer." *Nature, 209*, 241, 1966.

Frank, J. "Mind-Body Interactions in Illness and Healing." Presented at the May Lectures, "Alternative Futures for Medicine," April 4, 1975, Airlie House, Airlie, Virginia.

Freymann, J. *The American Health Care System: Its Genesis and Trajectory.* New York: Medcom Press, 1974.

Fuchs, V. "The Contribution of Health Services to the American Economy." *The Milbank Memorial Fund Quarterly, 44*, 65, 1966.

Fuchs, V. *Who Shall Live?* New York: Basic Books, 1974.

Harman, W. "New Images of Man: What to Do until the New Paradigm Arrives." Presented at the May Lectures, "Alternative Futures for Medicine," April 4, 1975, Airlie House, Airlie, Virginia.

Higginson, J. "A Hazardous Society? The Role of Epidemiology in Determining the Individual versus Group Risk in Modern Societies." Rosenhaus Lecture. American Public Health Association Annual Meeting, November 17, 1975, Chicago, Illinois.

Hoyman, H. "The Spiritual Dimensions of Man's Health in Today's World." In Belgum, D., Ed., *Religion and Medicine*. Ames, Iowa: Iowa State University Press, 1967.

Iliad of Homer. Translated by R. Lattimore. Chicago, Ill.: The University of Chicago Press, 1951.

Illich, I. "Medical Nemesis." *Lancet, 1*, 918, 1974.

Jago, J. " 'Hal'—Old Word, New Task—Reflections on the Words 'Health' and 'Medical'." *Social Science and Medicine, 9,* 1, 1975.

Kessner, D. et al. *Infant Death: An Analysis by Maternal Risk and Health Care.* Washington, D.C.: Institute of Medicine, National Academy of Sciences, 1973.

Koos, E. *The Health of Regionville.* New York: Hafner Publishing Co., 1954.

Kunitz, S. et al. "Changing Health Care Opinions in Regionville, 1946–1973." *Medical Care, 13,* 549, 1975.

Lalonde, M. *A New Perspective of the Health of Candians.* Ottawa, Canada: Government of Canada, 1974.

Lilienfeld, A. Personal communication. June 24, 1975.

Markley, O. "Changing Images of Man." Stanford, Calif.: Policy Research Report #4, Center for the Study of Social Policy, Stanford Research Institute, May, 1974.

Mather, H. et al. "Acute Myocardial Infarction: Home and Hospital Treatment." *British Medical Journal, 3,* 334, 1971.

McKeown, T. "A Historical Appraisal of the Medical Task." In McLachlan, G., and McKeown, T., Eds., *Medical History and Medical Care.* New York: Oxford University Press, 1971.

McLaughlin, C., and Sheldon, A. *The Future and Medical Care.* Cambridge, Mass.: Ballinger Publishing Company, 1974.

Mechanic, D. *Politics, Medicine, and Social Science.* New York: Wiley, 1974.

Millis, J. "A Rational Policy for Medical Education and Its Financing." New York: The National Fund for Medical Education, 1971, pp. 53–58.

Morris, J. "Uses of Epidemiology." Baltimore, Md.: Williams & Wilkins, 1964.

Mueller, M. "Private Health Insurance in 1973: A Review of Coverage, Enrollment, and Financial Experience." *Social Security Bulletin, 38,* 21, 1975.

Navarro, V. "The Industrialization of Fetishism or the Fetishism of Industrialization, a Critique of Ivan Illich." *International Journal of Health Services, 5,* 347, 1975.

Parsons, T. *The Social System.* Glencoe, Ill.: The Free Press, 1951.

Parsons, T. "Definitions of Health and Illness in the Light of American Values and Social Structure." In Jaco, E., Ed., *Patients, Physicians, and Illness.* Glencoe, Ill.: The Free Press, 1958.

Platt, J. "What's Ahead for Medical Research and Health Care." Presented at the Ninth Council for International Organizations of Medical Sciences Round Table Conference, August, 1974, Rio de Janeiro, Brazil.

Rosen, G. *A History of Public Health.* New York: MD Publications, 1958.

Schneiderman, M. "Cancer—A Social Disease?" Presented at the Interagency Collaborative Group on Environmental Carcinogenesis, June 11, 1975, National Institutes of Health, Bethesda, Md.

Sigerist, H. *Medicine and Human Welfare.* College Park, Md.: McGrath Publishing Co., 1970.

Skipper, J., and Leonard, R. "Children, Stress, and Hospitalization." *Journal of Health and Social Behavior, 9,* 275, 1968.

Stead, E. "Excellent Care: The Clinician's." In Walker, E. C. et al., Eds., *Evaluation of Care in the University and Community Hospital.* Hartford, Conn.: Connecticut Health Services Research Series, 1971.

Sun Valley Forum on National Health. "Medical Cure and Medical Care." *Milbank Memorial Fund Quarterly, 50,* 231, 1972. (Summary)

Susser, M. "Ethical Components in the Definition of Health." *International Journal of Health Services, 4,* 539, 1974.

Szasz, T. *The Manufacture of Madness.* New York: Harper & Row, 1970.

Thomas, L. *Lives of A Cell.* New York: Viking Press, 1975.

Weinerman, E. "Research on Comparative Health Service Systems." *Medical Care, 9,* 272, 1971.

Weinerman, E. R. "Anchor Points Underlying the Planning for Tomorrow's Health Case." *Bulletin of the New York Academy of Medicine, 41,* 1203, 1965.

White, K. "International Comparisons of Health Services Systems." *Milbank Memorial Fund Quarterly, 46,* 117, 1968. (Personal communication: Dr. White has stated in 1975 that he considered this estimate to be still generally accurate.)

White, R. *Right to Health: The Evolution of an Idea.* Ames, Iowa: The University of Iowa Press, 1971.

Wise, H. et al. *Making Health Teams Work.* Cambridge, Mass.: Ballinger Publishing Co., 1974.

World Health Organization. "The Constitution of the World Health Organization." *WHO Chronicle, 1,* 29, 1944.

Zaborowski, M. "Cultural Components in Responses to Pain." *Journal of Social Issues, 8,* 16, 1952.

3

Data for Health and Health Care

Steven Jonas

Introduction

Quantitative analysis provides a basic means of describing, and thus understanding, the population served by our health care delivery system. Quantitative analysis of populations—especially in terms of number, health status, and health care services utilization—serves to elucidate the populations' place in and relation to the delivery system.

Because of the nature of most data-gathering and reporting on the one hand, and book-writing and publishing on the other, most of the data in this chapter will be at least three years out of date by the time this book first appears. Some data will be presented, of course, particularly in relation to change and rates of change, major issues in any health care delivery system. However, it is intended that the reader should use this chapter (and indeed all sections of the book in which data appear) in conjunction with Appendix I, "Guide to Sources." Thus, when we discuss population, for example, the reader will not be dependent on estimated census data for 1974 or 1975; Appendix I tells him where the most current data may be found. We are concerned, then, not with numbers per se, but with the principles and purposes of using numbers in describing a population.

Quantitative Perspectives

There are three major quantitative perspectives from which a population can be viewed in relation to health and health care services. First is the *number* of people, and what are called "demographic" characteristics, from the Greek "describing the people." Among the important demographic characteristics are geographic distribution, age, sex and marital status, and such social characteristics as ethnicity, income, education, employment, and measures of social class. Second is the actual *health status* of the population, or conversely, the *sickness status*; these can be characterized in terms of mortality (death) and morbidity (sickness). Mortality and morbidity may be counted for the population as a whole, in which case the resultant numbers or rates are described as "crude," or may be counted by cause, or by demographic characteristics used in describing segments of the population. The third perspective is utilization of health services: who uses how many of what kinds of services. Utilization can be measured from the point of view of the consumer, i.e., what is the per-person physician visit rate, or from the point of view of the provider, i.e., how many visits does a particular physician give. When one knows how many people there are, what their health status is, and the levels at which they utilize services, one has quantitatively characterized a population in relation to health and health care fairly well.

Numbers and Rates

Population, health status, and utilization data all can be presented in two forms: as numbers and as rates. A *number* represents simply a quantity of conditions, individuals, events. A *rate* has two parts, a numerator and a denominator; the numerator is a number of conditions, individuals, events counted, while the denominator is a larger group (usually) of conditions, individuals, events from among which the numerator is drawn. It is customary to give the rate as applying during a particular time period. For example, one could count 1,000 deaths occurring in a particular population during a year. This *number* of deaths becomes a *rate* if one counts the population, finds that number to be 100,000 and then says that the mortality *rate* is 1,000/100,000, per year. The rate can be expressed as a percentage (in this case 1%), or as a rate per thousand (in this case 10), or any other whole number denominator that is useful. Denominators are usually in multiples of 10 and the magnitude of the denominator is usually chosen so as to make the numerator a number of reasonable size. Thus, the more infrequent the event being counted by the numerator, the greater the magnitude of the denominator. For example, crude death rates for a whole population, all causes, are usually given as per thousand population, whereas rarer cause-specific mortality rates are given as per 100,000 or even as per 1,000,000. This is done so that the numerator itself will not appear as a fractional number.

Denominators, as well as numerators, can be fairly specific. In discussing deaths from lung cancer related to cigarette smoking, for example, a rate can be determined for the number of deaths from lung cancer in males over age 45 who have smoked two or more packs of cigarettes per day for 20 years or more (the numerator), per all males over 45 who have smoked two or more packs of cigarettes per day for 20 years or more (the denominator), per year. The units of the numerator and the denominator in health indices, however, are usually different. For example, in cause-specific mortality rates, the unit for the numerator is deaths by cause, while the unit for the denominator is persons.

Although rates are usually fractions, they will occasionally be whole numbers. For example, in measuring total morbidity in a population, one may find that the number of diagnosed disease conditions is greater than the number of people. The rate then is usually given with a denominator of one, e.g., in the population of a central African city there are 2.5 disease conditions per person. This usage also occurs in utilization rates, e.g., the physician-visit rate in the United States is approximately 5.0 per person. A very important use of rates is to measure changes over time, e.g., the death rate for condition X went down from one year to the next. Health care service utilization rates are not usually given in terms of numerators and denominators. Hospital admission rates that are specific for a particular hospital, for example, are not usually given as per person, but simply as per unit of time, as follows: in 1975, the admission rate for hospital Y was 1000 per month. This practice prevails because the dimensions of the populations served by most providers are not known.

The Purposes of Quantification

Description. Quantification has two major purposes in relation to understanding a health care delivery system. First, quantification is descriptive. It describes the size of the population under consideration. Demographic characteristics such as location (Do many people live near marshes in which malaria-carrying mosquitoes live?) and age distribution (Are there many infants and/or old people?) give some indication of the population's relative disease risk. Disease-specific mortality and morbidity rates point out the major health and illness problems in the population. The infant mortality rate gives some indication both of general health levels and the availability of medical care.

Crude and disease-specific mortality and morbidity rates can be distributed by place, age, sex, ethnic group, and social class to show which population subgroups are being affected by which diseases. An analysis of such data reveals what diseases and conditions of ill health the population has, and which subgroups of the population are affected by what problems.

Utilization data also show how the population uses the health care system. As we noted above, utilization of health services can be viewed from the consumer's perspective—how many times the average person sees a physician per year, and what the sources of care are—or from the point of view of the provider—how many patient visits the average physician gives in a year. Again, these kinds of data can be subdivided according to the various demographic characteristics of the population—i.e., what is the average annual per-person physician visit rate by age, sex, geographic location, social class, and the like. From the provider side, the demographic makeup of the group of patients admitted to a particular hospital in the course of a year can be examined. In addition, there can be demographic analyses of the providers themselves, both individual and institutional; that is, one can determine the average number of visits provided annually by physicians according to their age, practice location, and specialty. Thus, descriptively, quantification tells us how many of what kind of people are at risk, what kinds of diseases and conditions of ill health they have, how those problems are distributed in the population, and, finally, who goes where for how many of what kinds of health services, delivered by which types of providers.

Program planning. The second purpose of quantification in health care delivery is prospective. Description can reveal the existence of problems; if there is a desire to do something about the problems, data can be used for prospective program planning. Once new programs are under way, data can be used to evaluate their effects and effectiveness. Thus data are necessary for logical program planning, as they are in most fields of human endeavor. However, it must be remembered that they are not sufficient: the agencies and institutions that control the health care delivery system must first make a policy decision to undertake program planning and to implement a suitable plan before the prospective use of data has any real meaning. We discuss the problems of health care program planning in the United States in some detail in Chapter 12.

To illustrate the use of data prospectively, let us take the hypothetical case of planning a hospital for a medical school in a suburban/semirural area. A program is to be designed for this hospital which will help meet the health care needs of the community as well as the educational and research needs of the medical school, since the three functions of any medical school, in theory at least, are patient care (service), teaching, and research. It is to be hoped, of course, that these three activities can be made congruent.

Let us look at some of the questions we would need to answer in undertaking intelligent, rational program-planning for a new medical school hospital. First, a proposed service area would be delineated by counting population, determining population density, examining modes of transportation, and evaluating existing health care resources, particularly the more complex and sophisticated ones already in use. Thus, the questions are defined. Among them are:

—How many people are there and where are they located?
—What are the rates of population change?
—What are the age, sex, and marital status distributions?
—What are the social class and ethnic makeups of the population?
—What diseases do they get?
—What diseases do they die of?
—What are the existing health care resources?
—How are they used?
—What do existing providers see as their needs?
—How do they view the new facility and how will they relate to it?

The answers to these and many other similar questions indicate the health and health care needs of the population to be served. Going a step further, taking into account existing health care services and what they do, the data identify the *unmet* health and health care needs of the population. An analysis of the provider utilization patterns shows what the providers are doing, and what they are not doing, and indicates what *their* needs are. In planning any new health care facility, it is essential to know how it is going to relate functionally to existing providers, both individual and institutional. Finally, as we noted above, educational and research needs must be taken into account.

Amalgamating, classifying, and analyzing all these data is the basis for rational program planning. The data enable us to make intelligent decisions on facility design, location, services, space allocation, administrative structure, community relations, staffing and personnel policies, teaching and research programs, capital cost, expense budget, and so on. In general one can say that intelligent decisions depend on intelligent use of data; unfortunately, such use does not always obtain in the United States.

Population
Number

A census enumerating the population of the nation is required at least once every 10 years by the Constitution of the United States (U.S. Bureau of the Census, p.1). Its original purpose was to provide the basis for the apportionment of seats in the House of Representatives of the United States Congress. A census has been carried out every 10 years since 1790. Although every effort is made for completeness, the Bureau has estimated that it undercounted in 1970 by 2.5% (U.S. Bureau of the Census, p.1). In addition to the decennial censuses, the Bureau makes interim estimates on various parameters based on information gathered from population samples and a variety of other sources. The resident population as of April 1, 1970 was officially reported as 203,235,298 (U.S. Bureau of the Census, Table 1). In addition, there were about one million armed service persons resident abroad. (By January 1, 1974, with the virtual end of American involvement in Vietnam, the number of armed service persons abroad has dropped to just over one-half million.) Births, deaths, immigration, and emigration produce change in population size. In the first half of the 1970s, the population growth rate averaged about 0.8% per year, whereas in the first half of the 1960s the population had grown at the rate of about 1.5% per year. This decline stems primarily from a decline in the birth rate, which we shall consider in more detail below. The bearing of such matters as population size, growth rate, and birth rate on health services planning should be obvious.

Demographic Characteristics

In 1970, 68.6% of the population lived in what are called Standard Metropolitan Statistical Areas (SMSAs) (U.S. Bureau of the Census, Table 16). The definition of a SMSA is determined by the federal Office of Management and Budget, an agency of the Executive Branch. As of November 1971, a SMSA had to include at least: (a) One city with a population of 50,000 or more (75,000 in New England), or (b) A city with a population of 25,000, plus surrounding areas with a population of at least 1,000 per square mile, to produce, "for general social and economic purposes, a single community with a combined population of at least 50,000." In addition, a SMSA must include the county in which the central city is located, and adjacent counties that are "determined to be metropolitan in character" (U.S. Bureau of the Census, p. 863).

In 1970, 68% of whites lived in SMSAs, 28% in the "central cities," while 74% of "Negroes" lived in SMSAs, 58% in "central cities" (U.S. Bureau of the Census, Table 16). In 1970, 74% of Americans lived in areas defined as "urban," as compared with 64% in 1950 and 46% in 1910 (U.S. Bureau of the Census, Table 17). As of 1970, the U.S. population was 48% male, 89% white (as contrasted with "Negro"), and had a median age of 28.0 (28.9 for whites, 22.4 for "Negroes") (U.S. Bureau of the Census, Table 25). In terms of age distribution, in 1970, 40% of the population was under 21, 50% between 21 and 65, and 10% 65 and over (U.S. Bureau of the Census, Table 34). In March 1970, about 75% of males and 70% of females over 14 were married (U.S. Bureau of the Census, Table 47). In 1970, more than 2 million Americans were inmates of institutions, nearly 1 million in homes for the aged, about 435,000 in mental hospitals, more than 325,000 in prison, more than 200,000 in homes for the mentally retarded, and approximately 85,000 in tuberculosis and other chronic disease hospitals (U.S. Bureau of the Census, Table 63).

Social class status is often thought to be a valuable parameter by which to cross-tabulate population, health and illness, and utilization data.* Unlike England, the U.S. Government has not developed a "social class" index by which it cross-tabulates its demographic data. Thus one is forced to use ethnicity and income as rough indicators of, at least, relative social class. This is unfortunate, because social class is really determined by the combination of a number of factors: income, education, employment, and dwelling-place. A great deal of such information is in fact collected by the government, but an index has not been created.

The information we have been presenting so far comes from

* A detailed discussion of this very important subject area, with an extensive bibliography, is presented in *The Health Gap*, ed. Robert Kane, M.D. (New York: Springer, 1975). See also: National Center for Health Statistics, "Selected Vital and Health Statistics In Poverty and Nonpoverty Areas of 19 Large Cities, United States, 1969–1971," *Vital and Health Statistics*, Series 21, No. 26, USDHEW, November, 1975.

Section 1 of *Statistical Abstracts*, "Population." Additional information, necessary to develop a comprehensive profile, is contained in these other sections of the *Statistical Abstract*: Education; Social Insurance and Welfare Services; Labor Force, Employment, and Earnings; and Income, Expenditures and Wealth.

Vital Statistics
How the Data Are Collected

Traditional in public health, the "Vital Statistics" consist of births, deaths, marriages, and divorces. In the United States, primary responsibility for collecting these data lies with the states. Not all states collect all categories of data. In most states that do collect these data, the Department of Health is responsible; where possible, state health departments rely on county and other local health departments to do the actual counting. The locally accumulated data are then organized at the state level and transmitted to the federal level. The District Government for Washington, D.C., carries out the above responsibilities in that city.

The collection of mortality data in the United States did not begin on an annual basis until 1900. At that time, 10 states and the District of Columbia became "death registration states" to carry out that task and forward the results to the federal government (U.S. Bureau of the Census, p. 49). (Until 1946, the Bureau of the Census assembled the vital statistics at the national level. From 1946 to 1960, the work was performed by the Bureau of State Services of the United States Public Health Service. Since 1960, the National Center for Health Statistics, USDHEW, has carried out the function.) Beginning in 1915, 10 states and the District of Columbia formed a "birth registration area," collecting birth data on an annual basis. By 1933, all states were in both the birth and death registration areas. Fetal deaths have been counted annually since 1922. The corresponding "marriage registration area," first formed in 1957, included 41 states and the District of Columbia by 1973. The "divorce registration" area was established in 1958, and by 1973 covered 29 states and the District of Columbia.

Vital statistics rates are calculated by the National Center for Health Statistics and are based upon the actual number of persons counted by the Bureau of the Census on April 1 of each decennial year, as well as the midyear estimates made by the Bureau of the Census for other years. Death statistics are based

on a 10% sample of all reported deaths. Fetal deaths and still-
births are not included, nor are deaths among Armed Service
persons abroad. Cause-specific mortality data are classified
according to the "Eighth Revision International Classification of
Diseases, Adapted for Use in The United States (1968)," the so-
called "ICDA." The use of a system at least parallel to the "International Statistical Classification of Diseases, Injuries, and
Causes of Death," produced by the World Health Organization, is
required for WHO membership (U.S. Bureau of the Census, p.
49), and the ICDA is such a system.

Natality

In mid-1975, babies were being born in the United States at the
rate of about 3.2 million per year (National Center for Health
Statistics, Aug. 1975). This represented an annual rate of 15.0
births per 1,000 population rate, up slightly from the 1974 rate of
14.8. That rate represented a low point in a birth rate that had
been steadily dropping from a post-World-War-II high of 25.2,
achieved in 1957 (National Center for Health Statistics, Aug.
1975; U.S. Bureau of the Census, Tables 9, 67). The fertility rate
(annual births per 1,000 resident females 15 to 44 years of age)
for 1973 was 69.3, down from the post-World-War-II high of
122.9 (U.S. Bureau of the Census, Table 9). This declining birth
rate still produces net population growth each year (U.S. Bureau
of the Census, Table 3).

Mortality

The crude death rate (total deaths per 1,000 population) in the
United States in mid-1975 was 9.1 (National Center for Health
Statistics, Aug. 28, 1975). This was an interesting drop for a
rate that had generally hovered between 9.4 and 9.5 from 1955
through 1974, going no higher than 9.7 (once, in 1968), and no
lower than 9.3 (three times, in 1955, 1971, and 1974) (National
Center for Health Statistics, Aug. 28, 1975; U.S. Bureau of the
Census, 1974, Table 67). Time will tell if the drop is significant.
    Mortality data are rather neatly reported. There is one pri-
mary reporting authority, the local health department, or, where
none exists, the state health department acting in its place. Death
is a well-defined event in the vast majority of cases, although
with recent advances in medical technology, the possibility of dispute has arisen. Determination of cause of death has presented
some problems from time to time, since it is left up to the physi-

cian certifying that the patient is dead, in most cases, and physicians do have varying diagnostic styles, opinions, and abilities. Furthermore, there have been changes in the technical definitions of causes of death over time. For example, is diabetes or coronary artery disease the cause of death in a patient who dies from a heart attack which resulted from complications secondary to diabetes? The reporting authorities have rules to cover these instances, however, and most physicians follow them, so that this last problem is not too serious. Finally, since both hospitals and funeral directors are legally required to report all deaths, with rather serious penalties for failure to comply, we can assume that most deaths are reported.

A great deal of data concerning differential death rates by the basic demographic variables of age, color, and sex can be found in *Monthly Vital Statistics Reports, Vital Statistics of the United States*, the *Statistical Abstract*, and special studies published in *Vital and Health Statistics*, Series 20 (in particular numbers 15 and 16).* We will only give a few representative numbers in Table 3.1. It can be seen that mortality is relatively high during the first year of life, drops to a relatively low level until the mid-40s, and then begins to climb again. For the total population, males have a higher mortality rate than do females, at all ages. As the population grows older *in toto*, the preponderance of females over males in the older age group increases. Although the crude death rate for nonwhites is lower than for whites, the age-specific death rates for nonwhites are higher than for whites at all ages until 80. The crude death rate is lower for nonwhites because the nonwhite population is younger.

Cause-specific mortality rates. Turning to cause-specific mortality rates, the 10 leading causes of death in 1973 (excluding the diagnostic categories of "Symptoms and Ill-Defined Conditions" and "All other diseases") were, in order: heart disease; cancer; stroke; accidents; influenza and pneumonia (primarily pneumonia); diabetes mellitus; cirrhosis of the liver; certain diseases of early infancy (primarily related to problems of delivery); bronchitis, emphysema and asthma (primarily emphysema); and suicide. Homicide was eleventh (National Center for Health Statistics, June 27, 1974, Table 8). In 1950, the 10 leading causes of death were heart disease; cancer; stroke; accidents; certain diseases of early infancy; influenza and pneumonia;

* For a description of these publications, see Appendix I.

Table 3.1

Deaths and Death Rates by Age, Color, and Sex, U.S., 1973

Age in Years	TOTAL			WHITE			ALL OTHER		
	Both Sexes	Male	Female	Both Sexes	Male	Female	Both Sexes	Male	Female
Number:									
All ages	1,977,000	1,097,830	879,090	1,731,010	958,130	772,880	245,910	139,700	106,210
Under 1	55,300	31,480	23,830	39,440	23,000	16,440	15,870	8,480	7,390
1–4	10,890	6,220	4,670	8,330	4,780	3,550	2,560	1,440	1,120
5–14	16,130	10,140	5,990	12,800	8,010	4,790	3,330	2,130	1,200
15–24	50,370	37,990	12,430	40,060	30,250	9,810	10,360	7,740	2,620
25–34	43,460	29,920	13,560	32,070	22,220	9,850	11,410	7,700	3,710
35–44	65,700	40,350	25,370	48,650	30,260	18,390	17,070	10,090	6,980
45–54	166,300	105,900	60,420	135,180	86,930	48,250	31,140	18,970	12,170
55–59	132,740	86,700	46,040	113,500	75,070	38,430	19,240	11,630	7,610
60–64	176,910	114,810	62,100	152,300	99,970	52,330	24,610	14,840	9,770
65–69	212,400	131,000	81,400	185,660	116,290	69,370	26,740	14,710	12,030
70–74	241,570	139,820	101,750	213,820	124,970	88,850	27,750	14,850	12,900
75–79	265,240	135,910	129,330	242,920	124,110	118,810	22,320	11,800	10,520
80–84	251,890	117,150	134,740	236,140	109,630	126,510	15,750	7,520	8,230
85 and over	284,380	108,650	175,770	267,040	101,130	165,910	17,380	7,520	9,860
Not stated	3,500	1,780	1,740	3,130	1,510	1,620	390	270	120

Rate:									
All ages^a	9.4	10.7	8.2	9.5	10.7	8.3	9.2	10.9	7.6
Under 1	18.0	20.0	15.8	15.3	17.5	13.1	31.2	33.0	29.4
1–4	0.8	0.9	0.7	0.7	0.8	0.6	1.1	1.3	1.0
5–14	0.4	0.5	0.3	0.4	0.5	0.3	0.5	0.7	0.4
15–24	1.3	2.0	0.6	1.2	1.8	0.6	1.9	2.9	0.9
25–34	1.5	2.1	0.9	1.3	1.8	0.8	3.3	4.8	2.0
35–44	2.9	3.6	2.2	2.4	3.1	1.8	6.1	8.0	4.6
45–54	7.0	9.2	4.9	6.4	8.4	4.4	12.3	16.1	9.0
55–59	13.1	17.9	8.7	12.3	17.0	8.0	20.6	26.7	15.2
60–64	19.4	27.0	12.8	18.5	26.1	11.9	27.7	36.2	20.4
65–69	27.9	38.7	19.2	27.1	38.1	18.2	35.6	44.0	28.8
70–74	43.1	59.1	31.4	41.7	58.1	29.8	58.5	68.8	49.8
75–79	67.7	87.2	54.9	67.3	86.9	54.4	73.7	90.1	61.2
80–84	98.1	123.7	83.2	99.8	126.7	84.3	78.0	91.7	68.6
85 and over	174.5	199.4	162.0	179.2	205.1	166.4	124.1	141.9	112.0

Source: Annual Summary, Vital Statistics of the United States; Monthly Vital Statistics Report, June 27, 1974, Table 6. (See Appendix I, A4 and A5.)

Note: Table based on a 10% sample of deaths. Rates per 1,000 population in specified group. Due to rounding estimates of deaths, figures may not add to totals.

^a Figures for age not stated included in "All ages" but not distributed among age groups.

51

tuberculosis; nephritis and nephrosis; diabetes mellitus; and congenital anomalies. Suicide was eleventh, but homicide was well down on the list (U.S. Bureau of the Census, Table 86).

The rates for heart disease and stroke remained remarkably stable from 1950 to 1973. The cancer rate has gone up over 20%. The overall accidental death rate has gone down 10%, owing to a drop of 25% in deaths due to accidents other than automobile, for which the rate has increased 15%. Tuberculosis, nephritis and nephrosis, and congenital anomalies dropped out of the "top 10," while cirrhosis of the liver, diabetes mellitus, and bronchitis, emphysema, and asthma moved up. Some of the changes are due to alterations of definitions and some to alterations of diagnostic style. However, the significant changes are due to improvements in tuberculosis control, increases in cigarette smoking (related to malignancy, in particular lung cancer, and chronic lung disease), increases in alcoholism (cirrhosis of the liver), and relative increases in violence in the society (automobile accidents, suicide, and homicide). Distributions of rates for the 15 leading causes of death in 1969, by age, sex and color, between 1950 and 1969, are presented in *Vital and Health Statistics,* Series 20, Number 16, "Mortality Trends for Leading Causes of Death: United States, 1950–69." For most causes, the death rates are higher for non-whites than for whites.

Infant Mortality

The *infant* mortality rate is the number of deaths under the age of one, among persons born alive, divided by the number of live births. Since infant mortality appears to be related to a variety of socioeconomic, environmental, and health care factors, as was pointed out in Chapter 2, some authorities (Morris, pp. 56 ff., 267; Rosen, p. 342) consider it to be a fairly sensitive indicator of general health levels in a population. In mid-1975, the infant mortality rate in the United States was 16.5 per 1,000 live births (National Center for Health Statistics, Aug. 28, 1975). The rate has been declining steadily since 1950, when it was 29.2 (U.S. Bureau of the Census, Table 84). In fact, the infant mortality rate has been falling since it was first recorded in this country at 99.9 in 1915 (Grove and Hetzel, Table 38).

The most striking feature of the U.S. infant mortality rate is that although it has consistently fallen over the years, the non-white rate has just as consistently remained almost double the white rate. A detailed examination of the relationship between ethnicity, other factors, and infant mortality is contained in *Vital and Health Statistics*, Series 22, Number 14, "Infant Mortality Rates: Socioeconomic Factors."

A brilliant, detailed contemporary study in New York City of factors related to infant mortality in 140,000 births is to be found in a comprehensive study sponsored by the National Academy of Sciences (Kessner et al.), mentioned in Chapter 2. It finds that in this time of relatively low overall infant mortality rates, with the infectious diseases that formerly took the lives of many infants in the main under control, "generally, adequacy of [health] care . . . is strongly and consistently associated with infant birth weight . . . and survival" (Kessner et al., p. 1). Kessner and his co-authors also concluded from their study that "the survival of infants of different ethnic groups varies widely; . . . there is consistent association between social classes as measured by the educational attainment of the mothers and infant birth weight and survival; . . . within categories of mother's educational attainment, there are consistent trends relating the adequacy of care . . . to infant survival; . . . there is a gross misallocation of services by ethnic group and care when the risks of the women are taken into account . . . " (pp. 2-3).

Marriage and Divorce

Turning to the remaining Vital Statistics, by the mid-1970s the marriage rate stood at 10.3 per 1,000 population (National Center for Health Statistics, Aug. 28, 1975), down from a pre-World-War-II high of 12.1 (U.S. Bureau of the Census, Table 93). The divorce rate, which had stood at 2.0 per 1,000 population in 1940 (U.S. Bureau of the Census, Table No. 93), had reached 5.0 in 1975 (National Center for Health Statistics, Aug. 28, 1975), almost 50% of the marriage rate! Detailed analyses of marriage and divorce statistics can be found in *Vital and Health Statistics*, Series 21, "Data on Natality, Marriage and Divorce."

Morbidity

Morbidity refers to sickness, illness, disease. Like mortality, morbidity data can be expressed as rates and can be cross-tabulated with the broad range of demographic characteristics. Morbidity data are extremely important in characterizing the health status of a population. Mortality data alone are not adequate for that purpose, for several reasons. Many diseases and conditions of ill health that are widely prevalent in the population—particularly in a country like the United States, in which communicable disease, with a few exceptions, is not a major problem—do not appear in mortality figures. The unreported conditions include arthritis, low-back pain, the common cold, mild emotional and sexual problems, and the like. Other diseases that do kill do so rarely in relation to their appearance in the population. Included in this category are duodenal ulcer and gall bladder disease. When looking at morbidity, one learns not only which are the important diseases and the patterns of their distribution in the population, but also how they affect people in terms of limitation of activity.

To understand morbidity data, we must understand the terms incidence and prevalence. *Incidence* is the number of new cases of the disease in question occurring during a particular time period, usually a year. *Prevalence* is the total number of cases existing in a population during a time period or at one point in time ("point-prevalence").

Reporting and Sources of Data

Reporting morbidity is not nearly so simple as reporting mortality. When is a person sick? Who decides? The physician? The patient? The problems of perception of illness, and of the sick role, were referred to in the previous chapter. Furthermore, although it is thought that the determination of cause of death by physicians is reasonably reliable, the accuracy of physician diagnosis in illness is more questionable (Koran).

Although the law requires that all deaths be reported, only certain categories of sickness, the infectious diseases, must be reported. The list appears in *Morbidity and Mortality Weekly Report*. Among the 36 such diseases only 12 can be considered significant in the United States: chickenpox; hepatitis A,B, and unspecified; measles; mumps; German measles; Salmonellosis; shigellosis; tuberculosis; syphilis; and gonorrhea (Center for Disease Control). Of these, four are common childhood viral diseases (for three of which there are vaccines available), while two are venereal diseases. Clearly many categories of disease important in the United States are not reported.

It is known that physicians fail to report certain diseases, even when legally required to do so. Some private physicians will not report venereal disease in private patients, on the grounds of avoiding "embarrassment." Tuberculosis reporting, other than from institutions, is inhibited by the possible economic consequences: some employers automatically fire persons with tuberculosis. (Although the disease is one of low infectivity, it is commonly thought to be highly contagious, even by some health professionals.) Many physicians fail to report cases of the common childhood viral infections because they consider them to be "inconsequential."*

In mortality, there is only one possible source of data, and it isn't the patient. In morbidity, however, both providers and patients can obviously be data sources; as a result, quite different pictures can be obtained. Providers can report morbidity in terms of diagnostic categories and also in terms of patient chief complaints; that is, what the patient reports to the physician as being the problem. (Patients don't usually come to a physician saying "I've got diabetes mellitus, Doc," but rather something like, "I've been feeling kind of weak, and I'm drinking a great deal of water and urinating a lot.") Patients can also report chief complaints directly in a survey. From a chief complaint profile for a population, obtained from either source, some estimates of the morbidity patterns can be obtained. One advantage of deriving information directly from patients is that certain patients with certain types of illnesses will never come to medical attention. Thus morbidity surveys that only gather information from providers will not give a complete picture.

Other than reportable communicable disease data published by the Center for Disease Control in *Morbidity and Mortality Weekly Report*, the regular sources of morbidity data in the United States are from the National Center for Health Statistics. They include the Health Examination Survey and the Health Records Survey, the results of which are published periodically in *Vital and Health Statistics*, and the Health Interview Survey, the Hospital Discharge Survey, and the National Ambulatory Medical Care Survey, the results of which are published in both *Vital and Health Statistics* and *Monthly Vital Statistics Report*. Together these activities constitute the National Health Survey

---

* For example, we can estimate that just before the introduction of the measles vaccine in the mid-1960s, the measles reporting was around 10%. Almost all children get measles before their fifth birthday. There were about 4,000,000 births annually in the U. S. at that time, but only 400,000 cases of measles were reported annually. Since, on the average, 4,000,000 children were getting the disease each year, the reporting rate was about 10%.

(National Center for Health Statistics, August 1963). Series 1 of
Vital and Health Statistics contains the general methodological
and historical accounts.

The Health Interview Survey is one of the ongoing activities of
the National Center for Health Statistics. The results are published continuously in Series 10 of *Vital and Health Statistics*.
Appendix I of most numbers in the Series, "Technical Notes on
Methods," describes the methodology in some detail. Using a sampling method, questionnaires are administered to members of
selected households concerning "personal and demographic characteristics, illnesses, injuries, impairments, chronic conditions,
and other health topics" (National Center for Health Statistics,
Sept. 1975, p. 31). This produces data on "incidence of acute conditions, limitation of activity, persons injured, hospitalization,
disability days, dental visits, and physicians" (National Center
for Health Statistics, Sept. 1975, p. 5). Thus both morbidity and
utilization data are collected from the population perspective.
Special studies produced details of conditions affecting the digestive system in 1968, skin and musculoskeletal systems in 1969,
the respiratory system in 1970, and the circulatory system in
1972. "Impairments" was the special topic in 1971 and "miscella-
neous conditions" in 1973 (National Center for Health Statistics,
Oct. 1974, p. 5). The cycle was recommenced in 1975.

Incidence of Morbid Conditions

In 1974, the incidence of acute conditions was 175 per 100 persons per year, down from 219 in 1971–72 (National Center for
Health Statistics, Sept. 1975, p. 2). Most common were upper
respiratory conditions (28%), followed by influenza (22%), and
injuries (18%). Acute conditions were associated with over 900
days of restricted activity per 100 persons per year (National
Center for Health Statistics, Sept. 1975, Table A). Details of the
data on acute conditions are contained in periodic publications in
Series 10 entitled "Acute Conditions: Incidence and Associated
Disability." It was found that 14.1% of the population experienced limitation in all activity owing to chronic conditions
(National Center for Health Statistics, Sept. 1975, Table B). The
major chronic conditions causing limitations in activity are heart
conditions, arthritis and rheumatism, impairments of lower
extremities and hips, impairments of back or spine, cerebrovas-
cular disease and paralysis, complete or partial (National Center
for Health Statistics, Nov. 1974, Figs. 2, 3). Details of the data

on chronic conditions are contained in periodic publications in Series 10 entitled "Limitation of Activity and Mobility Due to Chronic Conditions."

Turning to data collected from the provider perspective, the Health Records Survey has conducted three reviews of nursing homes and their patients in the United States, in 1963, 1964, and 1969. Sampling methods were used and information was collected about the institutions, the patients or residents, and personnel. The results of these surveys are published periodically in Series 12 of *Vital and Health Statistics*. The Health Examination Survey involves a series of direct examinations of population samples which have been carried out over the years by NCHS staff, from specially designed mobile units. To the early 1970s, there were three "cycles" of examinations: Cycle I on persons 18-79 years of age, conducted between 1959 and 1962; Cycle II on persons 6-11 years of age, conducted between 1963 and 1965; and Cycle III on persons 12–17 years of age, conducted between 1966 and 1970 (National Center for Health Statistics, Aug. 1975, p. 1). The voluminous data produced by the Health Examination Survey is published in Series 11 of *Vital and Health Statistics*. Some data from the HES also appears periodically in *Monthly Vital Statistics Report*.

The Hospital Discharge Survey reports on morbidity (and mortality) as it occurs in hospitals. These data do provide a rather accurate picture of the illness profile of those in hospitals. It must be remembered, however, that the overwhelming majority of ill persons do not require hospitalization; thus the morbidity profile of the population as a whole does not match that seen in hospitals. The results of the HDS through 1971 appear in *Vital and Health Statistics*, Series 13. Since then, they have been published in *Monthly Vital Statistics Report*. The HDS is carried out on a sampling basis in nonfederal, short-stay hospitals (hospitals with six or more beds and an average length of stay of 30 days or less). About 70% of hospital discharges from those hospitals are accounted for by six diagnostic groups: diseases of the circulatory system, 13%; diseases of the digestive system, 13%; complications of pregnancy, childbirth, and the puerperium, 13%; diseases of the respiratory system, 11%; diseases of the genitourinary system, 11%; and accidents, poisonings, and violence, 11% (National Center for Health Statistics, June 10, 1975, Table 1). The five most common specific diagnoses are: malignant neoplasms; ischemic heart disease; fractures, all sites; hypertrophy of tonsils and adenoids; and all other heart and hypertensive disease (National Center for Health Statistics, June 10, 1975, Table 1).

Finally, the most recent component of the National Health Survey is the National Ambulatory Medical Care Survey (National Center for Health Statistics, April, May 1974). Although the NAMCS will eventually cover all loci of ambulatory care, it began by concentrating on private physicians' offices, which in 1972 accounted for about 80% of all physician visits (National Center for Health Statistics, April 1974). The data are collected on a sampling basis from a stratified random sample of all office-based allopathic and osteopathic physicians in the United States, excluding anesthesiologists, pathologists, and

Table 3.2

Number, Percentage, and Cumulative Percentage of Visits to Office-based Physicians, by Diagnosis, U.S., May 1973–April 1974

Rank	Principal Diagnosis Classified	Number of visits (X 1,000)	% of Visits	Cumulative %
1	Medical or special examinations (Y00)	39,613	6.1	6.1
2	Medical and surgical aftercare (Y10)	32,345	5.0	11.2
3	Prenatal care (Y06)	25,359	3.9	15.1
4	Essential benign hypertension (401)	22,752	3.5	18.6
5	Acute respiratory infection (465)	21,514	3.3	22.0
6	Neuroses (300)	16,570	2.6	24.5
7	Observation, without need for further medical care (793)	15,893	2.5	27.0
8	Chronic ischemic heart disease (412)	15,487	2.4	29.4
9	Hay fever (507)	12,166	1.9	31.3
10	Otitis media (381)	10,523	1.6	32.9
11	Acute pharyngitis (462)	10,415	1.6	34.5
12	Obesity (277)	10,136	1.6	36.1
13	Refractive errors (370)	9,175	1.4	37.5
14	Other eczema and dermatitis (692)	9,152	1.4	38.9
15	Diabetes (250)	8,904	1.4	40.3
	All others diagnoses	384,889	59.7	100.0

Source: Monthly Vital Statistics Report, July 14, 1975, Supplement (2), Table 4. (See Appendix I, A4.)
Note: Diagnostic groupings and code number inclusions (in parentheses) are based on the Eighth Revision, International Classification of Diseases, adapted for use in the United States, 1965.

radiologists. Simple questionnaires on each patient seen during a given time period are filled out. Morbidity utilization data are collected, as well as data on practice characteristics.

Morbidity data were collected from two perspectives: patient chief complaint (reason for coming to the office) and physician's diagnosis. The first NAMCS Survey covered the period May 1973–April 1974 (National Center for Health Statistics, July 1974.) The 15 most common diagnoses are shown in Table 3.2. It is interesting to note the place of examinations, after care, prenatal care, neuroses, and observation. The patient's perspective on this situation is shown in Table 3.3. The morbidity profile in private physicians' offices is dominated by problems of a not too serious nature.

Table 3.3

Number, Percentage, and Cumulative Percentage of Visits to Office-based Physicians, by Complaint, U.S., May 1973–April 1974

Rank	20 Most Common Patient Problems, Complaints, or Symptoms	Number of Visits (× 1,000)	% of Visits	Cumulative %
1	Progress visits (980, 985)	75,673	11.7	11.7
2	Other problems, NEC (990)	37,126	5.8	17.5
3	Physical exam (900, 901)	26,117	4.0	21.5
4	Pain, etc.—lower extremity (400)	25,944	4.0	25.6
5	Pregnancy exam (905)	25,942	4.0	29.6
6	Throat soreness (520)	20,726	3.2	32.8
7	Pain, etc.—upper extremity (405)	18,956	2.9	35.7
8	Pain, etc.—back region (415)	18,824	2.9	38.7
9	Cough (311)	18,347	2.8	41.5
10	Abdominal pain (540)	16,418	2.5	44.0
11	Cold (312)	13,460	2.1	46.1
12	Gynecological exam (904)	13,154	2.0	48.2
13	Visit for medication (910)	13,103	2.0	50.2
14	None (997)	13,043	2.0	52.2
15	Headache (056)	12,314	1.9	54.1
16	Fatigue (004)	11,768	1.8	56.0
17	Pain in chest (322)	11,350	1.8	57.7
18	Well-baby exam (906)	10,699	1.7	59.4
19	Fever (002)	9,822	1.5	60.9
20	Allergic skin reaction (112)	9,458	1.5	62.4
	All other symptoms	242,650	37.6	100.0

Source: Monthly Vital Statistics Report, July 14, 1975, Supplement (2), Table 7. (See Appendix I, A4.)
Note: Symptomatic groupings and code number inclusion (in parentheses) are based on a classification developed for use in the NAMCS.

It should be clear that although we do know a great deal about how to characterize the health and illness status of our population, many aspects of this process are still not well understood. For example, we have yet to solve the problem of constructing a health status index for individuals (see Chapters 2 and 12), which could have broad usefulness and could be easily determined (Balinsky and Berger). There is still a great deal to be done.

Utilization
Introduction

We come finally to the third category of data concerning health—that is, how the population utilizes the health care delivery system. We have pointed out that in quantifying utilization of health services, the same series of events can be counted either from the patients' or from the provider's perspective. As we shall see below, the results of the two types of counts are not always the same; thus, when discussing utilization, one has to be very careful to distinguish the two approaches.

To understand this problem, compare the data on hospital ambulatory services utilization as reported by the Health Interview Survey (patient perspective) with that reported by the American Hospital Association (provider perspective). For 1971, the Health Interview Survey reported that patients said that they made about 102 million visits to hospital clinics and emergency units (National Center for Health Statistics, March 1975, Table 14). For the same year, the American Hospital Association's "Hospital Statistics" reported that patients made about 200 million visits to hospital outpatient services (American Hospital Association, 1972, Table 2A).

The causes of the discrepancy are open to conjecture (Jonas). It is probably fair to say that neither figure is valid. (About 10% of the difference is accounted for by the fact that the NHS does not count visits by members of the Armed Forces to Defense Department Hospitals, while the AHA does.) If this is so, the discrepancy is the result of underreporting by patients to the HIS on the one hand, and overreporting (double-counting) by the AHA on the other. One of course does not know the degrees of under- and over-reporting.

It must be borne in mind, however, that if the Health Interview Survey figures for hospital ambulatory visits are low, the comparable figures for private physician office visits may well be low, too. This could have a serious effect on health care planning, since it is customary to use the HIS figure for the average annual per-person physician rate (in the mid-1970s around 5.0) as a base-line datum. As more data become available from the National Ambulatory Medical Care Survey (NAMCS), which counts physician office visits from the provider perspective, it will be possible to validate the HIS data to some extent. Interestingly, in a paper on factors in the rise in health care costs, Nancy Worthington of the Social Security Administration estimated (without giving her sources) the average annual per-person physician rate for 1973 at over eight (1975, Table 4).

Utilization of Ambulatory Services

As we have noted, the Health Interview Survey provides patient-perspective data for this parameter. According to the HIS, in 1973, there were approximately 5.0 physician visits per person, and about 75% of the population made at least one visit (National Center for Health Statistics, Oct. 1974, Table 20). This figure had been showing a slight increase in recent years. In general, females made more visits than males, and, as might be expected, the visit rate increased with age. In the same year, the average number of dental visits per person was 1.6, with slightly less than one-half of the population making a dental visit in the year (National Center for Health Statistics, Oct. 1974, Table 18).

For place of visit, 1971 data, reported in a more detailed analysis of patient visits entitled "Physician Visits" (National Center for Health Statistics, March 1975), indicated that about 70% of the total visits took place in the physician's office, about 2% in the home, 10% in a hospital clinic or emergency room, 1.0% in an industrial health service, 13% over the telephone (telephone "visits" are included by the HIS in the annual total number of visits, which, when divided by the number of persons, gives the annual per-person visit rate), and 4% "other." "Physician Visits" also provides some interesting insights on the relationship between various sociodemographic variables and utilization variables.

There are several sources for provider data on the utilization of ambulatory services. The most comprehensive is the National Ambulatory Medical Care Survey, explained above, which appeared on the scene in the mid-1970s. For the period May 1973–April 1974, the NAMCS reported 645 million visits to what it called " 'office-based, patient care' physicians" (National

Center for Health Statistics, July 1975, p. 1). Because of differences in methods of sampling and data collection, and timeframe, it is difficult to determine if the results of the NAMCS are entirely consistent with those of the HIS (National Center for Health Statistics, Aug. 1963, April 1974). However, the two certainly give results for physician-office visits which are in the same order of magnitude. This consistency provides an interesting perspective on the disparity between the HIS and AHA results concerning hospital ambulatory visits. The NAMCS provides data on visits by age, color group, geographic region, metropolitan/nonmetropolitan living area, type of physician and duration of visit, as well as morbidity, as we saw above.

The other major source of provider-perspective ambulatory service utilization data is the American Hospital Association's annual publication *Hospital Statistics,* published each summer. Until 1970, it appeared as part of the AHA's "Guide Issue" to hospitals in the United States, but since 1971, it has been issued separately. For 1974, the AHA reported 108 million visits to hospital clinics, 71 million visits to hospital emergency units, and 71.5 million referred visits (American Hospital Association, 1975, Table 3). A clinic visit is an "outpatient visit to [an] organized subunit of the outpatient department." An emergency visit is an "admission to an emergency unit." A referred visit is to a "special diagnostic or therapeutic facility [and] service of the hospital upon referral of a physician" (American Hospital Association, 1975, p. xxiv). *Hospital Statistics* provides considerable detail on these data by such variables as hospital bed size, ownership, type, geographical region, and medical school affiliation (American Hospital Association, 1975, Tables 3, 5, 6, 8).

Utilization of Hospital Services

Turning to utilization of hospital services, patient-perspective data are provided by the HIS. For 1973, there were 13.9 reported discharges per 100 persons from short-stay hospitals* (National

---

* Note that the HIS definition of a "short-stay hospital" differs from that of the AHA. The HIS defines it as "one in which the type of service provided . . . is general; maternity; eye; ear, nose and throat; children's; or osteopathic; or it may be the hospital department of an institution" (National Center for Health Statistics, October 1974, p. 55). The AHA defines short-stay as a hospital in which average length of stay is less than 30 days (American Hospital Association, 1975, p. xxiv).

Center for Health Statistics, Oct. 1974, p. 4, Table 13). This amounts to about 29.2 million discharges. The average reported length of hospital stay was 8.1 days, representing a slight downward trend from 1971, while 10.7% of all persons were hospitalized one or more times. Further breakdowns by age and sex are also given (National Center for Health Statistics, Oct. 1974, p. 4, Tables 13, 14, 15).

The National Center for Health Statistics also provides provider-perspective hospital-utilization data through the Hospital Discharge Survey. The Center points out that because of "differences in collection procedures, population sampled, and definitions," the results from the HIS and the HDS are not entirely consistent (National Center for Health Statistics, Oct. 1974, p. 4). Other classes of data provided by the Hospital Discharge Survey are morbidity, discussed above, and an analysis of surgery (National Center for Health Statistics, May 30, 1975).

The other major source of hospital utilization data is the American Hospital Association. In addition to the annual *Hospital Statistics*, *Hospital Indicators* appears monthly in *Hospitals*, the Journal of the American Hospital Association. For 1974, the 7,174 AHA-registered hospitals, with a total of 1.5 million beds, reported 35.5 million admissions, an occupancy rate of slightly over 77%, and an average daily census of 1.15 million (American Hospital Association, 1975, Table 3). In the same year, the 6,450 hospitals that the AHA classifies as short-term admitted 34.7 million patients to their one million beds. The occupancy rate was 75.4% and the average daily census was just under 800,000. *Hospital Statistics* contains voluminous data on these variables and many others, including fiscal parameters, by hospital type, size, ownership, geographical location, and the like. *Hospital Indicators* covers similar parameters, and also publishes special studies. An advantage of *Hospital Indicators* is its frequency of appearance.

Certain provider-perspective hospital utilization data also appear in *Health Resources Statistics,* a National Center for Health Statistics data source published on an annual/biennial basis. The NCHS counts hospitals in a slightly more comprehensive manner than does the AHA (National Center for Health Statistics, *Health Resources Statistics,* p. 348). It also compiles hospital utilization data slightly differently.

Of course, it should be pointed out that, in addition to publishing provider-perspective hospital utilization data, *Hospital Sta-*

tistics, Hospital Indicators, and *Health Resources Statistics* are the major sources of hospital census data.

Conclusion

In the United States a great deal of data concerning the population, its health, and how it uses the health care delivery system are collected. Thus we know a great deal about health, disease, and illness in the United States, and about the functioning of the health care delivery system. There are gaps in our knowledge, to be sure; some of them will be filled if the provisions of the National Health Resources Planning and Development Act (P.L. 93–641, Sect. 1513, b, 1) relating to data are carried out. These requirements, which call for the mandatory, national collection of data on population health status, health care delivery system utilization, effects of the health care delivery system on health, health care delivery resources, and environmental and occupational exposure factors relating to health, will if met constitute the biggest step forward in health data assemblage since the organization of the Vital Statistics system. However, we already have a great deal of data. We need to remember that data mean little until they are put to use.

References

American Hospital Association. *Hospital Statistics,* for the years 1971 through 1975. Chicago, Ill., 1972–75.

Balinsky, W., and Berger R. "A Review of the Research on General Health Status Indexes." *Medical Care, 13,* 283, 1975.

Brook, R. H., and Williams, K. N. "Quality of Health Care for the Disadvantaged." *Journal of Community Health, 1,* 132, 1975.

Center for Disease Control. "Reported Morbidity and Mortality in the United States, 1974." *Morbidity and Mortality Weekly Report, 23,* for year ending December 28, 1974.

Grove, R. D., and Hetzel, A. M. *Vital Statistics Rates in the United States: 1940–1960.* Washington, D.C.: National Center for Health Statistics, USDHEW, 1968.

Jonas, S. "Physician Visits." *American Journal of Public Health, 64,* 204, 727, 1974. (Letters)

Kessner, D. M. et al. *Infant Death: An Analysis by Maternal Risk and Health Care.* Washington, D.C.: Institute of Medicine, National Academy of Sciences, 1973.

Koran, L. "The Reliability of Clinical Methods, Data and Judgments." *New England Journal of Medicine, 293,* 642, 695, 1975.

Morris, J. N. *Uses of Epidemiology.* Baltimore, Md.: Williams and Wilkins, 1964.

National Center for Health Statistics. "Origin, Program and Operation of the U.S. National Health Survey." *Vital and Health Statistics,* Series 1, No. 1, August, 1963.

――――. *Health Resources Statistics: Health Manpower and Health Facilities, 1974.* Rockville, Md.: USDHEW, 1974.

――――. "National Ambulatory Medical Care Survey: Background and Methodology: United States—1967–1972." *Vital and Health Statistics,* Series 2, No. 61, April, 1974.

――――. "The National Ambulatory Medical Care Survey: Symptom Classification." *Vital and Health Statistics,* Series 2, No. 63, May, 1974.

――――. "Provisional Statistics, Annual Summary for the United States, 1973." *Monthly Vital Statistics Report, 22,* June 27, 1974.

――――. "Current Estimates from the Health Interview Survey: United States—1973." *Vital and Health Statistics,* Series 10, No. 95, October, 1974.

――――. "Limitation of Activity and Mobility Due to Chronic Conditions: United States—1972." *Vital and Health Statistics,* Series 10, No. 96, November, 1974.

――――. "Physician Visits: Volume and Interval Since Last Visit—United States—1971." *Vital and Health Statistics,* Series 10, No. 97, March, 1975.

――――. "Hospital Discharge Survey Data: Surgery in Short-Stay Hospitals: United States, 1973." *Monthly Vital Statistics Report, 24,* No. 3 (Supplement), May 30, 1975.

――――. "Hospital Discharge Survey." *Monthly Vital Statistics Report, 24,* No. 3 (Supplement 2), June 10, 1975.

――――. "National Ambulatory Medical Care Survey." *Monthly Vital Statistics Report, 24,* No. 4 (Supplement 2), July 14, 1975.

――――. "Serum Uric Acid Values of Youths 12–17 Years: United States." *Vital and Health Statsitics,* Series 11, No. 152, August, 1975.

――――. "Hospital Discharge Survey Data: Utilization of Short-Stay Hospitals—Summary of Nonmedical Statistics: United States, 1973." *Monthly Vital Statistics Report, 24,* No. 5 (Supplement 2), August 19, 1975.

――――. "Provisional Statistics." *Monthly Vital Statistics Report, 24,* No. 6, August 28, 1975.

――――. "Current Estimates from the Health Interview Survey: United States—1973." *Vital and Health Statistics,* Series 10, No. 100, September, 1975.

P. L. 93–641. Health Planning Resources and Development Act of 1974.

Rosen, G. *A History of Public Health.* New York: MD Publications, 1958.

U.S. Bureau of the Census. *Statistical Abstract of the United States: 1974.* Washington, D.C.: Department of Commerce, 1974.

White, K. L. "Life and Death and Medicine." *Scientific American,* September, 1973, p. 23.

Worthington, N. L. "Expenditures for Hospital Care and Physicians' Services: Factors Affecting Annual Changes." *Social Security Bulletin,* November, 1975, p. 3.

4

Health Manpower

Ruth S. Hanft

Introduction

With this chapter, we begin our consideration of the personnel and institutional inputs to the health care delivery system in the United States. The health care industry is labor-intensive; consequently, the education and use of health manpower is a critical variable in determining the distribution, efficiency, economy, and cost of the industry and its products. Manpower is of course not a variable standing on its own: financing, organization and delivery of health services, biomedical research, and consequent technological developments all affect the size and use of the health manpower pool.

The health care field has enjoyed a long period of expansion with continuous growth in funding of services and programs from both the private and public sectors (see Chapter 9). Until recently, it was not really necessary to make hard choices among programs because more money always seemed to be available and resources were relatively unconstrained. Moreover, since World War II, both the number and types of health care workers have increased greatly. Because of the open-ended flow of third-party payments for certain types of health services, relatively few observers of the system raised questions concerning efficiency and efficacy or considered the cost implications of adding new types of personnel, new technology, or new services.

Overall, the health industry is labor-intensive. Many new health services require significant manpower inputs; as a result, they significantly affect costs. Furthermore, physicians, who are the centerpiece of the health care delivery system, create a major portion of the demand for their own services (Fuchs and Kramer, p. 2), as do certain other types of health manpower. Increases in the manpower pool and the development of new types of manpower tend to increase the total supply of services—

more physical therapists mean that more physical therapy services will be available. Since health manpower creates its own demand, by prescribing the use of services for patients, increases in supply may well increase the demand for services. The traditional constraints of the economic market do not operate in the health field (Fuchs). (See also Chapter 9.)

In the mid-70s, a number of health manpower problems were being discussed in government, by the public, and among experts in the field. These included the following:

—How large a manpower pool is needed? Is there a danger of producing, for example, too many physicians?

—Why is the manpower-to-hospital-bed ratio higher in the United States than it is in any other industrialized country?

—How can the distribution of manpower by both specialty and geography be improved?

—How many primary care physicians are needed? How many specialists?

—Should the trends toward further specialization of professional and allied health manpower be encouraged or halted? Should the various certification and licensure processes that have proliferated so rapidly since World War II be re-evaluated?

—Will "physicians' extenders" (e.g., physicians' associates and clinical nurse practitioners) be substitutes for physicians or will they be used instead to expand and enhance services and possibly add to health sector costs?

—Why are education costs for health professionals so high? Can the health care education enterprise operate more efficiently?

—Should the methods of financing health professional education be altered? Should the government continue to subsidize the education of high-earning professionals when it subsidizes other professions only minimally?

—What are the implications of the United States' dependence on foreign medical graduates?

In this chapter, we will deal with these questions and discuss the available information that can be used in answering them.

Types of Health Workers

For 1973, the National Center for Health Statistics recorded over 4.4 million active workers in the health field, as shown in Table 4.1. The total does not include the large, but unknown, number of housekeeping, kitchen, and maintenance personnel who work in the health care industry, primarily in institutions. The range of skills required in the industry is vast and overlaps those of many other industries. The sites of employment in the industry are also numerous; they include hospitals, nursing homes, private offices, ambulatory health care centers of various types, health maintenance organizations, research laboratories and foundations, patients' homes, elementary and secondary schools, colleges and universities, manufacturing plants, hospital supply companies, pharmaceutical companies, prisons, custodial institutions, ships and more.

In terms of mode of functioning, health care providers may be divided into three major groups: independent practitioners, dependent practitioners, and supporting staff, the lines separating the three groups being rather unclear at times.* The independent practitioner group consists of those health care providers allowed by law to deliver a delimited range of services to any persons who want them, without supervision or authorization of the practitioner's work by third parties. Among the independent practitioners are physicians (osteopathic and allopathic), dentists, chiropractors, optometrists, and podiatrists.

The dependent practitioner group is allowed by law to deliver a delimited range of services to persons, under the supervision and/or the authorization of independent practitioners, often of a particular type specified by law. The dependent category includes nurses, psychologists, social workers, pharmacists, physicians' assistants, dental hygienists, and the various therapists: speech, physical, and occupational. However, in certain situations, in relation to certain patients, many of the workers in those occupations may and can assume the role of independent practitioner. The definition of the line between the independent and dependent groups is the source of many conflicts at present.

Supporting staff, rather than providing a range of services to patients, carry out specific work tasks authorized by and under the supervision of independent and/or dependent practitioners. The work of supporting staff may or may not be regulated by laws directly pertaining to them, but if there are not special laws, they work under the legal sanctions provided for their supervisors. This group includes clerical, maintenance, housekeeping and food-processing workers, research workers, administrators,

---

* This model is similar to that described by Eliot Freidson in *Professional Dominance: The Social Structure of Medical Care* (New York: Atherton Press, 1970), especially Chapter 5.

Table 4.1

Estimated Number of Persons Active in Selected Occupations within Each Health Field, U.S., 1973

Health Field and Selected Occupations	Persons Active
Total[a]	4,403,450 to 4,448,250
Administration of health services	48,200
Anthropology and sociology	1,600
Automatic data processing in the health field	4,000
Basic sciences in the health field	60,000
Biomedical engineering	11,500
Chiropractic	15,500
Clinical laboratory services	162,800
Dentistry and allied services	274,400
Dentists	105,400
Dental hygienist	21,000
Dental assistant	116,000
Dental laboratory technician	32,000
Dietetic and nutritional services	68,000
Economic research in the health field	400
Environmental sanitation	17,000 to 20,000
Food and drug protective services	44,400
Funeral directors and embalmers	50,000
Health and vital statistics	1,350
Health education	22,500 to 23,000
Health information and communication	6,700 to 9.300
Library services in the health field	7,900
Medical records	54,000
Medicine and osteopathy	345,300
Physician (M.D.)	333,300
Physician (D.O.)	12,000
Midwifery	4,200
Nursing and related services	2,207,000 to 2,212,000
Registered nurse	815,000

recordkeepers, nurses' aides, dental assistants, and technicians, primarily laboratory and radiological. In certain situations, some of these persons may assume the role of dependent practitioner; the struggles over status and responsibility between certain categories of supporting staff and dependent practitioners sometimes mirror those between independent and dependent practitioners.

The largest categories of health worker are as follows: nursing and related services (over 2,000,000), physicians (approximately 350,000), dentists and allied services (about 275,000), secretarial services (about 300,000), clinical laboratory services (about 165,000), pharmacists (about 135,000) and radiological technologists (100,000) (Table 4.1). Most health care workers are female, but most physicians, dentists, other independent health

Table 4.1 (continued)

**Estimated Number of Persons Active in Selected Occupations
within Each Health Field, U.S., 1973**

Health Field and Selected Occupations	Persons Active
Nursing and related services (cont.)	
Practical nurse	459,000
Nursing aide, orderly, attendant	910,000
Home health aide	23,000 to 28,000
Occupational therapy	13,200 to 14,200
Optometry and opticianry	35,200 to 35,400
Orthotic and prosthetic technology	2,500 to 3,500
Pharmacy	132,900
Physical therapy	24,600
Podiatry	7,100
Psychology	27,000
Radiologic technology	100,000
Respiratory therapy (inhalation) technician	11,000 to 12,000
Secretarial & office services in the health field	275,000 to 300,000
Social work	33,800
Specialized rehabilitation services	11,050
Speech pathology and audiology	26,500
Veterinary medicine	26,900
Vocational rehabilitation counseling	17,000
Miscellaneous health services	252,950 to 258,450
Ambulance attendant	207,000
Animal technician	5,000
Electrocardiograph technician	9,500
Electroencephalograph technician	3,500 to 4,000
Operating room technician	11,400
Ophthalmic assistant	15,000 to 20,000
Orthoptist	450
Physician's assistant	900
Surgeon's assistant	200

Source: National Center for Health Statistics, *Health: United States,
1975*, Table B.I.1. DHEW Pub. No. (HRA) 76-1232. Derived from National Center for Health Statistics, *Health Resources Statistics, 1974*,
Table I. DHEW Pub. No. (HRA) 75-1509. (See Appendix I, A8.)
ᵃ Each occupation is counted only once. For example, all physicians
are in medicine and osteopathy.

care practitioners, administrators and other persons in policy-making positions are male (Navarro, 1975). (For further detail
on types and roles of nurses and physicians in the United States
health care system, see Chapters 5 and 6 respectively.)

Compared with other nations, the United States is amply supplied with health workers. The United States has one of the highest physician-population ratios in the world (Table 4.2); it has
increased substantially since 1970 and is expected to exceed 200
per 100,000 population by 1990. The types of health manpower in

Table 4.2
International Physician/Population Ratios

Country	Population per Physician	Physicians per 100,000
Australia	850	118
Belgium	650	154
Canada	690	146
Denmark	690	144
England & Wales	820	122
France	750	134
Germ. Dem. Rep.	630	160
Germ. Fed. Rep.	580	172
Ireland	980	102
Israel	400	250
Italy	550	181
Japan	880	113
Netherlands	800	125
New Zealand	1,230	81
N. Ireland	750	133
Norway	720	138
Scotland	770	130
South Africa	1,970	51
Sweden	730	136
Switzerland	700	142
USA	630	158
USSR	420	238

Source: World Health Statistics Annual, 1970, vol. 3
(Geneva: World Health Organization, 1974).
Note: Statistics given are all from 1970 annual; how-
ever, some are from earlier base years.

the United States are also more varied than elsewhere—in the
independent category for example, osteopaths, podiatrists, and
optometrists are virtually unknown in most other countries. The
number and variety of allied manpower categories is also unique
to the United States. In contrast, other nations have experi-
mented more widely with substitutes for physicians of a scope
and nature not found in the United States—for example, the
feldsher (Sidel, 1968), barefoot doctor (Sidel, 1972; Wang), and
other types of auxiliaries (Fendall).

Training of Health Manpower

The sites for health manpower training are numerous. Physicians, osteopaths, dentists, veterinarians, optometrists, pharmacists, podiatrists, and nurses are all trained in both independent
and university-based colleges and professional schools. Nurses
are also trained in hospitals and community colleges. These var-

ious schools are found in both the public and private sectors, with a growing trend toward public schools and university-based institutions. In the past 10 years, most of the expansion of medical and osteopathic schools has come through state university institutions and the expansion of nursing programs through state and locally supported community colleges (see also Chapter 5).

Many of the schools that train health professional manpower have multiple functions. In medicine, for example, most schools are also centers of major biomedical research activities; are responsible for training both Doctors of Medicine (M.D.s) and basic scientists (Ph.D.s); and are involved in the training of graduate physicians at the internship, resident, and fellowship (subspecialty) levels. Faculty of medical schools also instruct nursing, dental, and other students. In addition, their own or affiliated teaching hospitals provide patient care services. Some of these hospitals are tertiary care centers for a region or a state or multiple states. They are often the sole source of care for large indigent populations (Freymann, Section IV; Institute of Medicine, 1976).

The number of schools and hospitals engaged in health professional education increased substantially during the decade 1965–75. In the eight health professions financed directly by the federal government (medicine, osteopathy, dentistry, podiatry, optometry, nursing, pharmacy, and veterinary medicine), more than 1,600 schools in the United States provide education, of which over 1,300 are for nurses. In 1975, there were 116 medical schools graduating approximately 14,000 students a year. In 1976, more new health professional schools in medicine, dentistry, osteopathy, optometry, and veterinary medicine were on the drawing boards, including eight new medical schools sponsored by the Veteran's Administration, and a military medical school. (See also Chapter 10.)

More and more often, individual health professional schools on university campuses are being tied together into academic health science centers (Freymann, Ch. 26; Pellegrino, 1973). Increasingly, universities are creating the position of vice-chancellor for health services to whom deans of the individual schools report. These combinations are designed to facilitate the sharing of faculty and services, to reduce duplication in the basic science curriculum, and to provide unified management of the school and hospital. In some institutions, students in the different disciplines receive some of their clinical training together, in an effort to provide team-teaching and greater efficiency in the provision of services. These efforts have met with some but not uniform success (Pellegrino, 1975).

Allied health manpower are trained in four-year colleges, community colleges, proprietary technical schools, hospitals, and in on-the-job training programs (McTernan and Hawkins). There is no accurate count available of the number of institutions or programs training allied health manpower. Degrees in the allied field range from certificates of completion of less than a year of training for certain technicians and L.P.N.s, to associate degrees, baccalaureate degrees, master's, and in some cases Ph.D. degrees.

Many health workers receive training in institutions not regarded as health professional schools. Often programs are started without regard to national or local health manpower needs, thus leading to an oversupply of certain categories of technician and therapist. People are even trained for nonexistent jobs or taught skills too narrow to be transferable. This occurred in some training programs for local residents associated with Office of Economic Opportunity-funded Neighborhood Health Centers. Community colleges in the last 15 years have proliferated training programs in a wide variety of health and health-related fields without undertaking market research surveys.

In the professions, training can extend for many years beyond college degree and even the first professional degree. In some programs in surgery and the subspecialities of medicine, training is as long as six or seven years past the M.D. degree. In many of the professional and allied fields, the trend has been to extend the length of training. In the professions, the postgraduate trainee is also a provider of services. Controversy currently exists in medicine as to whether residents are employees or trainees. In 1976 the National Labor Relations Board ruled that they are trainees and thus do not have the legal right to bargain collectively with the managements of the institutions in which they work (American Hospital Association). After their first or second year, residents are licensed physicians; if they chose not to continue training, they would be practicing physicians. Osteopaths, for example, often enter practice after only a one-year internship (Institute of Medicine, 1976).

Foreign Medical Graduates

The manpower pool has been augmented by foreign-trained physicians and nurses. The United States is a major importer of phy-

sician manpower from abroad. This is a matter of major controversy (Association of American Medical Colleges; Williams and
Lockett; Haug and Stevens; Kleinman et al., 1974, 1975 (a),
(b) ; Goldblatt et al.). In 1974, the Immigration and Naturalization Service and the Department of State reported granting
immigrant visas to 4,537 foreign medical graduates, exchange
visitors' visas to 5,449 individuals, and 872 visas under non-
immigrant status (Immigration and Naturalization Service).
Between 1965 and 1973, 66,757 foreign medical graduates
entered the United States, while there were 76,041 new graduates
of American medical schools (Stevens, 1975). In 1974, 10,038
United States medical graduates and 6,485 foreign medical graduates were licensed to practice medicine.

The use of foreign medical graduates enter the United States medical
care system primarily at the graduate education level; they now
occupy about 30% of the filled residency positions in United
States hospitals (Institute of Medicine, 1976). Because the U. S.
Department of Labor has deemed that there is an undersupply of
physicians, special preference is granted to foreign physicians
under immigration requirements and quotas. At the same time
that large numbers of foreign medical graduates have been
coming to the United States to gain additional training and to fill
vacancies in house-staff programs, significant numbers of U. S.
citizens unable to gain admission to medical schools in this country are studying abroad (Lockett). In 1973, it was estimated that
more than 6,000 United States citizens were following this route.

The use of foreign medical graduates (FMGs) has provoked
considerable debate. Weiss (Kleinman et al., 1974) and Stevens
(1975), for example, disagree on so elementary a datum as the
number of FMGs in the country. Concern has been expressed in a
number of reports about the dependence of the United States
health care system on FMGs, the "brain drain" on under-
developed nations, and the quality of the education of FMGs
(Coordinating Council on Medical Education; National Advisory
Commission on Health Manpower; National Board of Medical
Examiners; Association of American Medical Colleges). Health
manpower legislation passed late in 1976 (P.L. 94–484) is expected to sharply reduce the influx of FMGs by changing certain
immigration regulations. This move was strongly supported by
the Institute of Medicine (1976), the Coordinating Council on
Medical Education, and the Association of American Medical
Colleges.

Costs of Education in the Health Professions

The cost of education in the eight major health professions exceeds that of virtually every other profession. The Institute of Medicine (1974) studied these costs at the request of Congress in 1973. The average annual cost per student by profession is shown in Table 4.3. The costs increased by 16% or more between 1973 and 1976. Part of the reason for the high cost of education is the training process itself, which includes not only instruction but also research and patient care essential for education. Indeed, the health professions are the only ones for which the training institutions must themselves deliver the professional product in order to carry out the education—that is, a medical school must practice medicine as a school, teaching its students through that practice, whereas no law school practices law, as a school, even though individual faculty members may do so.

No definitive studies have been undertaken to estimate the cost of the postprofessional degree training, but these costs are also thought to be high. In the health professions, postdoctoral training is carried out in osteopathy, dentistry, medicine, and podiatry through internships and residencies. The costs of training include the stipends or salaries and fringe benefits paid to the residents, as well as faculty costs. Furthermore, many observers of the education process believe that additional health care costs are

Table 4.3

**Average Annual Cost per
Student, Education in Selected
Health Professions, 1972–73**

Medicine	$12,650
Osteopathy	8,950
Dentistry	9,050
Optometry	4,250
Pharmacy	3,250
Podiatry	5,750
Veterinary medicine	7,500
Nursing	
Baccalaureate	2,500
Associate	1,650
Diploma	3,300

Source: Institute of Medicine, *Costs of Education in the Health Professions* (Washington, D.C.: National Academy of Sciences, 1974).

incurred through extra procedures and diagnostic tests that are part of the educational process; these require additional equipment and allied health manpower. The patient care services provided by the graduate trainees offset these costs. Approximately 84% of house-staff time is spent in patient care (Institute of Medicine, 1976). No national cost figures are available on the training of allied health manpower.

Unlike any other profession, the public sector is now preeminent in the support of health care provider education. Substantial increases in federal government support began in the late 1960s. In addition, the federal government served as a catalyst for the creation of a number of new types of health manpower, particularly physician and dental extenders of various types. It also indirectly encouraged the proliferation of allied manpower through research support and the introduction of new sophisticated technologies, which require various types of technician skills.

Until the 1960s, the federal government provided little direct support for the training of health manpower, which was regarded as a state and private responsibility. The government began to support the education of health professionals directly through institutional grants to the health professional schools in 1963. The support grew, and in 1971 the federal government began to provide "capitation" aid (grants based on the number of students) to educational institutions for eight health professions: medicine, osteopathy, dentistry, nursing, podiatry, pharmacy, optometry, and veterinary medicine. The federal government also supports graduate medical education and allied health manpower training in the Veterans' Administration, military, and other federal hospitals. In 1976, both the concept and size of capitation support for the professions was undergoing extensive review, particularly in Congress.

The government also indirectly supports the training of health manpower—both professional and allied—in hospital-based programs through the reimbursement formulas of Medicare and Medicaid. The major indirect support for the training of physician manpower and allied health manpower comes from third-party payments to hospitals. Hospital-based training programs include the training of interns and residents, diploma nurses, and a variety of technicians. The costs of these programs are included as part of hospital costs or charges paid through patient care revenues and thus they have been hidden.

Until the 1972 Social Security Act Amendments, reimbursement for these costs was essentially open-ended, since the original reimbursement mechanisms made Medicare and Medicaid "uncontrollable" expenditures. The 1972 amendments gave the Social Security Administration more authority to determine the "reasonableness" of reimbursement. The amendments also allowed Medicaid to deviate from the Medicare method of reimbursement of hospitals. In accordance with this legislative change, the Social Security Administration began to classify hospitals into groups and to put a ceiling on the amount paid for routine hospital costs, including graduate training costs (92-603, Sec. 223). At the same time, Blue Cross began to question some training costs, particularly in hospitals in Pennsylvania and Michigan, and to cut back the level of support. State rate-regulation commissions began to take a hard look at these costs as well. The rate-regulation commissions are expanding rapidly and are in at least partial operation in New York, New Jersey, Maryland, Connecticut, and Washington. (See also Chapter 9.)

The magnitude of hospital costs that can be attributed to the education of health professionals and allied health manpower is unknown. There are more than 1,200 hospitals in the country providing graduate medical education. In 1974, there were more than 48,000 residents in medicine and approximately 1,500 residents and interns in training in osteopathy (American Medical Association; American Association of Osteopathic Medicine). There is no accurate count of other health trainees in hospitals. Although most of the hospitals that provide medical education are associated with medical schools, the degree of control over the residency programs varies widely.

Tuition, except in nursing and podiatry, meets only a very small proportion of the cost of health sciences education, smaller than for any other professionals. There are no tuition charges for internship and resident training. As would be expected, tuition in the private institutions is substantially higher than in the public colleges and universities (Institute of Medicine, 1974). In all types of institutions, however, tax-levy money pays a significant proportion of the total costs. There have been several recent legislative proposals that would require health professions students either to work in underserved areas for specified periods of time after completing their training, or to pay back to the government the full tax-levy costs of their education (S. 3239). It is likely that some approaches of this nature will be gradually implemented.

Problems in Medical Education

The problems in the medical education process and in the educational institutions are linked to the problems in health manpower distribution and the delivery of services, particularly the distribution of physicians by specialty and geography, and costs. The medical education community and the public are now engaged in a serious debate regarding the role of medical schools in producing physicians.* The issues being debated include the medical schools' responsibility for training primary care physicians; the medical schools' responsibility for graduate medical education programs; the appropriate curricula and training sites for the development of primary care physicians; the medical schools' role in assuring that physicians locate in underserved areas; and constraining the rise in the costs of medical education.

Medical education evolves slowly and the changes it does make are only gradually reflected in the health care delivery system because of the length of the education process. The education of a physician takes from 10 to 15 years after graduation from high school. To affect the choices of physicians regarding specialty and geography, intervention would be needed at the college, medical school, residency, and practice levels.

Historical factors. Historically, several major trends influenced the current orientation of medical schools. The Flexner Report (1910) changed the methods of instruction to emphasize the scientific basis of medical education. As a result, there was a sharp decline in the number of proprietary medical schools, which had been very prominent until the time of the Flexner Report, as well as in the preceptorship-apprenticeship orientation of clinical medical education, while basic science instruction and clinical training in hospitals were strengthened.

Following World War II, the federal government decided to give financial support to biomedical research in the medical schools rather than in the science departments of parent universities. This decision was strongly influenced by the adamant opposition of the American Medical Association to direct federal aid to medical education. Supporting biomedical research in medical

* Much of this debate can be found in testimony related to Health Manpower Legislation presented in 1974 and 1975 before the Congress in the Health Manpower Hearings.

schools was one way that the federal government could indeed support medical education without appearing to do so directly. This approach had the effect of orienting the medical schools and their faculty toward research (Strickland, chs. 3 and 4). The availability of research grants to support faculty salaries allowed the medical schools to expand the scope of faculty capabilities in specialties and subspecialties. The technological breakthroughs achieved in the 1940s, 50s, and 60s, combined with the growing desire of World War II veterans to enter specialty training, changed the emphasis of graduate medical education toward greater specialization and training in highly sophisticated hospital settings.

State legislatures expected their medical school hospitals to be the source of tertiary care and skilled care for large regions or whole states, as in the cases of the Universities of Colorado, Washington, Iowa, and Mississippi. Both before and after Medicare and Medicaid, the states also expected the public medical school hospitals to care for their indigent populations. The university-owned and associated hospitals of many private medical schools found, as populations shifted from the city to suburbs, that they were located in low-income areas and were the principal source of outpatient and inpatient care for large low-income populations.

Need for community exposure. By and large, medical schools and their teaching hospitals are located in large cities, offering few opportunities for clinical training in rural areas. Because of the hospital-based, specialty-oriented nature of graduate medical education and teaching hospitals (Mumford), undergraduate and graduate medical students get little exposure to office-based or group practice. One of the problems in altering specialty and geographic distribution of physicians and in providing primary care training is the need to develop non–hospital-based training and training in small communities with close and adequate supervision of the trainees by medical school faculty (Petersdorf, Dec. 1975). Several experiments now underway aim to train undergraduate and graduate students in office-based sites, community hospitals, and small communities (Breisch; Steinwald and Steinwald). Some examples include the University of Indiana statewide system, the University of Illinois extensions in Rockford and Peoria (Evans et al.), the University of Washington WAMI (Washington, Alaska, Montana, Idaho) system, and the George Washington University HMO and preceptor-training programs.

Some of the newer medical schools are now being located or planned in smaller communities in the hope that students will be encouraged to locate in them and that a regional center for specialized care will be established for these areas.

Issues in Health Manpower

The major issues in health manpower under public and governmental discussion fall into two different categories: the size of the health care manpower pool and how it should be distributed.*

Size of the Health Manpower Pool

The health industry has expanded exponentially over the past 30 years, as pointed out above. The proportion of the GNP consumed has increased rapidly as has the manpower employed. Without external constraints, these trends could continue. The nature and magnitude of the expenditures and the nature of the medical care cost inflation are such that artificial constraints on expenditures are beginning to be imposed. (See Chapter 9.)

To determine rationally the size of the manpower pool, some measure of need or demand for services is necessary (Institute of Medicine, 1976), but need and demand alone cannot be the base for determining manpower. Patterns of practice vary (Wennberg and Gittlesohn, 1975), productivity varies (American College of Surgeons; Schonfeld), and supply affects demand (Lave et al.). One can alternatively try to rely on the force of an economic market to regulate the size of the pool. This is, in general. what has been tried to date; it has not been too effective (see Chapter 9). If market mechanisms were effective, the manpower pool would expand or contract, as it does in other sectors of the economy, in relation to changes in supply and demand. The market

---

* Health care manpower is but one major factor in the mix of resources that produces health services. Although the discussion that follows treats health care manpower as a separate issue, the reader should recognize that change in the organization and delivery of services and in their financing affect the size and distribution of the health care manpower supply (Davis). In addition, an increasing proportion of experts in the field (Anderson; McKeown and Lowe; Fuchs, ch. 2) are concluding that an increase in health services (and manpower) may have only marginal effects on health. (See Chapters 2 and 15.) It may well be more crucial to turn our attention to income support, environmental protection, housing, improved nutrition, and community rather than personal health services.

mechanism, however, falters because of lack of consumer information; artificial licensure and certification barriers; the nonprofit nature of most of the hospital sector; the ability of the
provider to influence the demand for services; rapid changes in
technology; and consumer expectations (Fuchs). Only in allied
health do market forces exercise some constraint.

The increase in physician specialization has serious cost implications (Worthington; Wennberg and Gittelsohn, 1975). For
example, dermatologists will demand and receive a higher price
for treating a rash than a family practitioner; more rashes will
be treated, but no improvement in health status will necessarily
result. The United States and Canada have the highest population
surgery rates in the world. Data show that where there is a high
surgeon/population ratio, there is a high surgery rate (American College of Surgeons).

Through the 1960s, there was a widespread opinion that the
United States faced a serious physician shortage (Surgeon General's Consultant Group; Peterson and Pennell; National Advisory Commission; Carnegie Commission on Higher Education;
Johnson). However, another view, increasingly adopted, identified the problem not in terms of absolute supply of physicians but
rather in terms of what they do, what specialties they are in, and
where they are geographically located (Fein, 1967; Castleton;
Senior and Smith; Navarro, 1974). Projections in the mid-70s, as
indicated earlier, are that physician-to-population ratios will
exceed those of most other countries by 1990 (Bureau of Health
Resources Development).

What effect will adding more physicians have on costs and utilization of services? Will more physician services or medical services create improved health outcomes? What has happened to
physician productivity? (With rising incomes, the number of
hours worked by physicians per week has decreased.) These same
questions can be raised about most of the specialties and subspecialties and many types of allied manpower. The answers of
course have implications for determination of the total manpower
pool and costs.

In allied health manpower, the fractionation of functions and
the increase in personnel per hospital bed should long ago have
raised serious questions about costs, efficiency, and productivity.
Part of the fractionation stems from the sophisticated technologies often introduced wholesale in the health industry without
any testing of their impact on personnel requirements or cost in
relation to changed health outcomes. The duplication of expensive

technologies leads often to infrequent use in individual institutions. This situation has major manpower consequences since standby personnel are needed to man the underutilized units, and quality consequences where infrequent use with resulting lack of practice may adversely affect morbidity and mortality.

As funds tighten, hospitals are beginning to look at their staffing patterns and practices. The trend has been toward fracturing functions, securing certification and, in some cases, state licensure, for very narrow fields. Also developing are a whole host of guild organizations and quasi-craft unions that bargain on individual bases with hospitals and other institutions and are beginning to fight each other over turf. In dealing with these problems, nonprofit institutions do not normally have the same economic incentives for efficiency as do competitive organizations. As long as funding is available, the incentive to bargain or reassess behavior is weak.

If a rational plan for the development of an optimal health manpower pool were to be developed. the following types of information would be needed (Kramer and Roemer) :

—Health care needs data. Needs cannot easily be measured, but adequate health care utilization data and national epidemiological data would be useful.
—Functional analysis of tasks to provide health care services and analysis of how these tasks could be distributed within the health manpower pool. Productivity data.
—Effects of different organizational models on the use of health manpower.
—Cost implications of manpower pools of different sizes and distributions.
—Effects of substitution of capital (machinery) for labor and analysis of whether in the health care industry new capital requires expansion of manpower rather than substitutes for it in a significant proportion of cases.
—The relationship of manpower distribution to health outcomes.
(Lave et al.; Institute of Medicine, 1976)

Data in all of these areas are limited and currently inadequate to develop optimal manpower numbers. It is hoped that the data collection and analysis required by the National Health Planning and Resources Development Act of 1974 (P.L. 93–641, Sec. 1513 (b)) will prove helpful in dealing with this problem area. In addition, a major study of physician productivity is underway at the University of Southern California. In fact, either dollar constraints or arbitrary numbers limitations rather than rational planning may well set the size of the manpower pool for the late 70s and early 80s.

Distribution of Physician Manpower by Specialty and Geography

In the mid-70s great attention was being devoted to the issues of specialty and geographic distribution (Hudson and Nourse). There is an apparent imbalance in the distribution of physicians between primary care and certain specialties, particularly general surgery and subspecialties in medicine and pediatrics (Institute of Medicine, 1976; Coordinating Council on Medical Education). There is little agreement as to what the right ratios are, and international data show that specialty ratios vary widely from country to country (Table 4.4).

Compared to other developed countries, the United States has fewer primary physicians and more specialists per population. In

Table 4.4

Physician Distribution by Contact and Specialty Areas, Selected Countries, 1970

Country	Total Physicians	General and Family Practice, Internal Medicine, Pediatrics[a]		Specialist Physicians		Others	
		N	%	N	%	N	%
Canada	31,166	15,557	49.9	9,556	30.7	6,053	19.4
England & Wales	59,791	29,304	49.0	18,217	30.5	12,270	20.5
France	68,000	48,408	71.2	19,592	28.8	—	—
German Fed. Rep.	105,976	74,067	69.9	25,597	24.1	6,312	6.0
Israel	7,281	5,386	73.9	2,029	27.9	168	2.3
Japan	117,195	52,904	45.1	43,400	37.1	20,891	17.8
Netherlands	16,292	6,632	40.7	4,401	27.0	5,259	32.3
New Zealand	3,232	1,648	51.0	919	28.4	665	20.6
N. Ireland	2,015	1,097	54.4	807	40.1	111	5.5
Norway	5,361	3,942	73.5	1,674	31.2	6	.1
Scotland	6,769	4,255	62.9	2,168	32.0	346	5.1
S. Africa	10,912	8,925	81.8	1,943	17.8	44	.4
Sweden	10,950	8,568	78.2	4,039	36.9	—	—
Switzerland[b]	8,890	3,578	40.3	2,140	24.1	3,382	38.0
USA	323,203	150,932	46.7	152,537	47.2	19,734	6.1
USSR	577,300	239,300	41.5	212,500	36.8	125,500	21.7

Source: World Health Statistics Annual, 1970, vol. 3. (Geneva: World Health Organization, 1974).
[a] Includes subspecialties of internal medicine and pediatrics.
[b] Some multispecialty physicians are included in more than one category.

1973, according to the AMA and AOA, 46% of United States physicians could be designated as primary care physicians. In the National Health Service of England and Wales, 58% of all physicians were considered to be primary physicians. Distribution of physicians in Canada was similar to that in the United States. Only in radiology did Sweden exceed the United States in the proportion of specialists in a particular field, and only in orthopedics and anesthesiology were the British proportions of specialists greater than in the United States. Although the health care systems of these countries differ significantly from that of the United States in their organization and financing, this country's relative dependence on physician specialists is nonetheless striking. Another unusual aspect of physician organization in the United States is that a high proportion practice both inside and outside the hospital; such dual practice is unusual in most other countries.

Complicating the problem is the lack of a firm agreement on the definition of primary care or the distribution of tasks among health professionals, including physicians. For example, the AMA regards obstetricians and gynecologists as primary care providers; the Institute of Medicine does not. There is an extensive literature on the definitional problems (Alpert and Charney; Draper and Smits; Jonas; Parker; Petersdorf, Dec. 1975; Rogers; Silver and McAtee; White, 1967; Hudson and Nourse). Definitional problems and overlap exist among the specialties and the various professional organizations, with little agreement as to the use of specialists, subspecialists, and generalists for a wide range of conditions—fractures, rashes, emotional upsets, childbirth, and others. Even less agreement exists as to the transfer of certain functions from physicians to other manpower, such as nurse-midwives and clinicians. (See also Chapter 6, on primary care.)

The geographic distribution of practicing physicians is uneven (Table 4.5).* In 1973, in Mississippi and South Dakota there

* Note that Table 4.5 does not take into account house-staff and physicians not in active practice who are in teaching, research, or administration, who are not working in a health-related field, or who are retired. In 1976, the overall physician/population ratio in the United States was about 170 per 100,000. When house-staff and physicians not in active practice are added into the state-by-state ratios, the imbalances in the direction of the large industrial states with the major medical centers obviously become even more marked.

Table 4.5

**Active Patient Care Physicians, Civilian Population,
Physician to Population Ratios, 1973**

State	Civilian Population, July 1, 1973 (× 1,000)	MDs per 100,000 Population	DOs per 100,000 Population	Total Physicians Per 100,000 Population
Total	208,094	130	7	137
Alabama	3,514	82	0	82
Alaska	303	78	2	80
Arizona	2,030	131	20	151
Arkansas	2,029	81	1	82
California	20,285	168	1	169
Colorado	2,387	150	11	161
Connecticut	3,061	169	1	170
Delaware	570	121	8	129
D.C.	737	339	1	340
Florida	7,587	127	12	139
Georgia	4,732	102	3	105
Hawaii	776	140	3	143
Idaho	764	87	3	90
Illinois	11,200	125	3	128
Indiana	5,303	92	3	95
Iowa	2,903	89	14	103
Kansas	2,248	104	9	113
Kentucky	3,309	94	1	95
Louisiana	3,735	105	1	106
Maine	1,018	101	20	121
Maryland	4,013	159	1	160
Massachusetts	5,795	177	3	180
Michigan	9,029	114	27	141
Minnesota	3,894	133	2	135
Mississippi	2,256	77	0	77
Missouri	4,731	115	24	139
Montana	714	96	4	100
Nebraska	1,530	104	2	106
Nevada	539	102	5	107
New Hampshire	786	123	2	125
New Jersey	7,326	131	12	143
New Mexico	1,089	97	13	110
New York	18,236	195	3	198
North Carolina	5,181	100	1	101
North Dakota	626	85	1	86
Ohio	10,716	119	12	131
Oklahoma	2,635	90	17	107
Oregon	2,223	130	8	138
Pennsylvania	11,890	132	15	147
Rhode Island	945	151	9	160
South Carolina	2,657	88	0	88
South Dakota	678	71	4	75
Tennessee	4,106	107	1	108
Texas	11,628	107	8	115
Utah	1,153	126	1	127
Vermont	464	151	9	160
Virginia	4,665	113	1	114
Washington	3,383	134	6	140
West Virginia	1,793	93	5	98
Wisconsin	4,568	109	4	113
Wyoming	349	89	3	92

Source: AMA *Distribution of Physicians in the U.S., 1973*, American Osteopathic Association.

were fewer than 80 practicing physicians per 100,000 population. In New York, California, Massachusetts, and Arizona, the practicing physician-to-population ratio far exceeded that of the nation as a whole, which was about 130 per 100,000. Part of these differences can be explained by the location in the high physician/population ratio states of major tertiary care medical centers serving patients who reside out-of-state. However, the most important source of these differences lies in the complex set of factors that make some areas of the country particularly attractive to physicians and others particularly unattractive.

Comparing physician-to-population ratios for areas as large as states can blur the magnitude of the geographic inequities in physician distribution within states by averaging out high- and low-distribution areas. These disparities can be truly enormous. For example, a recent study of the variation in physician-to-population ratios among counties in Maryland showed a range of physician concentration from 308 per 100,000 population to 30 per 100,000 population between the most physician-rich and physician-poor counties in that state (Alexander and Bowden).

In 1974, the Secretary of the DHEW designated more than 900 areas (including rural and inner-city areas) in which the physician-to-population ratio was less than one physician for 4,000 people as having critical physician shortages.

In the past several years, efforts have been made to alter the specialty and geographic imbalances, but the data on factors that influenced specialty and geographic distribution are not clear. The following factors have contributed to the imbalances:

—The content of the training programs at the undergraduate and graduate medical education levels, including the site of clinical training and the types of faculty models to which students are exposed (Mason; Weber)
—The selection of medical students; where they were raised; and their interests
—The social and cultural amenities of given geographic areas (Sloan; Hambleton; Steinwald and Steinwald)
—For location choice, the peer contact available in different areas, including the existence of medical schools, area health education centers, and contact with other physicians, particularly through organized group-practice arrangements

Study of economic influences has just begun. Data on physicians' income are not available geographically or in small regions by specialty. A recent analysis of physician fee levels shows that high prevailing charges and high fees tend to correlate with high physician-to-population ratios (Institute of Medicine, 1976). There is some evidence that shifts in physician distribution are correlated with shifts in the geographic distribution of relative per capita income (Clark and Koontz). There is also some evidence that the fee structure may be biased in favor of procedure-oriented specialties (Institute of Medicine, 1976).

Since graduate medical education is critical in altering specialty distribution, the support available to the different specialty training programs is important. It is more difficult to support ambulatory care-oriented graduate medical education programs in primary care specialties than programs in other specialties. The reasons include the benefit packages under insurance programs and the way outpatient hospital services are reimbursed under private health insurance programs, Medicare, and Medicaid (Institute of Medicine, 1976).

During the last several years, the federal and state governments have tried to ameliorate specialty and geographic imbalance. In the area of increased primary care training, the federal government provided special project grant support for family practice residencies (P. L. 92-157, 1971). Some state governments are providing direct appropriations for training in primary care.

To encourage physicians to locate in underserved areas, the federal government is supporting two major programs, the National Health Service Corps and Area Health Education Centers (P. L. 92-157, 1971). The first is designed to place physician and nonphysician health manpower in areas designated as health manpower scarcity areas. This thrust was greatly strengthened by provisions of H.R. 94–484 (1976). Area health education centers are designed to provide peer contact, continuing education, and remote-site training in rural areas. Since these programs are quite new, it is too early to assess their impact.

Congressional testimony by the AMA based on 1975 residency data indicated that changes are beginning to occur in the distribution of residency positions (Nesbitt). These data show increases in filled positions in primary care positions, defined by the AMA as internal medicine, pediatrics, family practice, and obstetrics and gynecology, and a decline in surgical residencies. However, the data include obstetrics/gynecology and subspecialty training in internal medicine and pediatrics. Some other groups do not regard these as primary care specialties. One year's data are inadequate to determine whether there is an actual change in trends. Furthemore, data are not yet available on the question of the educational content in those specialties which have been labeled "primary care." Many programs in internal medicine have been designed principally to prepare physicians for further subspecialty fellowship training. If this situation is not altered, such a program cannot be considered primary care training.

While there will be a substantial increase in physician-to-population ratios in the 1975–85 decade, there are no current control mechanisms to assure that the increases will provide better ratios in true primary care or in underserved areas. An extensive debate is under way as to whether the medical profession can exert the internal discipline to provide more equitable geographic and specialty distributions of physicians without direct federal government intervention.

Several recent reports have recommended that commissions be established to determine the number of residency positions needed by specialty (Institute of Medicine, 1976; Macy Foundation). Bill S. 3239 would have established a commission to determine residencies by specialty and region. Expansion of National Health Service Corps scholarships to supply more health manpower in underserved areas is provided for in H.R. 94–484. The Senate proposal also would have required that a certain proportion of medical students contract to enter primary care specialties. This was not included in the final law (H.R. 94–484). The role of the Health Systems Agencies (see Chapter 12) in manpower distribution is unclear. For many of the agencies the first priority will be control of facilities expansion.

The state of the art of manpower planning in terms of total numbers and distribution by function, specialty, and geography is still primitive. Fine tuning of manpower and its distribution is decades off; yet some of the imbalances appear so serious that a variety of external control and financing decisions aimed at influencing distribution will be made in the next several years.

Trends in manpower in the industry have been toward greater specialization of both professional and allied health manpower (Freymann, chs. 5, 11, 12; Stevens, 1971). While the recent debate has focused on the imbalances of specialists and generalists in medicine, these same trends exist in the allied health field, with a proliferation of new technician and nursing categories and new allied health professions. The nation rarely heard of an oncologist or an inhalation therapist 20 years ago. Functions previously performed by one person are assigned to more than one. With every new technological development, one or several new allied health titles are born, as are physician specialties. As cost constraints continue, attention will be focused on allied manpower as well.

Conclusion

Health manpower has expanded rapidly in the past 20 years in response to increased expenditures for health care and new technology. Combined with this expansion, an accelerating trend toward specialization developed. In the past several years, concern has grown regarding inequities in distribution of manpower by specialty and geography and the influence and cost of the training process for health professional manpower.

A major public policy discussion is taking place regarding the size of the manpower pool; a change in the balance between primary care manpower and specialty manpower; greater equity in the geographic distribution of health professional manpower; the role of training in influencing specialty and geographic distribution; and the role of the public and private sectors in affecting change. The sources of support of undergraduate and graduate medical education are being re-evaluated. The constraints on economic resources and the inflation in the medical care sector of the economy require analysis of choices in the health manpower field that were hitherto unscrutinized.

References

Alexander, C. A., and Bowden, G. R. *Physician Manpower in Maryland, 1973.* Baltimore, Md.: University of Maryland School of Medicine, 1974.

Alpert, J., and Charney, E. *The Education of Physicians for Primary Care.* Washington, D.C.: Bureau of Health Services Research, USDHEW Pub. No. (HRA) 74-3113, Autumn, 1973.

American Association of Osteopathic Medicine. *Directory of Internships and Residencies.* Selected years.

American Hospital Association. "Headlines: Housestaff Are Students." *Hospitals, J.A.H.A.*, April 16, 1976, p. 17.

American Medical Association. *Directory of Internships and Residencies.* Selected years.

American College of Surgeons and the American Surgical Association. *Surgery in the United States: A Summary Report of the Study on Surgical Services to the U.S.* Chicago, Ill., 1975.

Anderson, O. W. *Health Care: Can There be Equity?* New York: Wiley, 1972.

Association of American Medical Colleges. "Graduates of Foreign Medical Schools in the United States: A Challenge to Medical Education." *Journal of Medical Education, 49,* 809, 1974.

Breisch, W. F. "Impact of Medical School Characteristics on Location of Physician Practice." *Journal of Medical Education, 45,* December, 1970.

Bureau of Health Resources Development. *The Supply of Health Manpower: 1970 Profiles and Projections to 1990.* Washington, D.C.: USDHEW, December, 1974.

Carnegie Commission on Higher Education. *Higher Education and the Nation's Health.* New York: McGraw-Hill, 1970.

Castleton, K. B. "Are We Building Too Many Medical Schools?" *Journal of the American Medical Association, 216,* 1989, 1971.

Clark, L. J., and Koontz, T. L. "Analysis of the Impact of the Hill-Burton Program on the Distribution of the Supply of General Hospital Beds and Physicians in the United States, 1950–1970." Paper delivered at the annual meeting of the American Public Health Association, November, 1973, San Francisco, Calif.

Confrey, E. A. "The Logic of a 'Shortage of Health Manpower.'" *International Journal of Health Services, 3,* 253, 1973.

Coordinating Council on Medical Education. Chicago, Ill. Unpublished report on foreign medical graduates, 1976.

Davis, K. "Financing Medical Care: Implications for Access to Primary-Care." In Andreopoulos, S., Ed., *Primary Care, Where Medicine Fails.* New York: Wiley, 1974.

Draper, P., and Smits, H. "The Primary-Care Practitioner—Specialist or Jack-of-All-Trades." *New England Journal of Medicine, 293,* 903, 1975.

Evans, R. L. et al. "The Community-Based Medical School: Reactions at the Interface between Medical Education and Medical Care." *New England Journal of Medicine, 288,* 713, 1973.

Fein, R. *The Doctor Shortage.* Washington, D.C.: Brookings Institute, 1967.

Fein, R. "Some Health Policy Issues: One Economist's View." *Public Health Reports, 90,* 387, 1975.

Fendall, N. R. E. *Auxiliaries In Health Care: Programs in Developing Countries.* Baltimore, Md.: Johns Hopkins Press, 1972.

Field, M. G. "American and Soviet Medical Manpower: Growth and

Evolution, 1910–1970." *International Journal of Health Services,* *5*, 455, 1975.

Flexner, A. *Medical Education in the United States and Canada.* The Carnegie Foundation for the Advancement of Teaching, 1910. Reprinted, Washington, D.C.: Science and Health Publications, 1960.

Freymann, J. G. *The American Health Care System: Its Genesis and Trajectory.* New York: Medcom Press, 1974.

Fuchs, V. *Who Shall Live?: Health Economics and Social Change.* New York: Basic Books, 1974.

Fuchs, V., and Kramer, M. J. "Determinants of Expenditures for Physicians' Services in the United States 1948–1968. Washington, D.C.: USDHEW Pub. No. (HSM) 73–3013, December, 1972.

Goldblatt, A. et al. "Licensure, Competence and Manpower Distribution." *New England Journal of Medicine, 292,* 137, 1975.

Hambleton, J. W. *Main Currents in the Analysis of Physician Location.* Health Economics Research Center, Research Report Series No. 8. Madison: University of Wisconsin Department of Economics, May, 1971.

Haug, J. N., and Stevens, R. "Foreign Medical Graduates in the United States in 1963." *Inquiry, 10,* March, 1973.

Hudson, J. I., and Nourse, E. S., eds. "Perspectives in Primary Care Education." *Journal of Medical Education, 50,* Part 2, December, 1975.

Immigration and Naturalization Service. *1974 Annual Report.* Washington, D.C.: G.P.O., 1974.

Institute of Medicine. *Costs of Education in the Health Professions.* Washington, D.C.: National Academy of Sciences, 1974.

Institute of Medicine. *Medicare-Medicaid Reimbursement Policies.* Washington, D.C.: National Academy of Sciences, 1976.

Johnson, R. L. "Physician Shortage Threatens Health Proposals." *Hospitals, J.A.H.A.,* July 1, 1972, p. 53.

Jonas, S. "Some Thoughts on Primary Care: Problems in Implementation." *International Journal of Health Services, 3,* 77, 1973.

Kleinman, J. C. et al. "Physician Manpower Data: The Case of the Missing Foreign Medical Graduates." *Medical Care, 12,* 906, 1974.

Kleinman, J. C. et al. "Postgraduate Training and Work Experience of Non-ECFMG Certified Physicians in the U.S." *Medical Care, 13,* 305, 1975. (a)

Kleinman, J. C. et al. "A Reply to Stevens, Goodman and Mica." *Medical Care, 13,* 445, 1975. (b)

Kramer, C., and Roemer, R. "Health Manpower and the Organization of Health Services." Mimeographed. Institute of Industrial Relations: University of California at Los Angeles, 1972.

Lave, J. R. et al. "Medical Manpower Models: Need, Demand and Supply." *Inquiry, 12,* June, 1975.

Lockett, B. A. "U.S. Citizens Studying Medicine Abroad." *Journal of Medical Education, 49,* 985, 1974.

McKeown, T., and Lowe, C. R. *An Introduction to Social Medicine.* 2nd ed. Philadelphia, Pa.: Lippincott, 1974.

McTernan, E. J., and Hawkins, R. O., eds. *Educating Personnel for the Allied Health Professions and Services.* St. Louis, Mo.: C. V. Mosby, 1972.

Macy Foundation. *Physicians for the Future: Report of the Macy Commission.* New York, 1976.

Mason, R. "Medical School, Residency, and Eventual Practice Location: Toward a Rationale for State Support of Medical Education." *Journal of the American Medical Association, 223,* 49, 1975.

Mumford, E. *Interns: From Students to Physicians.* Cambridge, Mass.: Harvard University Press, 1970.

National Advisory Commission on Health Manpower. *Report.* Vols. I and II. Washington D.C.: G.P.O., 1967.

National Board of Medical Examiners. "Evaluation in the Continuum of Medical Education." *Report of the Committee on Goals and Priorities of the NBME.* Philadelphia, Pa., 1973.

National Center for Health Statistics. *Health Resources Statistics: Health Manpower and Health Facilities, 1974.* Washington, D.C.: USDHEW, 1974.

Navarro, V. "A Critique of the Present and Proposed Strategies for Redistributing Resources in the Health Sector and a Discussion of Alternatives." *Medical Care, 12,* 721, 1974.

———. "Women in Health Care." *The New England Journal of Medicine, 292,* 398, 1975.

Nesbitt, T. Testimony before Subcommittee on Health, Committee on Labor and Public Welfare. U.S. Senate, Washington, D.C., November 18, 1975.

Parker, A. W. "The Dimensions of Primary Care: Blueprints for Change." In Andreopoulos, S., Ed., *Primary Care: Where Medicine Fails,* pp. 15–77. New York: Wiley, 1974.

Pellegrino, E. D. "The Regionalization of Academic Medicine: The Metamorphosis of a Concept." *Journal of Medical Education, 48,* 119, 1973.

Pellegrino, E. D. "The Academic Role of the Vice President for Health Sciences: Can a Walrus Become a Unicorn?" *Journal of Medical Education, 50,* 211, 1975.

Petersdorf, R. G. "Health Manpower: Numbers, Distribution, Quality." *Annals of Internal Medicine, 82,* 694, 1975.

Petersdorf, R. G. "Issues in Primary Care: The Academic Perspective." *Journal of Medical Education, 50,* December 1975, Part 2, pp. 5–13.

Peterson, P. Q., and Pennell, M. Y. "Physician-Population Projections

1961–1975: Their Causes and Implications." *American Journal of Public Health, 53,* 163, 1963.

P. L. 92–157. *Amendments to Title VII of the Public Health Service Act.* U.S. Congress, Washington, D.C.

P. L. 92–603. *National Health Planning and Resources Development Act of 1974.* U.S. Congress, Washington, D.C.

P. L. 93–641. *Social Security Act Amendments of 1972.* U.S. Congress, Washington, D.C.

P. L. 94–484. *Health Professions Educational Assistance Act of 1976.* U.S. Congress, Washington, D.C.

Roback, G. A. *Distribution of Physicians in the U.S., 1973.* Chicago, Ill.: American Medical Association, Center for Health Services Research and Development, 1974.

Rogers, D. E. "The Challenge of Primary Care." Mimeographed. Princeton: Robert Wood Johnson Foundation, 1975.

S. 3239. "Health Professions Educational Assistance Act of 1976." U.S. Senate, Washington, D.C., 1976.

Schoenfeld, H. K., Heston, J. F., and Falk, I. S. "Numbers of Physicians Required for Primary Medical Care." *New England Journal of Medicine, 286,* 571, 1972.

Senior, B., and Smith, B. A. "The Number of Physicians as a Constraint on Delivery of Health Care." *Journal of the American Medical Association, 222,* 178, 1972.

Sidel, V. W. "Feldshers and Feldsherism." *New England Journal of Medicine, 278,* 934, 981, 1968.

Sidel, V. W. "The Barefoot Doctors of the People's Republic of China." *New England Journal of Medicine, 286,* 1292, 1972.

Silver, H. K., and McAtee, P. R. "A Descriptive Definition of the Scope and Content of Primary Health Care." *Pediatrics, 56,* 957, 1975.

Sloan, F. "Economic Models of Physician Supply." Ph.D. dissertation, Harvard University, 1968.

Steinwald, B., and Steinwald, C. "The Effect of Preceptorship and Rural Training Programs on Physicians' Practice Location Decisions." *Medical Care, 13,* 219, 1975.

Stevens, R. *American Medicine and the Public Interest.* New Haven, Conn.: Yale University Press, 1971.

Stevens, R. "Physician Migration Reexamined." *Science, 190,* 440, 1975.

Strickland, S. P. *Politics, Science and Dread Disease.* Cambridge, Mass.: Harvard University Press, 1972.

Surgeon General's Consultant Group on Medical Education. Report. *Physicians for a Growing America.* Washington, D.C.: Public Health Service, USDHEW, 1959.

Wang, V. L. "Training of the Barefoot Doctor in the People's Republic of China: From Prevention to Curative Service." *International Journal of Health Services, 5,* 475, 1975.

Weber, G. I. *An Essay on the Distribution of Physicians Amongst Specialties.* Washington, D.C.: USDHEW Pub. No. (OS) 171-71, 1973.

Wenneberg, J. E., and Gittlesohn, A. "Small Area Variations in Health Care Delivery." *Science, 182,* December 14, 1973.

Wenneberg, J. E., and Gittlesohn, A. "Consumer Characteristics and Physician Choice as Determinants of Health Care Consumption." Mimeographed. Burlington: University of Vermont, 1975.

White, K. L. "Primary Medical Care for Families—Organization and Evaluation." *New England Journal of Medicine, 277,* 847-852, 1967.

White, K. L. "Health and Health Care: Personal and Public Issues." Michael M. Davis Lecture, May 29, 1974, University of Chicago School of Business, Center for Health Administration, Chicago, Illinois.

Williams, K. N., and Lockett, B. A. "Migration of Foreign Physicians to the United States: The Perspective of Health Manpower Planning." *International Journal of Health Services, 4,* 213, 1974.

Worthington, N. L. "Expenditures for Hospital Care and Physicians' Services: Factors Affecting Annual Changes." *Social Security Bulletin, 38,* 3, November, 1975.

5

Nursing

Nancy R. Barhydt

Introduction

This chapter considers some aspects of the development of the nursing profession, its present status and problems, and its prospects for future change and growth. In discussing this largest single health manpower category, we are actually dealing with a wide range of health care provider groups which are gathered together under the single rubric, "nursing." The related groups are distinguished from one another by title, training, job description, salary, requirements for credentials, and educational background. For example, the licensed practical nurse (L.P.N.) with one year of training in a hospital; the registered nurse (R.N.) with a two-year associate degree or a diploma from a hospital-affiliated school; the R.N. with a baccalaureate degree from a four- or five- year collegiate program; and the R.N. with a master's degree or doctorate, representing up to nine years of training, are all "nurses." There are also numerous nurses' aides, assistants, and nursing technicians with a variety of training programs and job descriptions whom patients, not knowing the fine distinctions, often call "nurse."

In nursing, which is both an art and a science, certain principles are applied in the delivery of quality health care to the sick and to the well. It involves highly complex relationships with a multitude of health care providers and increasingly depends on technology. Nursing is equally concerned with the prevention of disease and the conservation of health and uses a holistic approach. The profession, or at least its leading elements, has been engaged for many years in a struggle to broaden its role. According to Bonnie Bullough:

> 30 states have now revised their nurse practice acts to facilitate
> role expansion for registered nurses. Several approaches are being
> used in these laws including mandating new board regulations,

expanding the definitions of nursing, increasing the power of physicians to delegate, and mandating the use of standardized protocols to guide the practice of nurses who are accepting new responsibilities. (1976, p. 249)

As is well known, the vast majority of nurses are female—in fact, as was pointed out in the previous chapter, the vast majority of all health workers are female (Ehrenreich). Of course, most independent health professionals, as the term is used in the preceding chapter, and administrators are male, and this fact lends an added significance to the conflict over "the expanding role of the nurse."

Historical Development of Nursing*

The nursing profession, which was shaped by the apprentice system as an arm of hospital administration rather than as a clinical department, developed during an era when relatively few women attended college (O.W. Anderson). As early as the colonial period, women were serving as autonomous healers or general practitioners, as well as midwives (Ehrenreich). Anne Hutchinson, the religious reformer, was a general practitioner, and Harriet Tubman, the black leader who guided many slaves to freedom, worked as both nurse and doctor. Practice by these female "lay" healers was suppressed and outlawed when physicians established themselves as the legal and official medical profession and relegated women to a subsidiary position. During the mid-nineteenth century it was a rare woman indeed who was accepted into medical school; those few who were, were excluded from medical associations and from the male collegial referral system (Kushner, 1973). Most women were left with only one career choice in health care—nursing.

The evolution of the medical and nursing professionals were thus complementary. Two distinct occupations emerged where there had once been a single generalized "healer": nurses took on the responsibility for "caring"; physicians were concerned with "curing" and the technical functions. The sexism pervading the health care delivery system in this country has its roots in early nineteenth-century medicine. The division of labor accomplished then also had economic implications: technology could be profita-

* A useful history of the nursing workforce in the United States is found in Kathleen Cannings' and William Lazonick's "The Development of the Nursing Labor Force in the United States: A Basic Analysis," *International Journal of Health Services, 5,* 185, 1975.

bly used in private enterprise, caring could not. Thus, the medical division of labor contributed to the downgrading of the nurse (Ehrenreich).

During the Victorian era hospital nursing was considered by many to be a disreputable occupation; nurses were often depicted in the literature as lewd, drunken, and dishonest (Kushner, 1973). Florence Nightingale (1820–1910) deserves a great deal of credit for encouraging "well-bred" young women to emancipate themselves from their subservient role in the home by providing scientifically based nursing at the hospital. But, in fact these women, lowly paid and forced to do menial tasks, were being freed from one straightjacket only to be strapped into another (Bullough, 1975).* In the disciplined environment of the nursing school, nurses were taught the traditional feminine qualities, submissiveness and obedience. Thus, a conventional existence, complete with a set of social values—curfew, dress, rules, lights out—certainly did not support individual initiative or self-confidence in nursing (Kushner, 1973).

Florence Nightingale's philosophy for those dedicated women perpetuated the "feminine mystique" in the nursing profession. Nurses were expected to treat doctors with wifely obedience, to devote a mother's loving care to patients, and to supervise hospital personnel with the condescension of the household manager dealing with maids, butlers, and grocery boys (Navarro, 1975). However, this stereotype is dying as a new breed of nurses emerges, aided by the women's movement and changes in the health care delivery system. Nurses now are able to function more creatively. The end result of this creativity may well be to make the nurse's role separate from but equal to that of the physician, which would not only raise nurses' status but would also ultimately improve patient care.

Educational Programs in Nursing
Introduction

There are hundreds of training programs for nurses at all levels of proficiency in many different types of institutions, including hospitals, two- and four-year colleges, universities, and a wide

* Nightingale did, however, suggest that nurses, like doctors, be required to take examinations and be licensed. State licensure throughout the United States was finally achieved in 1923, on a voluntary basis, at least, but it did not remove the stigma of "women's work."

variety of graduate programs. Of 20,000 nurses employed as faculty members in nurse education programs, 46% are in diploma programs, 32% in baccalaureate and higher degree programs, and 22% in associate degree programs. Approximately 5,000 faculty members are employed in training licensed practical nurses (American Nurses' Association). The United States Office of Education recognized the National League for Nursing as the official accrediting agency for master's, baccalaureate, associate degree, diploma, and practical nursing programs (Walsh).

Practical Nursing

Practical nursing programs prepare men and women to give nursing care under the supervision of a registered nurse or a physician to patients in simple nursing situations. In more complex situations, the licensed practical nurse (L.P.N.) functions as an assistant to the registered nurse (National League for Nursing, 1974–75(d)). Preparation for licensure as a L.P.N. is usually completed in a one-year program, although programs range in length from 8 to 24 months. Each program establishes its own admission requirements; academic requirements as well as tuition and fees vary from state to state. Satisfactory completion of a state-approved program in practical nursing is required before the nurse is permitted to take the examination for licensure, given by state Boards of Nursing. Licensed practical nurses are employed in a wide variety of health care facilities, including hospitals, extended care facilities, nursing homes, and clinics. The number of L.P.N.s is growing rapidly. More than 45,000 were graduated from schools of practical nursing in 1974 alone.

Registered Nursing

Registration in nursing means licensure for nurses who have completed a higher level educational program than that for the L.P.N. All states had enacted legislation providing for voluntary registration by 1923 (Bullough, 1975) : under this system a registered nurse was defined in terms of educational requirements met and examinations passed, not in terms of work tasks performed. Registration merely conferred the privilege of using the letters R.N. after one's name, much like contemporary certification in other health care occupations (see Chapter 13). The first mandatory licensing law, which did define a body of work, was not passed until 1938, in New York State.

Associate degree programs. Among the available academic

preparations for registered nursing is the community college offering an associate degree program. First instituted in 1952, these programs are now proliferating more rapidly than any other type of nursing program (National League for Nursing, 1974–75 (c)). With some variations, a number of features are basic to the associate degree programs. Most are conducted or controlled by public, junior, or community colleges. They vary in length from two academic years to two calendar years, with the program of study combining nursing courses and related college courses. The students must meet requirements of the college to be admitted to the nursing program and on completion are granted the Associate in Arts degree. The associate degree nursing programs prepare students to take state board examinations to become registered nurses. College credits earned in the associate degree programs often can be applied toward a baccalaureate degree in nursing should a graduate decide to pursue further education (National League for Nursing, 1974–75 (c)).

Registered nurses with A.A. or A.A.S. degrees work for the most part in hospitals or other institutions as general-duty or staff nurses engaged in giving direct care to the sick. They are sometimes referred to as "bedside" nurses. Since these nurses give direct care to patients, they must possess considerable technical knowledge and skill, and must understand the scientific principles of nursing care. It should be noted, however, that associate degree nurses are not prepared for teaching on a collegiate level or for total patient management. Unfortunately, many nurses now carry out the latter functions by default, since agencies and institutions place these nurses in positions for which they are not fully trained. Consequently, institutions and health care providers are often not altogether happy with the performance of the associate degree graduate.

A recent innovation in the education of nurses at the associate degree level leads to an external degree in nursing. This degree, authorized by the New York State Board of Regents in 1971 and approved by the State Department of Education in 1973, makes it possible for candidates to earn an external degree with or without formal in-residence courses and entirely on the basis of independent study. During the course of study, the student must take seven high-quality, standardized examinations. If the student passes these examinations, a final Clinical Performance Nursing Examination is administered, in which nursing knowledge equal to that of students who complete the associate degree program in a collegiate institution must be demonstrated. The student is then qualified to take state board examinations for licensure as an R.N. The first class graduated in 1974. The New York Board of Regents is now developing a program to grant an external bachelor of science degree in nursing (Lenberg, 1976).

Diploma programs. Another setting for preparation as a registered nurse is the school that awards its graduates a diploma in nursing. These schools, which may apply for accreditation by the National League for Nursing, are usually under the control of a hospital, although in some instances they are independently incorporated. They currently prepare more than 40% of the registered nurses needed to meet the demands of American society. The diploma programs suit the qualified high school graduates who want a program centered in a community institution identified with the care of patients. As opposed to the situation in a college-based program, students who want an early opportunity to be with patients and health services personnel and who want to prepare for beginning staff positions in hospitals and similar institutions also find such programs attractive (National League for Nursing, 1974 (a)).

The school of nursing may enter into cooperative relations with collegiate or other institutions to provide certain courses of study needed to meet the requirements for graduation. The nursing courses combine theory with practice, reinforcing learning through experience with caring for medical and surgical patients, mothers, children, and the mentally ill. According to the National League for Nursing (1974 (a)), graduates of accredited diploma programs in nursing

1. know basic scientific principles, and utilize them in planning and giving quality nursing care to people;
2. recognize the indications of diseases and disabilities, and the psychological, social, and physical needs of patients;
3. have the understanding and the skills necessary to organize and implement a plan of nursing care that will meet the needs of groups of patients and promote the restoration of health;
4. are qualified to plan for the care of patients with other members of the health care team and to direct other members of the nursing team;
5. are qualified for general duty nurse positions in the medical, surgical, obstetrical, pediatric, and psychiatric nursing areas of the hospitals and similar community institutions;

6. need to be oriented to new work situations as beginning practitioners and to be given time and opportunity to become increasingly effective in the practice of nursing.

Graduates of a school offering a program approved by a state board of nurse examiners are eligible to take the state examination for licensure to practice as a registered nurse (National League for Nursing 1974 (a)).

Baccalaureate degree programs. A baccalaureate degree program in nursing prepares graduates for the general practice of professional nursing. The student earns a B.S. degree and also becomes eligible to take a state licensing examination. The program must include all the learning experiences required to prepare the student to practice professional nursing in all environments where health care is offered and in any setting where the need for nursing care manifests itself (Ozimek). That is, a baccalaureate degree program prepares the beginning practitioner of professional nursing as a generalist, capable of providing health care to persons, families, and groups in a variety of settings through the utilization of a nursing process that incorporates both scientific and humanistic concepts. Moreover, it provides an educational base upon which graduate study for specialization as a clinician, teacher, administrator, or researcher in nursing may be built. The program emphasizes intellectual skills such as problem solving, critical thinking, and decision making, as well as interpersonal and technical skills.

In these four-year programs, the nursing major is concentrated in the last two years and is built upon a broad general education in natural and social sciences. The nursing major focuses on the entire life span and total health care needs of persons and families rather than solely on an individual and acute episode of illness. Emphasis is on prevention, teaching, intervention, restoration, and rehabilitation (Ozimek).

Advanced Education Programs

Advanced education consists of "sequences of professional courses aimed at developing specialized qualifications characterized by formal academic recognition of completion, such as the awarding of a degree" (Bullough and Bullough, 1977).

Graduate programs. Graduate programs in nursing education prepare the registered nurse for more complex practice as a clinical specialist, a nurse practitioner, a nursing administrator, or a teacher. Many nurses prepare for such positions by completing a course leading to a master's degree. One well-known area of study at this level is public health. Most baccalaureate undergraduate programs prepare their students for beginning level staff positions in public health agencies, but those who hold a master's degree provide the backbone of nursing administration in public health departments at state and local levels throughout the country.

Doctoral level work in nursing offers preparation for careers in research, teaching, and educational administration. Increasingly, these specially qualified nurses are engaging in both basic and clinical research—particularly the latter, which aims at providing improved practice and better patient care. For example, some find positions as research consultants, assisting nurses who have not been trained in research methods to carry out small studies that may have implications for the improvement of patient care or may inspire more sophisticated studies of specific problems (Notter, 1974).

Continuing education programs. Continuing education (C.E.) for nurses is defined as "formalized learning experiences or sequences designed to enlarge the knowledge or skills of practitioners. As distinct from advanced education, continuing education tends to be more specific, of generally shorter duration, and may result in certification or completion of specialization, but not formal degrees" (Bullough and Bullough, 1977).

Continuing education is an increasingly important aspect of professional life, both for active nurses and for returning inactive nurses. State nursing associations and groups of such associations have set up committees to deal with the many problems involved in ensuring that C.E. programs maintain certain standards. One such committee, appointed by the Midwest Continuing Educational Professional Education for Nurses (MCEPEN), had as its objectives the identifying of local C.E. needs and the setting up of mechanisms for planning and coordinating C.E. efforts in their area (Forni and Bolte, 1973).

One of the current issues in regard to C.E. is whether it should be mandatory for continued licensure. Some states have enacted such legislation and several others are considering doing so; nursing leaders are divided on this question. Other important issues are how the costs of presenting high-grade programs can be met, whether and by what standards credits should be given for various offerings, how to obtain uniformity in quality of programs, and how to secure adequately trained faculty.

Continuing education does not necessarily have to take place in a classroom setting. For example, one young psychiatric nurse practitioner working in a mental health center in a small town taped her conferences with a group of outpatients, added her comments and questions to the tapes, and mailed them to a more experienced clinician in a distant city. The clinician listened to the tapes, gave her own reactions and advice and sent the tapes back in time for the practitioner to have them before her next meeting with the group (Lego, 1973).

Nurse internship programs are developing to help new graduates bridge the gap between being a student and being an independent practitioner. Because of the differences in preparation of nurses coming from three distinct types of nursing education programs, internship programs have proven popular and successful (Martel and Edmunds, 1972). Internship programs may also be integrated into undergraduate curriculums. One such experiment, in which the investigator dubbed the course "Technoterm," has been reported in detail (Treece, 1974).

Inservice education programs. Programs that are administered by an employer and are "designed to upgrade the knowledge and skills of employees for their functioning in that agency" are referred to as inservice education programs. But active and inactive returning nurses benefit from these courses which are usually given in the work setting. Many hospitals and other care agencies employ a full-time inservice education director.

Federal Government Support for Nursing Education

The first federal support program for nonmilitary nursing education—developed to meet war needs—lasted from July 1941 to July 1943. It provided funds for refresher courses for inactive nurses, grants for teachers and other nursing personnel, the preparation of nurses for advanced administrative positions, and increased enrollment in nursing schools (Bullough and Bullough, 1974). The United States Cadet Nurse Corps, which was directly related to the military, provided nursing students with free education and uniforms, as well as a small monthly stipend for a maximum of 30 months. In return, the students had to promise to serve in the armed forces after graduation or in a critical civilian nursing capacity.

Broad federal support for nursing education became available under the Nurse Training Act of 1964 (P.L. 88-581), which aimed to increase the number of nurses capable of providing quality nursing care. Federal assistance programs authorized direct support for students, operating expense money for nursing schools, funds for construction of nursing education facilities, and support for demonstration projects to improve nurse training. The act allowed hospital training programs and schools of nursing to raise educational standards, expand facilities, and reorganize curricula to implement the developing new philosophies in nursing education and to provide expanding career ladders (Bullough and Bullough, 1974). Open curriculum, independent study, and self-paced learning are all curriculum innovations designed to encourage people to enter nursing and to be free to change career goals without penalty. The Health Manpower Act of 1968, Title II, broadened the programs for all three major types of schools of nursing. The Nurse Training Act of 1971 further expanded federal aid in the form of capitation grants to schools of nursing for the purpose of increasing enrollments and providing advanced education for certain categories of nurses and nursing practitioners. The 1971 Act, with continuing resolutions through 1975, also makes grants to schools in financial distress as well as special project grants for new nurse-training programs (Report to the Congress).

In 1975, the National Commission for the Study of Nursing and Nursing Education cited the following figures for the average cost per student per year for nursing education: diploma programs—$4,345; associate degree programs—$2,590; baccalaureate degree programs—$3,411. In comparing these costs, we must take into account their varying length, amount of nursing service provided while in training, and what cost items are included in these figures (National Commission, 1975).

Supply of Nursing Personnel

The ratio of nurses to population has increased steadily from 249 per 100,000 in 1950 to 338 per 100,000 in 1968. In contrast, during the same period the physician to population ratio went from 141 to 150 per 100,000 (National Commission for Study of Nursing and Nursing Education, 1971).

In 1972, of 1,127,657 registered nurses who held licenses to practice, 778,470 (69%) reported employment in nursing, while 316,611 (28%) did not. In January 1973, about 815,000 registered nurses, 390 per 100,000 population, were employed—a 4% increase over the previous year (Report to Congress). It is significant that so many qualified R.N.s do not work in nursing; clearly, shortages of nurses in many areas could be at least partly dealt with by attracting inactive nurses back to work—even if only on a part-time basis during the childrearing years—providing refresher courses and continuing education as needed.

In 1973 there were 459,000 licensed practical nurses in the United States, 80% of whom were employed in hospitals, nursing homes, and other health care institutions. In addition, 19% were practicing in doctor's offices and 1% in community settings (Report to the Congress). There are approximately one million nurses' aides, working primarily in institutions.

Distribution of Nursing Personnel

The geographic distribution of nurses in the United States is uneven. New York had the largest number of active registered nurses in 1972, with California second. In general, the New England states had the highest nurse-population ratios while the south-central states had the lowest. The District of Columbia had the highest registered nurse ratio—673 nurses per 100,000 population—followed by Massachusetts with 640 per 100,000. Arkansas had the lowest nurse-population ratio with 190 per 100,000 population (American Nurses' Association).

Work Settings

In 1972, about 70% of registered nurses were employed in institutional settings—64% in hospitals and the balance in nursing homes (American Nurses' Association). Mental health facilities employed 34,139 registered nurses in 1972, with state and county mental hospitals employing 40% of these nurses. In the same year, 7,571 professional nurses were working in 180 osteopathic hospitals. In 1971, 66,434 registered nurses were employed in nursing and personal care homes, the majority in the northeast; 66% worked in proprietary facilities and 24% in facilities run by church-related and other nonprofit groups.

The proportion of nurses working in private duty (one nurse working full-time taking care of one patient on a private-pay basis) has declined steadily over the years. In 1962, 12% of employed nurses were working in private duty; this figure declined to 9.7% in 1966 and to 5% in 1972. One reason for this decline has been the growth of intensive-care and special care units, making it less necessary for the seriously ill or postoperative patient to employ a "special" nurse. These units have also created a demand in the hospital for highly trained, clinically specialized nursing personnel. Increased salary commensurate with the advanced training needed have made these positions competitive (American Nurses' Association), and they have siphoned off nurses from private duty.

In early 1970 there were 53,969 registered nurses working in community health agencies; two years later there were 58,241. These figures reveal emerging patterns of health care: more nurses have advanced preparation to give primary care and direct community services in areas currently underserved.

In 1973, 10,000 registered nurses were serving in the three military nurse corps, with the attrition rate at 11% during the years 1968–73. The United States Civil Service Commission estimates that 26,104 registered nurses were employed full-time by the federal government in 1972, an increase of 7% over the previous year. This increase has been attributed largely to the additional nurses employed by the Veteran's Administration (American Nurses' Association).

Nursing Research and Quality Assessment

Because nursing is a practice profession, nurses and nurse educators have traditionally stressed its practical aspects. Therefore, the earliest research studies—those done in the 1920s and 1930s —were either time studies or concentrated on nursing techniques or procedures. Those of the 1940s were concerned with various aspects of nursing education. It was not until programs for nursing education were established within the framework of colleges and universities that nurses could be adequately prepared to do research. From the 1950s onward, the growth of collegiate education for nurses and the support of national nursing leaders, national nursing organizations, and government at various levels have made research a major movement in the profession (Notter, 1974). It is important to note that, whereas in the past most courses in research methods (for nurses) were limited to persons studying at the master's or doctoral level, such courses are now included in the curriculums of all four- and five-year programs and in those of some of the other types of nursing education programs.

Nursing research is now taking on new directions as the profession attempts to develop a practical system for assessing the role and functions of the nurse. In addition, the clinical expertise of nurses is being utilized in research activities that are developing systems of evaluating the quality of patient care. The American Nurses' Association has established standards for practice, and recommends the use of the nursing audit as one tool for measuring the quality of care delivered by nurses (Carter et al., 1976). Such audits are accepted practice in most institutions and health agencies (Report to Congress, 1974).

In "Methodology for Monitoring the Quality of Nursing Care," by Jelinek et al. (1974), the quality of care given is assessed by monitoring a set of nursing activities. These activities are components of the nursing process and include assessing the patient's needs and problems, formulating a plan of nursing care, implementing the plan of care, and evaluating the patient's progress as well as the achievement of nursing goals. These components constitute the basis against which the quality of nursing care is measured.

Components for Change
Nurse Practitioners: Role and Conflict

The impetus behind the development of the nurse practitioner has been cogently expressed:

> While most of the country goes around shaking its head about the doctor shortage, I am impressed by the existence of considerable waste. The waste is evident when you see so many physicians spending so much of their time at tasks that could be performed as well or better by someone with considerably shorter, more specialized training. The pediatrician providing well baby care, the gynecologist attending normal delivery, internists treating common colds are just a few of the examples of this phenomenon. (Fuchs, 1969)

As early as 1943, Frances Reiter, the nursing educator, used the term "nurse clinician" to describe a superior kind of nurse, distinguished by the depth of her clinical knowledge and by her ability to form interdependent working relationships with physicians and other health care providers. Reiter proposed that the nurse clinician or clinical nurse specialist be prepared at a graduate level. One of the distinguishing characteristics of this clinical nurse specialist is the high degree of discriminative judgment the nurse uses in assessing nursing problems when determining priorities of care.

Since this early definition, some confusion has arisen over titles, for over the years many new terms arose for the "nurse practitioner." Primary care nurse, primary care nurse clinician, family nurse practitioner, clinical nurse practitioner, were titles that began to be used interchangeably around the country. For the purpose of this chapter, the clinical nurse specialist and the nurse clinician are nurse practitioners with training at the master's degree level. Titles such as primary care nurse practitioner or family nurse practitioner will be applied to nurses in clinical practice (defined below) who do not necessarily have graduate degrees. The generic term, however, is "nurse practitioner," N.P.

The nurse may be prepared for the expanded role in several ways. Programs across the country vary from four months to two years in length. Currently, most of them are at the post-R.N. level, involving either programs leading to a certificate, or full-time graduate work leading to an advanced degree.

All these professionals learn history-taking, physical assessment, interpretation of laboratory procedures, and selected aspects of clinical medicine (including diagnosis and treatment) ; they also gain an understanding of the utilization of community resources needed to deal with patients' total health care needs (Ross, 1973).

A review of the duties and responsibilities of nurses throughout the twentieth century reveals that while the formal academic education being provided to prepare nurses for the expanded role is new, the role itself has a long history. The public health nurse, the nurse midwife, the private duty nurse, the frontier nurse in the hills of Kentucky (Kirk et al.), and the nurse anesthetist have long functioned well beyond the limits traditionally considered to constitute nursing practice as it became necessary and when physicians were not readily available (Lees, 1973). Nonetheless, an aura of newness surrounds the expanded role; there is an impression that a revolutionary process is taking place (Lees).

The term "expanded role" as applied to the N.P. refers to the nurse's potential for performing functions not traditionally considered within his/her domain. Direct patient care by nurses goes beyond the technical activities traditionally assigned to nursing. In the past, nurses usually found themselves primarily accountable to the physician and the institution, and only secondarily accountable to their patients.

Typifying N.P. training is a one-year education program for the registered nurse who is trained to exercise initiative and judgment in providing comprehensive health care to both children and adults. Usually, four months of intensive didactic and clinical instruction are followed by an eight-month supervised clinical internship. During the four-month didactic and clinical period, the student acquires basic skills in the physical assessment of the adult and child and is taught to differentiate the normal from the abnormal. During the internship period, the student applies acquired clinical knowledge in the three primary disciplines—medicine, pediatrics, and obstetrics-gynecology—and refines her clinical judgment (Albany Medical College). Successful completion of the course leads to certification as a primary care nurse practitioner.

Numerous reports from professional organizations and governmental agencies on the numbers and kinds of N.P. programs have been published (Report to the Congress). Recent directories list 135 continuing education programs and over 50 master's degree programs. These programs offer courses in child care (with such titles as Pediatric Nurse Practitioner or Pediatric Nurse Associate) ; in adult care (with such titles as Adult Health Care Practitioner, or Medical Nurse Associate) ; in maternal care (with such titles as Nurse-Midwife, Midwife–Family Nurse Practitioner, or Ob-gyn Nurse Practitioner).

The following outline summarizes the skills all such programs aim to teach :

A. *Collection of the Data Required for Making Nursing Judgments*
   1. Obtaining a comprehensive health history.
   2. Performing and recording a physical examination and assessing the patient's mental status.
   3. Obtaining appropriate laboratory and X-ray studies.
B. *Application of Clinical Judgment from Data Base*
   1. Recognizing and identifying major departures from normality on the basis of observations made during history-taking and physical examination.
   2. Preparing a complete write-up of the health history and physical examination as well as formulating a problem and planning for management.
   3. Analyzing and interpreting laboratory data in the management of common episodic and chronic illnesses.
   4. Recognizing, appropriately assessing, and prescribing and/ or managing treatment programs according to the established protocols mutually developed by the nurse practitioner, the physician, and/or the pharmacist.

5. Referring or consulting with another member of the health care team when indicated.
6. Interpreting to the patient and/or relatives the symptoms, disease, treatment, and prognosis appropriate to each patient.
7. Providing counseling, anticipatory guidance, and appropriate health education to the patient regarding the particular disease entity.
8. Recommending preventive health measures when appropriate.
9. Coordinating care by correlating pertinent clinical and social information from a variety of sources.

According to the American Nursing Association's former executive director, Eileen Jacobie, one of the greatest barriers to the expanded role is "attitudinal" (Kushner, 1973). The physician is reluctant to relinquish functions because having another individual make decisions under the general cover of the physician's license could increase his liability in the case of malpractice litigation; and the nurse is reluctant to take on increased responsibilities and accountability. The male/female role caricature, a barrier to role expansion, has been called the doctor-nurse game (Bullough, 1975). The object of the game is to make the doctor feel in control at all times. For example, nurses make recommendations so that they appear to have been initiated by the physician. If the N.P. is to function effectively, this game must be given up, a sad prospect for certain players on both sides.

The nursing profession has always valued the qualities of tact, gentleness, and patience. However, in order to be effective, nurses who move into the expanded role must also be self-assertive and decisive. The knowledgeable primary care nurse practitioner must communicate directly rather than obliquely with the physician and other members of the health care team. Indeed, the present trend is to educate nurses to become competent and more independent practitioners, rather than obedient handmaidens (Rothenberg, 1973), but relationships may become strained if male physicians do not accept the judgments of self-assertive and competent women.

Two important concepts inherent in the expanded role are "foreseeability" and accountability to the patient (Anderson et al.). "Foreseeability" means that the N.P. has adequate scientific preparation to predict with considerable accuracy the outcome and consequences of her acts. Accountability entails her recognizing and being responsible for her actions. As pointed out above, physicians who work with this new type of practitioner often experience identity crises (Bullough, 1975). First, the physician as principal provider is responsible personally for each of the traditional steps in the diagnosis and therapeutic process. As he relinquishes portions of his conventional role, he often has trouble trusting another health worker's data base (Bates). The physician has been taught in medical school that any good doctor does his own history and physical. Often he finds it difficult to share the decision-making process and to accept and trust the judgments and decisions of others. Physicians are sensitive to the potential for competition that the existence of the nurse practitioner implies (Pickard; Burrows and Traver).

There has been a widespread trend toward developing protocols which can be used by N.P.s as well as by physicians' assistants (see below) for diagnosis and treatment of minor acute diseases and other well-defined conditions. These must be developed by the physician and nurse working together as a cooperative team. However, disease protocols have limited value in that they do not always take into account every possible variation, and can impose a counterproductive cookbook approach.

The clinical work of various types of N.P. has been extensively evaluated. In an internal medicine clinic "nurse care was judged to be adequate in dealing with 98 percent of old problems (defined by the physician) and 85 percent of new problems (detected by the nurse)" (Spector et al., 1975, p. 1234). A pediatric nurse practitioner program was studied and found satisfactory (Yankauer et al., 1972). A Canadian study found that for randomly allocated patients, the quality of care provided by nurse practitioners was similar to that provided by physicians in a primary care practice (Spitzer et al.; Sackett et al.). A study undertaken in a university hospital medical clinic randomly allocated a small group of patients with chronic diseases between an experimental nurse practitioner clinic and the regular medical clinic. They found that there were no differences in deaths or severity of disease between the two groups of patients, and that the nurses did better in terms of reduction of disability and patient satisfaction (Lewis et al., 1969). The problems of instituting widespread use of N.P.s of various kinds thus seem much more related to history, attitudes, psychology, economics, and male-female role definition than they do to the technical content of the N.P.s' work and the quality of their performance.

The Physicians' Assistant

One proposed solution to the health manpower shortage (if indeed there is a shortage—see Chapter 4) has been the development of programs to train an additional health care provider called the physicians' assistant or associate. The educational preparation for the physicians' assistant seems to vary even more than that for the clinical nurse practitioner. Programs range from eight weeks to five years. Eugene Stead, of the Duke University Physicians' Assistant Program, one of the originators of the concept, describes the intended role of physicians' assistants:

> The Physicians' Assistant is seen as a new category within the structure of the health field, designed to provide a career opportunity for men functioning under the direction of doctors, with greater capabilities and growth potential than informally trained technicians. As the title implies, these individuals will be trained to assist the doctor in his clinical or research endeavors in such a way as to facilitate better utilization of available physicians and nurses. Graduates of the program at Duke are viewed as the individuals capable of performing responsibly and reliably certain of the skills currently practiced by doctors, nurses, and technicians. (1966, p. 1108)

The role of the physicians' assistant (P.A.) differs from that of the nurse in that P.A.s do not make nursing diagnoses or do bedside nursing care (Estes, 1971). Other differences are:

1. P.A.s work for an individual physician who assumes responsibility for the validity of all activities.
2. They work in several physical locations depending on the doctor's needs, over a workday whose length coincides with that of the doctor.
3. They carry out data gathering and treatment functions, using the tools of the physician—the stethoscope, the ophthalmoscope, the sigmoidoscope, and so on.

The P.A. is responsible first to the physician and then, through the physician, to the patient. His role and function are personally defined by the employing physician (Stead, 1966).

It is important to note that the masculine pronouns are often used in descriptions of P.A.s and their training. This is no accident: P.A. programs were originally designed to take advantage of and provide useful, interesting careers for medics returning from the Vietnam War in the 1960s, who were of course mostly male.* Women are now generally admitted into P.A. programs, but the male orientation remains.

The National Academy of Sciences has developed three classifications of P.A.s. The Type A assistant is capable of approaching the patient, collecting historical and physical data, and organizing and presenting data so that the physician can visualize the medical problem and determine appropriate diagnostic and therapeutic steps. The Type B assistant, while not equipped with the general knowledge and skills relative to the whole range of medical care, possesses exceptional skill in one clinical specialty, or more commonly in certain technical procedures within such a specialty. The Type C assistant is capable of performing a variety of tasks over a whole range of medical care under the supervision of a physician, although he does not possess the level of medical knowledge necessary to integrate findings. He is comparable to the practical nurse. Type A is qualified to act as the primary patient contact; Type B is characterized as the "assistant specialist," and Type C resembles the Type A assistant in the range of supporting services, but his formal training is more limited in depth and breadth (Estes, 1970).

Both P.A.s and N.P.s have demonstrated that they can "extend" the role of the physician in the delivery of health care. Certain aspects of their duties do overlap. The N.P. assumes some responsibilities as an associate of the physician providing primary and follow-up health care to patients. The degree of independence or interdependence varies, but the nurse is independent as a licensed professional when functioning within the scope of nursing. Physicians' assistant training programs prepare P.A.s to assume a dependent position under supervision by the physician. However, there is no specific or clear definition of "supervision"—it can be direct, with the physician on site, or it can be indirect, with a connection by telephone or other electronic means to the physician with whom the P.A. works.

* At the Annual Meeting of the American Public Health Association in Atlantic City in November, 1972, there was a panel presentation on new health care delivery developments in Canada. One speaker's topic was nurse practitioners and their use. A questioner asked if there were P.A. programs as well in Canada. The answer came back: "We don't need to have P.A. programs. We have had no Vietnam War with the large number of returning medics to use and provide for. We need only nurse practitioner programs" (Jonas).

The overlapping and indistinct lines of work distribution between N.P.s and P.A.s is an area needing more examination. There is a great deal of potential and actual conflict between the two groups, who seem to be fighting over the same turf (Bullough, 1975). In fact, the struggle is really three-sided, with the physicians involved as well: both the P.A.s and the N.P.s are struggling to move from the dependent to the independent health care provider group, against the resistance of the physicians. Unfortunately, as often happens in cases of parallel struggle against the same adversary, the P.A.s and N.P.s sometimes fight with each other harder than either fights with the physicians. The fact that most of at least the earlier generation of P.A.s are men and can earn salaries considerably higher than nurses with a great deal more training contributes significantly to the rivalry and animosity, where it does exist. It should be noted, however, that there are instances in which P.A.s and N.P.s work very well together.

In reality, it is as hard to see real differences between the work of P.A.s (at least Type A P.A.s) and N.P.s as it is to see differences between their work and the majority of tasks carried out by most primary care physicians. These difficult conflicts must be resolved; if they are not, in the end only the patients—and the taxpayers—will suffer.

Current and Future Trends

The National Health Planning and Resources Development Act of 1974 (P.L. 93-641) established a national network of local planning agencies called Health Systems Agencies (see Chapter 12). One of the major provisions and priorities of the act is the training and increased utilization of nurse practitioners. Designating N.P.s as important providers of primary care, the act included them in the category of physicians' assistants and in some cases physician extenders (National League for Nursing, 1974 (b)).

Within the nursing profession, too, the role of the independent practitioner is being assessed. Steps are being taken to define who the nurse practitioner is and what qualifications she or he must possess (Kinsella; Murray and Ross; Rosasco). It is the responsibility of the profession to present a unified front and come to a common agreement as to who will have the authority for accreditation and certification and who will set the educational standards for this new category of nursing professional.

Much has been written about the confusion regarding roles

that exists within nursing itself. The changing roles of health care professionals have created serious concern about possible shortages of nurses in the traditional roles (Anderson, 1968). In the past, nursing education has placed much emphasis on the psychosocial aspects of patient care whereas the physician has focused primarily on the pathophysiological aspects of illness. The trend today is toward educating both doctors and nurses to view the patient as a whole and unique individual within a complex social framework. The physical diagnosis component traditionally dominant in medical schools has now found its way into the curricula of N.P. programs at the baccalaureate and master's degree levels. In these new educational programs, students are oriented toward providing care to patients, not service to institutions. They are educated to make more decisions, to take more responsibility, to become accountable for their actions. Unfortunately, upon graduation many nurses accept employment in institutional health care settings where the bureaucratic structure operates by means of hierarchical restraints: obedience to rules and authority is valued more than independence and initiative. The resulting conflict between educational ideals and job realities —a kind of role deprivation—may be the most significant reason why so many R.N.s are not active in nursing.

Nursing, a young profession, has come a long way in a little over 100 years. But there is much to be done. Nursing is at the crossroads of its development and its future will be determined by the commitments its professionals make and the attitudes they adopt. Nurses must decide who they are, which directions they will follow, how they will interact with other health care professionals in determining the quality of patient care. Nursing not only has the right to share in the planning, delivery, and evaluation of health care, but also the responsibility to do so. At present, securing this professional right and assuming this professional responsibility represent nursing's principal challenge.

References

Albany Medical College. *Preparing the Primary Care Nurse*. Albany, N.Y., 1975.

American Nurses' Association. *Facts about Nursing, 72–73*. Kansas City, Mo.: American Nurses' Association, 1974.

Anderson, J. et al. "The Expanded Role of the Nurse: Independent Practitioner or Physician's Assistant." *The Canadian Nurse,* September, 1975, p. 34.

Anderson, O. W. *Toward an Unambiguous Profession? A Review of Nursing.* Health Administration Perspectives No. A6. Chicago: University of Chicago, 1968.

Bates, B. "Physician and Nurse Practitioners: Conflict and Reward." *Annals of Internal Medicine, 82,* 702, 1975.

Bullough, B. "Barriers to the Nurse Practitioner Movement: Problems of Women in a Woman's Field." *International Journal of Health Services, 5,* 225, 1975.

Bullough, B. "The Law and the Expanding Nursing Role." *American Journal of Public Health, 66,* 249, 1976.

Bullough, B., and Bullough, V. L. *The Emergence of Modern Nursing.* New York: Macmillan, 1974.

Bullough, B., and Bullough, V. L. *Expanding Horizons for Nurses.* New York: Springer Publishing Co., 1977.

Burrows, B., and Traver, G. A. "Nurse Practitioner Programs." *Annals of Internal Medicine, 80,* 268, 1974.

Carter, J. et al. *Standards of Nursing Care: A Guide for Evaluation.* New York: Springer Publishing Co., 1976.

Ehrenreich, B. "Where Women Work, The Health Care Industry. A Theory of Industrial Medicine." *Social Policy,* Nov./Dec., 1975, p. 74.

Estes, E. H. Quoted in Carlson, C. L., and Athelstan, G. T., "The Physician's Assistant: Versions and Diversions of a Promising Concept." *Journal of the American Medical Association, 214,* 1857, 1970.

Estes, E. H. "Physician's Assistants, The Health Manpower Dilemma." Papers presented at the fourth annual meeting of the Council of Hospital and Related Institutional Nursing Services, October, 1971. New York: National League for Nursing, 1971.

Forni, P. R., and Bolte, I. M., "Planning for Continuing Education." *American Journal of Nursing, 73,* 1912, 1973.

Fuchs, V. R. "Improving the Delivery of Personal Health Services." *Journal of Bone Joint Surgery, 51,* 407, 1969.

Jelinek, R. C. et al. *A Methodology for Monitoring Quality Nursing Care.* DHEW Publication No. (HRA) 74–25. Washington, D.C.: Government Printing Office, 1974.

Jonas, S. Personal communication. July 1, 1976.

Kinsella, C. R. "Who Is the Clinical Nurse Specialist?" *Hospitals, J.A.H.A.,* November 1, 1973, p. 93.

Kirk, R. F. H. et al. "Family Nurse Practitioners in Eastern Kentucky." *Medical Care, 9,* 160, 1971.

Kushner, T. D. "Nursing Profession." *Ms. Magazine,* September, 1973.

Lees, R. E. "Physician Time-saving by Employment of Expanded-role

Nurses in Family Practice." *Canadian Medical Association Journal, 108,* 871, 1973.

Lego, S. "Continuing Education by Mail." *American Journal of Nursing, 73,* 840, 1973.

Lenberg, C. B. "The External Degree in Nursing: The Promise Fulfilled." *Nursing Outlook, 24,* 423, 1976.

Lewis, C. E. et al. "Activities, Events and Outcomes in Ambulatory Patient Care." *New England Journal of Medicine, 280,* 645, 1969.

Martel, G. D., and Edmunds, M. W., "Nurse-Internship Program in Chicago." *American Journal of Nursing, 72,* 940–943, 1973.

Murray, R. H., and Ross, S. A. "Training the Family Nurse Practitioner." *Hospitals, J.A.H.A.,* November 1, 1973, p. 93.

Navarro, V. "Women in Health Care." *The New England Journal of Medicine, 293,* 398, 1975.

National Commission for the Study of Nursing and Nursing Education. *Nurse Clinician and Physician's Assistant: The Relationship between Two Emerging Practitioner Concepts.* New York: National League for Nursing, 1971.

National Commission for the Study of Nursing and Nursing Education. *Cost of Nursing Education and a Case for its Greater Support.* Rochester, N.Y.: National League for Nursing, 1975.

National League for Nursing. *Education for Nursing—The Diploma Way.* Pub. No. 16–1314. New York, 1973–74. (a)

National League for Nursing. *Health Policy Making in Action: The Passage and Implementation of the National Health Planning and Resources Development Act of 1974.* Papers by the NLN Summer Study Fellows in Public Policy. Pub. No. 41–1600. New York, 1974. (b)

National League for Nursing. *Associate Degree Education for Nursing.* Pub. No. 23–1309. New York, 1974–75. (c)

National League for Nursing. *Practical Nursing Career.* New York, 1974–75. (d)

Notter, L. E. *The Essentials of Nursing Research.* New York: Springer Publishing Co., 1974.

Ozimek, D. *Initiating a Baccalaureate Degree Program in Nursing—Asking the Essential Questions.* New York: National League for Nursing, Pub. No. 15–1536, 1974.

Ozimek, D., and Yura, H. *Who Is the Nurse Practitioner.* New York: National League for Nursing, Department of Baccalaureate and Higher Degree Programs, Pub. No. 15–1555, 1975.

Pickard, C. G. "Family Nurse Practitioners: Preliminary Answers and New Issues." *Annals of Internal Medicine, 80,* 267, 1974.

Report to the Congress. *Nurse Training 1974.* USDHEW Pub. No. [HRA] 75–41. Rockville, M.D.: USDHEW, 1974.

Rosasco, L. C. "Of Nursing Practice and Nurse Practitioners." *Hospitals, J.A.H.A.,* June 1, 1973, p. 72.

Ross, S. "The Clinical Nurse Practitioner in Ambulatory Care Service." *Bulletin of the New York Academy of Medicine, 49,* 393, 1973.

Rothenberg, J. S. "Nurse and Physician's Assistant: Issues and Relationships." *Nursing Outlook, 21,* 154, 1973.

Sackett, D. L. et al. "The Burlington Randomized Trial of the Nurse Practitioner: Health Outcomes of Patients." *Annals of Internal Medicine, 80,* 268, 1974.

Spector, R. et al. "Medical Care by Nurses in an Internal Medicine Clinic: Analysis of Quality and Its Cost." *Journal of the American Medical Association, 232,* 1234, 1975.

Spitzer, W. O. et al. "The Burlington Randomized Trial of the Nurse Practitioner." *New England Journal of Medicine, 290,* 251, 1974.

Stead, E. A. "Conserving Costly Talents—Providing Physician's New Assistants." *Journal of the American Medical Association, 198,* 1108, 1966.

Treece, E. W. *Internship in Nursing Education: Technoterm.* New York: Springer Publishing Co., 1974.

Walsh, M. E. *Why Nursing Education Programs Should be Accredited.* New York: National League for Nursing, Pub. No. 14–1597, 1975.

Wozniak, D. "External Degrees in Nursing." *American Journal of Nursing, 73,* 1014 (June), 1973.

Yankauer, A. et al. "The Outcomes and Service Impact of a Pediatric Nurse Practitioner Training Program—Nurse Practitioner Training Outcomes." *American Journal of Public Health, 62,* 347, 1972.

6

Ambulatory Care

Steven Jonas and Barbara Rimer

Introduction

Ambulatory care is commonly defined in terms of whom it excludes. It is personal or combined health care service given to a person who is not a bed patient in a health care institution. Thus the term ambulatory care covers all health services other than community health services and personal and combined services given to institutionalized patients (see Chapter 2).

Since there are about three times as many visits to physicians on an ambulatory basis annually as there are hospital days of care (Danchik, Table B; American Hospital Association, 1974, Table 1), it can be concluded that the majority of physician-patient contacts in the United States take place on an ambulatory basis. As White points out, "The vast bulk of care is provided by physicians in ambulatory settings. Only 10 percent of the people [seen] are admitted to a hospital . . ." (White, 1973b).

There are two major categories of ambulatory care. One, by far and away the largest, is care given by private physicians in solo, partnership, or private group practice, on a fee-for-service basis. The other may be called ambulatory care in organized settings. An organized setting here is taken to mean a locus of medical practice with an identity independent from that of the particular individual physician(s) working in it. This category includes hospital-based ambulatory services (primarily clinics and emergency care), emergency medical services systems, health department clinics, prepaid group practices, Foundations for Medical Care, Health Maintenance Organizations (HMOs), Neighborhood Health Centers (NHCs), organized home care, Community Mental Health Centers, industrial health services, school health services, and prison health services. In this chapter we will deal with the first eight categories, which have a common

base in a medical institutional setting. Community Mental Health
Centers are dealt with in Chapter 8. Unfortunately, we do not
have the space to deal with organized ambulatory services provided in nonmedical institutional settings. However, suggested
readings on those topics will be found in Appendix 2.

Private Practice

The primary mode of organization of physicians in the United
States (and, indeed, of most other health care providers who are
licensed to practice independently, such as dentists, chiropractors, podiatrists, and optometrists) is what is called private practice. The physician in private practice provides a range of health
care services limited only by the licensing laws of the state in
which he/she may be operating as an independent entrepreneur.
The physician, in effect, contracts directly with patients
(although almost never in writing) to provide a set of services in
return for payment of a fee. This arrangement is appropriately
enough called the fee-for-service system. Physicians in private
practice provide care on a fee-for-service basis in settings that
include premises owned or leased by the physician, the patient's
home (on rare occasions), or an institution. Under this arrangement, a patient hospitalized under the care of his/her private
physician pays the hospital for all services other than physician
care. The physician's fee is paid directly. Thus, even when working in a hospital setting, the private practitioner's relationship to
the patient remains that of an independent contractor.

About 60% of all active U.S. physicians are in office practice
(Warner and Aherne, Table 23). About 20% are house staff
(interns and residents in training), 12% full-time hospital-based
practitioners (including those in federal service), and the balance in non-patient-care positions (Warner and Aherne, Table
24). Of those in office practice outside hospitals, about 95% are in
private practice, the balance working in prepaid group practices,
federal service, public health centers, neighborhood health centers,
and other organized settings (Warner and Aherne, derived from
Tables 23, 24, 34). Thus, taking into account all physicians who
are in active practice, including hospital-based physicians but
excluding house staff, about 80% are in private practice (Warner
and Aherne, derived from Tables 23, 24, 34). Clearly, the dominant mode of physician organization in American medicine is private practice.

The majority of ambulatory patient visits are made to physicians in their private offices, as one would expect. The National Health Survey, counting from the patient side (see Chapter 3), reported that in 1971 about 80% of all visits to a physician were made to private practices, a total of about 585 million visits (Danchik, Table 15). The National Ambulatory Medical Care Survey (NAMCS), counting from the provider side, reported for the period from May 1973 to April 1974 that 644.9 million visits were made to "office-based, patient-care" physicians, the vast majority of whom were private practitioners (NAMCS). Taking into account estimates of the volume of visits to other sources of ambulatory care (American Hospital Association, 1974), the proportion of the total made to private offices remained about the same between 1971 and 1973. It is unlikely that the proportions have changed much since those counts were made.

Although there are reasonably good measures of the number of private practioners and of the volume of their practices, we are much less certain about exactly what physicians do. Private practice is at once the most important and the least studied sector of the U.S. health care delivery system. This is not surprising, since private practitioners of any profession are loath to have outside researchers looking into their work. Thus it is difficult to describe, other than by anecdote and personal experience, the typical workday of a private practitioner. Wolfe and Badgley (1972, pp. 4–7) do offer an interesting picture of what is, in their estimation, the typical work-week of a Canadian private family practitioner. The description is of only the one specialty, however, and was not based on a randomized research study. Nevertheless, the insights are useful, and probably apply to the United States.

Little is known about how a doctor distributes his/her time among history-taking and examination, diagnosing, giving or explaining therapy, talking with patients, supervising staff, doing paperwork, traveling, teaching, attending meetings, reading, and what have you. There is little idea of what the vaunted "doctor-patient relationship" really consists. It is not known what doctors really talk about with their patients. Although there have been some studies of intradoctor referral mechanisms (Shortell), we do not know very much about how private physicians interact. The decision-making methods in private practice are not well understood and the ability to measure the quality of care in that setting is limited (see Chapter 13). Also, little information is available about the business aspects of private practice.

Some facts *are* available, however. About 75% of all physicians in office practice classify themselves as being in a specialty other than general practice (Warner and Aherne, Table 24). Thus, American medical practice is heavily specialized. Among physicians in active office practice, the highest proportions specialize in general internal medicine (about 12%), general surgery (about 9%), obstetrics and gynecology (about 7%), and pediatrics (about 5%). In all, about 25% of physicians are in a medical specialty or subspecialty (internal medicine, cardiology, dermatology, etc.), about 30% in a surgical specialty or subspecialty (general surgery, neurosurgery, orthopedics), about 20% in "other" specialties (psychiatry, radiology, pathology, etc.), and the balance in general practice (Warner and Aherne, Table 24). This high degree of specialization is one of the major problems confronting American medicine (Terris; White, 1974).*

Patients, particularly those who use the private sector and thus can pick their own points of entry, face a bewildering array of physicians from which to choose. The question has not been studied on a national scale, but many patients using the private sector seem to have what might be called a "group-practice-in-the-head," having, perhaps, "my" internist, "my" psychiatrist, "my" neurologist, "my" allergist, "my" surgeon, "my" obstetrician-gynecologist, and so on. (Fortunately, only a few patients have "my" pathologist, choosing to go to him/her at the appropriate moment, but you never can tell.) This means that when a new symptom (something a patient feels or experiences) or a new sign (something a patient or other observer notices objectively) appears, it is the patient, a usually untrained observer, who evaluates its meaning and picks an entry-point in the spectrum of specialists. Unfortunately for many patients, few if any members of the particular "group-practice-in-the-head" know each other. Thus communications between them are poor.

Specialists tend to concentrate on their own organ or organ system, and it is easy for the whole patient to get lost in a tangle of organs. The forest is indeed obscured by the trees. Patients may well suffer because there is no trained individual who can: (1) see them as a whole person, (2) put together a variety of

---

* A particularly erudite and detailed history of the development of specialization in American medical practice is presented by Rosemary Stevens in her book, *American Medicine and the Public Interest* (New Haven, Conn.: Yale University Press, 1971).

complaints into one clinical picture, (3) guide the patient through an intelligent utilization of specialists' knowledge, and (4) establish an organized means for communication among specialists. This is not an argument against specialization per se; the tremendous expansion of medical knowledge requires such specialization, at least for a certain proportion of the profession. It *is* an argument for a more rational approach to the organization of specialists (White, 1973a). (Aspects of the problems of specialization are also discussed in Chapter 4.)

An important feature of the private practice sector in the United States is that the majority of physicians see patients both on an ambulatory basis in their own offices and as hospital inpatients. (There is a small percentage of doctors who do not have hospital appointments, but the magnitude is unknown. Most of them are probably in urban areas.) In most other countries, physicians either see ambulatory patients only or work full-time in hospitals. The unusual American arrangement offers some significant advantages. For conditions for which one physician is technically competent to provide both ambulatory and inpatient care, as in many medical specialties, there is continuity of physician care for the hospitalized patient. For surgical conditions, in many cases the nonsurgical physician who referred the patient for surgery will participate in the pre- and postoperative phases of care in the hospitals, or at least will follow his/her hospitalized patient.

The average American physician spends about 50 hours per week working (Warner and Aherne, Table 44), the rural physician working slightly longer hours than his/her urban counterpart, for about 48 weeks per year (Warner and Aherne, Table 52). About 90% of this time is spent in direct patient care (Warner and Aherne, Table 48). During this time, the average American physician provides about 100 visits per week (Warner and Aherne, Table 60). The range is rather broad, from about 35 for psychiatrists through approximately 80 for surgeons to 135 for pediatricians and 145 for general practitioners. For all specialties, rural physicians see about 30% more visits than urban physicians. At the same time, the average American physician made about 40 hospital visits per week, ranging from 50 for rural physicians to 30 for urban physicians (Warner and Aherne, Table 61), again confirming the primacy of ambulatory care in the system. As might be surmised, surgeons made the highest average number of hospital visits per week (about 50), and psychiatrists the fewest (about 15). These figures, all for 1973, but still probably valid, confirm that the American physician does both hospital and nonhospital work. They also portray him/her as being rather busy. For this level of work, the average physician's income, as reported by themselves in 1973, was around $50,000 per annum (Warner and Aherne, Table 62).

Ambulatory Services in Organized Settings
Hospital Ambulatory Services

Introduction. The institutional center of the American health care system is the hospital. For a variety of historical reasons (Freymann, Ch. 3), the majority of American hospitals focus the bulk of their efforts and activities on patients who are acutely ill and confined to bed. Hospitals have also had to deal with a variety of other types of patients, however. Among them are those who do not immediately require admission to a bed. These patients are called "outpatients," as opposed to "inpatients."

Outpatients may require either immediate treatment for an acute, and often serious, illness or injury, or care for a more routine matter calling for medical attention, but not necessarily immediately. Very often, the services required by the latter type of patient are very similar to those needed by patients who attend private practitioners' offices. Although there are some exceptions, the patients needing immediate attention go to one of the two major divisions of hospital ambulatory services, the "Emergency Unit," while those who do not go to the "Clinics." Increasingly, hospital staffs and administrations are confused as to the differences in role and function of the two divisions, and they and the patients themselves have trouble deciding who should go where for what.

Historically, it apparently has been easier for hospitals to determine that emergency services should be provided than that clinic services should be. About 85% (4,713 in 1973) of community hospitals in the United States (by the American Hospital Association definition: "non-federal, short-term, general, and other special hospitals"; see Chapter 7) have emergency units (American Hospital Association, Table 12A). The original intended function of emergency units was to take care of people acutely ill or injured, particularly with life-threatening or potentially life-threatening problems that require immediate attention, personnel and/or equipment not found in private practitioners' offices, and, potentially, prompt hospitalization. Most hospitals have found it desirable or necessary to provide such services.

Historically, on the other hand, two kinds of hospitals have paid the most attention to clinic services: those located in areas where patients could not or would not attend private practitioners' offices for more routine care, usually for economic reasons (Roemer, 1971), and/or those that have teaching programs. Only about one-quarter of community hospitals (1,424 in 1973) have clinics (American Hospital Association, Table 12A). It is probably not coincidental that emergency outpatient services, particularly for critically ill patients, are not among those services that private physicians can easily provide in their own offices, whereas the type of service provided in clinics can usually be given by the private physician, economic considerations aside.

In the nineteenth century, clinic service was part of the functions of most hospitals serving the poor in urban areas (Freymann, Chs. 3,4). Until the late nineteenth century, hospitals were relatively uncommon in the United States. In 1875, there were fewer than 200 of them (Stevens, p. 52). A building boom then took place and, by 1909, there were 4,359 hospitals with a bed capacity of 421,000. Local government hospitals were established for the sole purpose of taking care of the poor, both inpatients and outpatients; care of the sick poor was separated from the general custodial functions provided for persons not self-sufficient for all reasons by the poorhouse/workhouse system. (For additional material on the history of hospitals, see also Chapter 7.) Nonprofit "voluntary" hospitals were also established, at least in part, to fulfill charitable purposes. One way they did so was by providing free clinic care to the poor. However, the voluntaries, which were much more important in setting the style for the organization of medical practice than were the local government hospitals, established clinics on their premises only grudgingly.

Dispensaries. So uninterested were the voluntaries in providing clinic services within the hospital walls that their corporations often established related but physically separate institutions to carry out that function. They were called "dispensaries" (Rosenberg). There were also nonaffiliated charitable dispensaries, as well as local government ones. Dispensaries were an important factor in urban medical care at one time (Rosenberg, p. 33). In 1900, there were about 100 in the U.S.; in New York City alone in that year, dispensaries provided facilities for more than 800,000 visits. However, they were poorly staffed, poorly financed, and viewed with displeasure by private practitioners, who saw them as competing for patients. Most of them had disappeared by the 1920s (Rosenberg, p. 49).

Hospital Clinics. Clinic services started growing in the voluntary hospitals themselves in the latter part of the nineteenth century. By 1916, 495 hospitals had clinics, in many cases serving an educational as well as a charitable function (Roemer, 1975a). However, the clinics certainly shared the second-class status of the dispensaries. When, for example, a clinic was built onto the archetypal nineteenth-century voluntary hospital, the Johns Hopkins in Baltimore, it was added at the back (Freymann, p. 56). This typified the approach. As Freymann says (p. 200): "It was and still is an appendix tacked on the periphery of the bed-filled tower that soaks up the pride and wealth of the community. The ambulatory services huddle at the nether end of the pecking order...."

In considering problems of hospital ambulatory services, it should be kept in mind that they vary in type and are found in several categories of hospitals. Most of the literature on hospital ambulatory care in the United States deals with university and other teaching hospitals and thus probably presents a distorted picture. Excluding Veterans' Administration hospitals (about which we also know little), approximately 65% of emergency department visits and 40% of clinic visits take place in hospitals not affiliated with medical schools (American Hospital Association, 1974, derived from Tables 3 and 8). Still, medical school-affiliated hospitals do set a great deal of the hierarchical tone in the United States, and thus it is useful to look at what goes on in them.

In 1965, the then Director of the Massachusetts General Hospital described the scene cogently in terms that still largely apply:

Turning to the outpatient department of the urban hospital, we find the stepchild of the institution. Traditionally, this has been the least popular area in which to work and, as a result, few advances in medical care and teaching have been harvested here for the benefit of the community. Ever since the day of the Flexner report, university hospitals have treated outpatients and outpatient departments as if they all had the plague. Heads of departments and professors have never toiled in these vineyards, preferring the prostrate inpatient with florid disease and the convenience of multiple test results for obvious reasons: the situation was easier to grasp, diagnosis and treatment were simpler, and all the not-so-easy to settle social and mental diseases were screened out or not admitted. Similarly, the practicing, part-time, and courtesy staff were given the outpatient labor assignment while the full-time department men (academicians) were given two rewards: they were: 1) excused from going to the outpatient department and 2) given choice of times for visiting the wards filled with inpatients. Those on the "inside" saw inpatients; the "outs" worked with the "outs." (Knowles, p. 70)

Clinics today still play their historical role of caring for the poor, although little "free" care remains. At best, patients have some third-party coverage; at worst, they are faced with a means-test–related sliding fee scale. Then, despite their second-class status, clinics do have a teaching function for medical students and house staff. Finally, many clinical researchers have found the outpatient clinics to be a useful place to work. However, the last function, and, to a considerable extent, the second one, have led to organizational problems resulting in confusion and conflict.

Clinic Organization and Staffing. The best way of organizing outpatient clinics to provide opportunities for teaching and research—especially in view of the way contemporary medical education is structured—is to have a large number of disease-, organ-, or organ-system-specific clinics (Freymann, p. 255). The typical contemporary teaching hospital has three groups of clinics: medical, surgical, and other. The medical clinic group, which may or may not have a "general medical clinic" approximating the function of the general internist, includes cardiology, neurology, dermatology, allergy, gastroenterology, and so on. Patients may stay in one or more specialty clinics for long periods of time, particularly in the typical situation in which the general medical clinic is small or nonexistent and specialty clinics admit patients directly without referral from a general clinic. The surgical clinic group includes general surgery, orthopedics, urology, plastic surgery, and the like. Since surgical care is usually more episodic than is medical care, patients are not as likely to remain in these clinics for long periods of time. The third group includes pediatrics and the pediatric subspecialties, obstetrics-gynecology and its subspecialties, and other specialties such as rehabilitation medicine.

Teaching hospital clinics are staffed by four categories of physician. Voluntary attending staff may draw clinic duty as part of their obligation to the hospital in return for receiving admitting privileges. Full-time, inpatient physicians, usually more junior ones, may be assigned, generally to carry out teaching, supervisory, and research functions. House staff, usually residents but occasionally interns, may be assigned to clinics on a rotating basis. In most hospital clinics the stress is on teaching and research rather than patient care. Since house staff are usually rotated frequently between various subspecialty clinics for teaching purposes, patients with stable conditions coming to a subspecialty clinic, say, once every three months, may see a different physician each time. Finally, for very busy clinics, hospitals may hire outside physicians on a sessional or salaried basis, exclusively to work in the clinics. They are usually not part of the regular hospital staff, do not participate in the educational program, and are truly what Knowles calls the "outs."

Most hospital outpatient departments are open all day every day, but many individual clinics, particularly when they are highly subspecialized, meet once or twice a week. Some teaching hospitals have over 100 different specialty and subspecialty clinics. Thus, a hospital-based physician working in the usual hospital clinic organization can concentrate on diabetes, peripheral vascular disease, or stroke in his/her teaching and/or research. This is advantageous to the provider who has a focus confined to a particular disease or condition. It may also be advantageous to the patient who has a single disease problem of a rather complex or unusual nature.

Three kinds of patients face difficulties in using such clinics. First is the patient with the ordinary problem for which no specialty clinic exists; few hospitals, for example, have "sore throat" clinics. Second is the patient with a categorical disease, like diabetes, which, however, is uncomplicated. Going to a diabetes clinic, such a patient is likely to have to take a back seat to a diabetic patient who has complications. Third is the patient with multiple problems. These patients, often elderly, may end up attending diabetes clinic on Tuesday, stroke clinic on Wednesday, peripheral vascular clinic on Thursday, and cardiology clinic on Friday. (Fortunately, Monday is a free day.) This is distinctly disadvantageous for two major reasons: it necessitates multiple trips to the clinic and precludes looking at the patient as a whole person rather than as a collection of diseased organs and organ systems.

Thus the basic conflict in hospital ambulatory services is established, between the needs of specialty-oriented providers on the

one hand and patients with either ordinary problems or several
different problems on the other. This situation is not new; neither is professional recognition of it. In 1964, at a conference on
"The Expanding Role of Ambulatory Services in Hospitals and
Health Departments" held at the New York Academy of Medicine, Cecil Sheps, M.D., said:

> As I sat through the sessions yesterday and today I had a per-
> sistent feeling of *déjà vu*. I possess a book written by Michael M.
> Davis [Clinics, Hospitals and Health Centers (New York:
> Harper, 1927)] and published in 1927. In it there is quoted a
> statement prepared in 1914 that describes the purpose of an out-
> patient department just as clearly as anything said at this confer-
> ence: that the focus must be on the patient, that care must be
> organized around the patient, and that the hospital must take the
> community as its venue and not simply the patients who come to
> it. (Sheps, p. 148)

At the same conference, John Knowles, M.D., outlined his
view of what comprehensive ambulatory care in the hospital
setting would mean:

> Comprehensive medicine in this context means the coordination of
> all the various caring elements in the community with those of
> the medical profession by a team of individuals representing all
> disciplines, with all the techniques and resources available to the
> physician and his patient. The aim of these individuals would be
> to provide total care—somatic, psychic, and social—to those in
> need, and to study and research the expanding social and eco-
> nomic problems of medical care with the intent of improving the
> organization and provision of health services. (Knowles, p. 73)

As Freymann says, "Instead of dividing diagnoses among doctors, doctors should be divided among patients" (p. 255).

The goal of these proposals is primarily to make hospital clinics more responsive to community needs than they are now. A
secondary goal, or certainly effect, of such changes would be the
education of physicians who would perforce develop an entirely
different view of hospital ambulatory services. It must be remembered that the essential difficulty is the contradiction between the
needs of the majority of clinic patients to receive comprehensive
care and the needs of the majority of physician staffs to carry out
their teaching and research functions as they see fit. At present,
the latter requires a disease orientation and generally an orienta-

tion toward diseases requiring hospitalization at one point or another. If teaching and research were to be reoriented toward an emphasis on the more common rather than on the more uncommon, if hospitals were to define their roles and responsibilities in terms of community needs, the contradiction would be resolved straight away and hospital clinics would be on the road to first-class status (Jonas, 1968, 1971; Freymann, ch. 18).

It must be borne in mind that these conflicts over clinic services affect only a minority of American hospitals, the 25% or so of all hospitals that have clinics (American Hospital Association, Table 12A). Of these, over half are in medical school affiliated hospitals (American Hospital Association, derived from Tables 10A, 12A). Other problems, concerning emergency services, affect the majority of American hospitals, since about 75% of them have emergency departments, as do 85% of community hospitals and over 95% of community hospitals with more than 200 beds (American Hospital Association, Table 12A).

Hospital emergency services. The hospital emergency unit serves a variety of functions. It does, of course, take care of critically ill and injured patients. In many hospitals, it serves as a secondary, well-equipped private doctor's office, in which staff physicians can see their own patients for whom more sophisticated care than that available in the doctor's own office is required. A third role, particularly for emergency departments in local government hospitals, is that of primary admitter of patients to the hospital. In one hospital in New York City, a busy emergency department was responsible for about 75% of hospital admissions (Jonas et al., 1976). A fourth, increasingly important role is the provision of care to persons who are not injured or critically ill, who do not have or cannot reach a private physician, and/or who do not use the hospital clinic, if one exists, or another organized ambulatory service, or find that it is not open when needed.

Weinerman et al. defined three categories of patient presenting themselves to emergency units: nonurgent, urgent, emergent (1966, p. 1040). Nonurgent is defined as: "Condition does not require the resources of an emergency service; referral for routine medical care may or may not be needed; disorder is nonacute or minor in severity." Urgent is: "Condition requires medical attention within the period of a few hours, there is possible danger to the patient if medically unattended; disorder is acute but not necessarily severe." Emergent is: "Condition requires immediate medical attention; time delay is harmful to patient; disorder is acute and potentially threatening to life or function." It should be borne in mind that these are professional definitions, from the point of view of the provider. Patients are not as likely to make these kinds of distinctions. Most patients presenting themselves for care to emergency departments are there because they feel that they need attention immediately, however their problem might be classified by a provider.

By the early 1960s, studies had shown that the proportion of patients in the nonurgent category had been on the increase since World War II (Weinerman and Edwards). A more recent review of data on categorical patient distribution showed that the average is approximately 5% emergent, 45% urgent, and 50% nonurgent (Jonas et al., 1976). There can be variations around these figures by type, role, and location of hospital, of course (Torrens and Yedvab).

Weinerman and Edwards pointed out that:

> A variety of medical and sociological factors are involved in these trends. The role of the general hospital has changed from that of a last resort for the seriously ill to a community resource for a broad spectrum of general medical care services to ambulatory patients. As medical practice has become more specialized, more highly structured and less personal, physicians are not as readily available for sudden call and not as willing to handle a wide variety of acute problems. An increasingly mechanized, synthetic, and high-speed environment engenders steadily rising rates of accidental injury, toxic reaction, and hypertensitivity. Higher costs of medical care and health insurance coverage for care in, but not out of, the hospital contribute to the popularity of the emergency service. Also, alert patients soon learn the advantages of the quick care offered in the emergency department over the long waits for a clinic or private office appointment.
>
> Perhaps most important of all is the steady trend toward concentration in the urban center, around the large hospitals, of economically dependent, socially isolated, minority population groups, who are often recent arrivals to these old communities and have only remote connections to the "usual" pattern of private medical care. (1964)

One problem faced by hospital emergency units is thus that of the "nonurgent" patient (G. Gibson, 1971). A variety of solutions has been proposed (Spencer, ch. 1), ranging from virtually barring the door to nonurgent patients, to providing a sorting or triage system (Weinerman and Edwards, Beloff, Albin et al.) to screen for nonurgent patients and refer them to alternative sources of care after making certain that no acute illness is in fact present, to treating patients as they come, with equanimity (Hannas, 1975), becoming a sort of community general clinic that happens to be open 24 hours a day (Satin and Duhl). The final word on this subject has not yet been written; rational solutions to the problem involve not only emergency departments but ether sectors of the health care delivery system as well. What Weinerman and Edwards said in 1964 is still true today:

> The ultimate solution must be found *outside* the walls of the hospital. It must encompass an integrated system of medical care for the entire community assuring availability of appropriate medical care at all hours and to all classes of the population. When this dream is realized, the emergency service will again be appropriately named, and triage will no longer be necessary.

There are a variety of physician staffing patterns for emergency departments (Webb and Lawrence). In teaching hospitals, it has been customary to staff emergency departments primarily with the least experienced members of the house staff, the interns. In many hospitals, they are being replaced with residents. Some teaching hospitals find that they cannot fully meet the needs from house staff and supplement them with full-time or sessional hired physicians. More often than not they occupy a similar "out" position in relation to the regular hospital staff as do hired clinic physicians. A small but increasing number of teaching hospitals, however, are assigning regular full-time staff to some responsibility in the emergency department.

The staffing situation is different in non-teaching hospitals. In those with light patient loads, members of the hospital attending staff may cover, in person or on call, on a rota system. In certain states there are legal staffing requirements. For example, Section 720.17 of the New York State Hospital Code requires that all hospitals with 40,000 emergency patient visits annually provide for full-time physician coverage. An increasingly popular approach to the solution of this problem is the full-time emergency department group practice, which has taken a variety of forms (Hannas, 1971; Gersonde; *Medical World News*, 1974).

The organization of hospital ambulatory services. There are at least as many modes of organization of hospital ambulatory services as there are types of hospitals, and, in the United States, that is many indeed. We will examine, briefly, one of the major patterns of organization, that found in a typical teaching hospital with both an emergency unit and clinics.

In many such hospitals, there are three vertical organizational lines: one for the medical staff, one for the nursing staff, and one for business administration, support services, and hotel operations. (The latter includes housekeeping, dietary, and maintenance. It is interesting to note that "hospital" and "hotel" both derive from the same Latin word.) Sometimes these vertical lines meet in the director's office; sometimes they never meet; occasionally they are well integrated.

This organizational structure is reflected in the ambulatory services. Generally each medical department is responsible for physician services in its own clinics. The pattern may extend to the emergency unit as well, or it may be the primary responsibility of one department, say, surgery. Alternatively, physician staffing in the emergency unit may be entirely the responsibility of a separate entity, an Emergency Department, which may stand on its own, may be part of a Department of Ambulatory Services or Community Medicine, or may be attached to the office of the hospital's director. In teaching hospitals, Departments of Ambulatory Services, when they exist, may exert some control over emergency unit physicians but only rarely have any true control over clinic physician staffing.

The Nursing Department generally controls the nursing services for both clinics and emergency units, sometimes designating an Associate or Assistant Director of Nursing for Ambulatory Care. Likewise, the hospital's administration runs the clerical and other support services, often through an associate or assistant administrator or director.

This tripartite approach works well as long as one is not particularly interested in establishing one coordinated *program* in ambulatory care. When there is not one person, or office, in charge of all the resources required to provide ambulatory services, it is very difficult indeed to mount such a unified program (Jonas, 1973). If one wishes to provide ambulatory services of a comprehensive nature in which the patient, rather than the disease or injury, is the focus (as discussed above), coordination of physician, nursing, and support services under unified leadership is essential.

Hospitals around the country are wrestling with this problem. Its resolution will require major changes in the way in which hospitals are administratively structured, and those structural changes will in turn require major changes in the way people think and feel. With a few exceptions, hospitals are not used to mounting coordinated *programs*, but rather to delivering *services*, each component putting in its piece more or less as it sees fit. To establish an ambulatory care program with a single director having ultimate responsibility for the whole means that the medical, nursing, and support services each must surrender some sovereignty, something each is loath to do. Furthermore, even if a *functionally decentralized* program in ambulatory care could be developed, offering coordinated, comprehensive care to patients, other problems are created. Does one end up with duplicated departments of medicine, pediatrics, surgery, nursing, and clerical services for inpatient and outpatient services for the very important functions of hiring, firing, discipline, quality control, setting patient-care policies, education, research, and the like? This question is still being debated. However, many of the problems are created by the present contradictions evident in the role and work of hospitals, as discussed above, between service, teaching, and research. Resolution of these contradictions along the lines of Freymann's *"mission-oriented hospital"* (1974) would solve many problems, as will be further discussed in the next chapter.

Emergency Medical Services*

Ambulance services are the key linkage in transporting victims of accidents and acute, overwhelming illnesses safely and quickly to an appropriate emergency medical facility and in rendering indicated first aid at the site and in transit (Gibson, 1973; Yolles). They are seriously deficient in many parts of the United States. Historically, ambulance services developed from a for-profit enterprise established by funeral directors. In this system, sometimes the same vehicle has been able to serve more than one purpose, on occasion consecutively. Since ambulance services tend to be unprofitable, funeral directors have gradually abandoned this service, leaving it for communities to provide (*Medical World News*, Dec. 4, 1970). However, in many communities there is an absence of defined responsibility for ambulance services. The deficiencies in emergency services in many communities are particularly disturbing given that accidents are among the leading

---

* An excellent and more detailed treatment of this problem is contained in R. Roemer et al., *Planning Urban Health Services: From Jungle to System* (New York: Springer Publishing Co., 1975).

causes of death in the productive age groups. Many of these deaths could be prevented if high quality emergency services were readily available (*Medical World News,* Dec. 4, 1970).

Ambulance services must be able to respond quickly to calls. The vehicles must be appropriately designed and they must be adequately staffed and organized so that the patient is taken to the most appropriate hospital emergency department. The success of an emergency medical services system is dependent upon a series of communication links, including victim and ambulance service, dispatcher and ambulance, and ambulance and hospital (Gibson, 1971).

There is a dearth of research evaluating the patient outcomes related to ambulance services. But Gibson (1973) has suggested some of the criteria by which ambulance services can be evaluated. These include the availability of ambulances, ambulance utilization rates, the types of medical aid that ambulance personnel are capable of administering, emergency rating and extent of injuries of ambulance cases, response time, appropriateness of patient disposition, and level of unmet need.

Any viable EMS requires adequate financing, manpower, equipment, and facilities, with strict standards for each, and the willingness of professions, agencies, institutions, and units of local government to work together and coordinate their resources (Hanlon; Gibson, 1974). Some solutions have focused on upgrading facilities, equipment, and/or personnel. Two pieces of federal legislation have been important. The Federal Highway Safety Act of 1966 contained performance criteria for EMSs and required the States to submit EMS plans. The Emergency Medical Services System Act of 1973 authorized $185,000,000 over three years to states, counties and other nonprofit agencies to plan, expand, and modernize EMSs (Harvey). Section 1201 of the Act defined an EMS as a "system which provides for the arrangement of personnel, facilities, and equipment for the effective and coordinated delivery in an appropriate geographic area of health care services under emergency conditions . . . and which is administered by a public or nonprofit private entity which has the authority and the resources to provide effective administration of the system" (EMS Act).

Three conditions of the law are significant. It requires that special consideration be given to rural areas applying for assistance, as well as to applications that will coordinate local system with statewide EMSs. In addition, the Act provides that the EMS be "organized in a manner that provides persons who reside in the system's service area and who have no professional training or financial interest in the provision of health care with an adequate opportunity to participate in making of policy for the system" (EMS Act). The law also stipulates that emergency services must be provided without prior inquiry as to ability to pay. In terms of community need, EMS is one area of the U.S. health care delivery system in which significant improvements can and should be made.

Health Department Services

Ambulatory personal health services are provided by government at the local level in most parts of the United States (see also Chapter 10). Information on these services is limited; they have not been frequently or extensively studied. The most recent national survey of local health department services was carried out in 1966 (Myers et al.). A study entitled "What Thirteen Local Health Departments Are Doing in Medical Care" was published in 1967 (Cashman).

Provision of direct personal health service by local health departments has been a subject of controversy since the practice began in the nineteenth century (Rosen; Winslow, ch. 17). Private physicians almost always regarded local health departments as competing for their fee-paying patients and therefore threatening their practices, particularly since local health departments—in contrast to local hospital departments—traditionally offered their services free to all persons, regardless of ability to pay. Battles over the role of local health departments were especially fierce during the 1920s as the organizational representatives of American physicians, having successfully reduced medical school enrollments (following implementation of the Flexner Report) and blocked the passage of any kind of national health insurance program (in which there had been broad national interest during and after World War I; see chapter 15), struggled to further limit competition and government control over private practice. They were successful in the local health department arena as well, since local health department personal services are generally limited to those areas in which private physicians are either not very interested (routine well-baby examinations) or not especially competent (treatment, case-finding, and contact-investigation of venereal disease and tuberculosis).

Local health services are provided by a variety of government jurisdictions (Myers et al.). It is not known if every section of the country is indeed provided with government local health services, at least on paper, but of approximately 1,700 government local health jurisdictions identified in 1966, about half were covered by county government health departments, 20% by city government health departments, and the balance by city-county units, local service units of state health departments, and independent local health districts. In 1975, it was estimated that less than 3% of all ambulatory personal health services were being provided by local health departments, excluding school health services (Roemer, 1975a).

The most frequently offered personal health services are tuberculosis control, venereal disease control, well-baby care, crippled children's care, prenatal and family planning services, adult screening programs for chronic disease, mental health diagnostic and follow-up service and general home public health nursing and homemaker services.* About one-half of local health departments run the school health services in their jurisdictions, the balance being run by boards of education on their own (25%) or in cooperation with the local health department. These are so-called *categorical* programs, in which categories of diseases or persons are taken care of.

There have been efforts since World War I to involve local, and sometimes state, health departments in the delivery of general personal health services (Rosen; Winslow, ch. 17). These have generally been unsuccessful. Although optimism is still expressed that this change in role can be accomplished (Roemer, 1975a), given the history of local health departments, their bureaucratic, categorically oriented administrative structure, continuing opposition from the private sector, and their close involvement with politically sensitive, financially pressed local governments (Jonas, 1975), it is unlikely that much headway will be made in this direction.

Group Practice and Health Maintenance Organizations

Group practice, in its simplest sense, means three or more physicians working in the same facility. However, there are a number of different types of group practice defined by different characteristics—the types of providers included, types of specialties

---

* For an excellent, detailed description of one type of local public health service, maternal and child health, see R. Roemer et al., *Planning Urban Health Services: From Jungle to System* (New York: Springer Publishing Co., 1974), especially Chapter 4.

included, mode of association between physicians, patterns of medical practice, mode of physician reimbursement, and mode of patient payment (Terris, 1968).

In terms of types of providers included, some groups can be defined as multidisciplinary, i.e., other health care providers besides physicians are included, in a health care team. Multidisciplinary groups, the most inclusive type, are also the newest in the United States; they are usually found operating in community-based, government-funded neighborhood health centers (see below), although this pattern is now to be seen in some independent prepaid group practices, and also in some hospital ambulatory services.

Physician-only groups may be single-specialty or multispecialty. Single-specialty groups are particularly popular in fields in which out-of-regular-hours calls tend to be fairly frequent. Multispecialty groups usually divide the physicians into two ranks, primary and referral. The primary care rank may consist of internists and pediatricians doing frontline medical practice, or general practitioners, or both. In the referral rank are the medical subspecialists and the surgeons.

The mode of physician association in group practice varies widely. In some groups, physicians may simply share space and perhaps a common billing procedure, but not patients. This sort of arrangement becomes a bit more sophisticated with the addition of a partnership arrangement among the participating physicians. Beyond that some groups are based on a corporation. The AMA defines group practice as "the application of medical services by three or more fulltime physicians, formally organized to provide medical care consultation, diagnosis, and/or treatment through joint use of equipment and personnel, and with the income from medical practice distributed in accordance with methods previously determined by the members of the group" (Rorem, p. 6). This definition excludes any combination of physicians that simply shares space, but does not exclude fee-for-service groups.

The pattern of medical practice may be true group or essentially solo. In the latter, physicians have complete responsibility for their own patients with no other physician ever involved, except on formal referral for consultation, or for night or weekend coverage, which is usually shared by group members on a regular rotation basis. In true group practice, physicians share patient-care responsibility.

The mode of physician reimbursement may be fee-for-service

(paid either directly by the patient or by the group even if the patient does not pay the group on a fee-for-service basis), capitation (a flat rate for each individual patient in return for agreeing to provide all needed medical services during a specified time period), or salary. The mode of payment to the group by the patient may be fee-for-service or what is called prepayment, in which the patient or, more usually, the patient's employer or union health fund, pays a premium to cover a set of agreed-to services for a particular time period. Almost every possible combination of the three methods of physician reimbursement and the two methods of patient payment is used somewhere, but the three most common combinations are fee-for-service patient payment with fee-for-service physician reimbursement, patient prepayment with physician reimbursement by capitation, and patient prepayment with physician reimbursement by salary.

The numbers of groups and of doctors working in groups have been rising gradually since the first one was founded by the brothers Mayo in Rochester, Minnesota, in 1887 (Silver; Roemer, et al.). In 1969, the most recent year for which complete figures are available, within the AMA definition, there were 6,371 groups of all kinds, single specialty, multispecialty, and prepaid, with 40,093 physicians (Warner and Aherne, Table 32). The rate of growth of the institution of group practice is increasing; still, less than 15% of all physicians are engaged in it. The five most popular specialties for single-specialty grouping (excluding "unspecified") are radiology, anesthesiology, orthopedics, internal medicine, and pediatrics (Warner and Aherne, Table 33).

Prepaid group practices (defined below) form a special category. There are few of them. The AMA listed only 85 prepaid groups nationally in 1969, of which one-third were associated with the Health Insurance Plan (HIP) in New York City, involving 3,912 physicians on a full-time and/or part-time basis and in which at least 50% of patients were covered by prepayment (Warner and Aherne, Table 34). Thus, prepaid group practice involved less than 2 percent of active physicians in the United States, even on a part-time basis, in that year. With the development of HMOs, the figure is somewhat higher now.

To make an estimate of patient visits to group practices, Roemer (1975a) used the 1969 AMA figure for the number of physicians in group practice, and, postulating an annual average visit rate of 4,600 for each physician, calculated that there were 185,000,000 visits all told to group practices that year. Turning to prepaid group practice, using the Roemer technique (based on the number of physicians in prepaid group practice, not all of them full-time), it could be estimated that in 1969 10 to 18 million visits were made to physicians in such practices. This would amount to 2 to 3% of all physician office visits. Again, with the development of HMOs, this figure has risen somewhat.

Prepaid group practice. Prepaid group practice (PPGP) is a relatively small phenomenon, but it receives a great deal of attention, particularly from persons who believe that the U.S. health care delivery system needs significant improvement. The first PPGP was created by Dr. Michael A. Shadid in Elk City, Oklahoma, in 1929 (MacColl, pp. 20-24). Many authorities have for a long time considered PPGP to be the wave of the future. Rorem thought so in 1931 (1971), and his thinking strongly influenced the Committee on the Costs of Medical Care (1970). Axelrod agreed (1956), as did Silver et al. (1957), and Silver again (1963), Falk (1963), MacColl (1966), Weinerman (1968), Saward (1969), the *Harvard Law Review* (1971), Roemer and Shonick (1973), the *Consumers Reports* (1974), Auger and Goldberg (1974), and Roemer (1975b).

A good working definition of PPGP is provided by the *Harvard Law Review*:

> Pre-paid group practice may be broadly defined as a medical care delivery system which accepts responsibility for the organization, financing, and delivery of health care services for a defined population. Essentially, it combines a financing mechanism—prepayment—with a particular mode of delivery—group practice—by means of a managerial-administrative organization responsible for ensuring the availability of health services for a subscriber population. (1971)

There are a number of different prepaid group practices in various parts of the country. Two of the most prominent ones are Kaiser-Permanente (Saward; Williams; Fleming; Carnoy, et al.), which operates primarily on the West Coast, and the Health Insurance Plan of Greater New York (Silver et al.; Brindle; Bates; Levy and Fein). Prepaid group practices generally make a special effort to provide as broad a range of services as possible, aiming toward comprehensive care.

Health Maintenance Organizations. In 1971, the term "Health Maintenance Organization" (HMO) was introduced to the American health care scene (Ellwood et al., 1971; Center for

Health Administration Studies; Myers). Although many persons thought, and some still think, that HMO is the same as PPGP, this is not the case, as the 1971 statement of the USDHEW on HMOs, based on the work of Paul Ellwood and his colleagues, made quite clear:

> An HMO can be organized and sponsored by either a medical foundation (usually organized by physicians), by community groups who bring together various interested leaders or organizations, by labor unions, by a governmental unit, by a profit or nonprofit group allied with an insurance company or some other financing institution, or by some other arrangement. The HMO may be hospital based, medical school based, or be a free standing outpatient facility or group of such facilities. (USDHEW, 1971)

The statement went on to say that an HMO is (1) an organized system of health care that accepts the responsibility to provide or otherwise assure the delivery of (2) an agreed-upon set of comprehensive health maintenance and treatment services for (3) a voluntary enrolled group of persons in a geographic area and (4) is reimbursed through a prenegotiated and fixed periodic payment made by or on behalf of each person or family unit enrolled in the plan. This is all basic to "the health maintenance strategy [which] envisions a series of government and private actions designed to promote a highly diversified, pluralistic, and competitive health industry" (Ellwood et al., 1971).

One of the practice forms alternative to PPGP that can qualify as an HMO under this definition is the "Foundation for Medical Care" (FMC) (Harrington; Blake and Carnoy; Egdahl; Brian; Newport and Roemer) in its "comprehensive" form. The Comprehensive FMC combines a prepayment mechanism for patients with fee-for-service solo practice for the physicians. The FMC is an agency that enrolls physicians who agree to a central billing mechanism, peer review of quality, and cost controls. It then contracts, usually with employers and/or union health and welfare funds, to provide a stipulated package of health care benefits to covered persons in return for a per-person payment to the FMC from the contracting entity. No money changes hands between individual patients and physicians. However, the physicians, working in their own offices, bill the FMC on a fee basis for each item of service provided. There is a maximum amount for which physicians can bill, of course; it is related to the total amount of money paid in by the contractee, and the FMC does monitor billing closely. Thus, although physicians charge on a fee-for-service basis, they are actually on a quasi-salary system. Comprehensive FMCs also are concerned with the medical quality of the product that their member physicians are delivering. There is also a "claims review" type FMC that simply provides peer-review services, for cost and/or quality of care, to insurance companies.

In 1972–1973, a few organizations received federal money for HMO development under various provisions of the Public Health Service Act and other federal legislation (Center for Health Administration Studies) while specific HMO legislation was being developed. Congress forced a halt in that kind of activity however until a specific HMO Act could be passed.

The reaction of the medical profession to the emerging HMO legislation affected its shaping considerably. In August, 1972, the *American Medical News,* which generally represents the views of the American Medical Association, said the following:

> For those who lived through the Great Depression the current diaologue over health maintenance organizations must sound like a not-so-instant replay of the debate that surrounded the 1932 report of the Committee on the Costs of Medical Care . . . the . . . majority recommended the development of an organized system of health care delivery. . . . In the view of organized medicine . . . the committee seemed to advocate a system that would be vulnerable to the evils of both contract practice and government intervention. . . . The AMA House of Delegates . . . adopted a hardline stand against unwarranted federal competition in the practice of medicine, and it urged opposition to any scheme that would allow corporations to sell physician services to the public. . . . (*American Medical News,* August, 1972).

In November, 1972, the House of Delegates of the AMA adopted a resolution stating that "there is a danger in experimenting with HMOs, an arrangement which could lead to a monolithic system in spite of experimental results" (*Medical World News,* December, 1972).

The first HMO Act was passed in December, 1973 (P.L. 93-222). It authorized $325 million over five years for grants and loans to help HMOs get underway (Starr). To qualify as an HMO, an organization had to provide or contract for the following services: physician care, inpatient and outpatient hospital care, medically necessary emergency health services, short-term evaluative and crisis intervention mental health services, medical treatment and referral services for the abuse of or addiction to alcohol and drugs, diagnostic laboratory and diagnostic and therapeutic radiological services, and preventive health services. Such supplemental services as dental care and prescription drugs could be contracted for as well. But services had to be available and accessible on a 24-hour-a-day, 7-day-a-week basis. The subscriber was to pay nothing, or only a minimal copayment, at time of service.

By mid-1975, it was estimated that nationally there were 181 HMOs in operation, 164 in active formation and 151 in the early planning stages (Wetherille and Nordby).

The HMO Act of 1973, which has since been amended, created an interesting contradiction (Dorsey, 1975). In its attempt to set a model for what comprehensive health care should be, the Act prescribed such a broad range of benefits that many organizations that were interested in sponsoring HMOs declined to do so because the benefit package would carry a very high price tag, in practice making it noncompetitive with existing plans like Blue Cross/Blue Shield, even though the benefits were better. This situation, plus a rather complex set of USDHEW regulations written pursuant to the Act, served to inhibit initiative in HMO development. If HMOs are indeed to flourish, some balance is required.

Prepaid group practice in perspective. In the end, the HMO Act of 1973 and its successors may or may not foster the expansion of PPGP in the United States. Further development of PPGP may or may not be encouraged by national health insurance legislation. Nevertheless, since prepaid group practice developed over the years in the United States, albeit slowly, in the absence of any legislation, and at times in the face of legislative roadblocks, it will doubtless continue to grow. One reason is that PPGPs have repeatedly demonstrated that their subscribers have significantly lower hospitalization rates than do comparable groups of Blue Cross/Blue Shield subscribers, generally by 40% (Roemer and Shonick; Reidel et al.). This, accomplished without discernible differences in quality of care in terms of patient outcomes, results from performing services on an outpatient basis wherever possible, encouraging preventive care, discouraging unnecessary surgery, and, most importantly, unifying hospital and ambulatory physician costs.

Silver summarized the advantages and disadvantages for physicians of group practice, including PPGP, in comparison to solo practice (1963). The advantages include a regular work schedule, reasonable competitive income, provision of malpractice insurance, the opportunity for collegial medical practice, better access to ancillary personnel and services, and freedom from concern with the business aspects of medical practice. Disadvantages include possible deterioration of the "doctor-patient relationship," limited professional contacts and choice of consultants, and a possible rigidity in practice modes and conduct. Advantages for patients include no or low charges at time of service, one-stop shopping for 24-hour, 7-day service, continuity of care, and protection against unnecessary surgery. Disadvantages center around the possibility of the development of a clinic atmosphere (Baehr), impersonality, long waits for service, and, particularly in profit-making group practices (Comptroller General of the United States, 1974), abuse of patients through overenrollment and understaffing, the result of overselling in relation to service capabilities.

However, the most serious problems of prepaid group practice may be ideological rather than practical. Weinerman, an early, strong advocate of prepaid group practice, reviewed the experience and was disappointed (1968). His observations, although made some time ago, are still pertinent. In essence, he said that PPGP looks great on paper, but the practical results are inconclusive; moreover, the idea really has not caught on to a great extent. He concluded that the mechanical-financial elements of the list of advantages cited above have been implemented, particularly for the physicians, but that the ideological aspects of true group practice have not. Most groups maintain physician elitism. "Group conferences," he said, "medical audits and informal office consultations are, in my experience, more common in the descriptive literature than in daily practice."

Perhaps most disappointing has been the hesitation on the part of most medical groups to effect changes in the "way of life" of the medical team itself. This would involve acceptance by the group as a whole of collective responsibility for the health of its patients or members . . . would mean actively reaching out into the community for . . . early detection . . . [and] identification and special protection for those at specific risk of disease . . . [and] would imply particular concern for those patients who do not use the service. . . . It implies as much concern with rapport as with diagnostic labels, as much with education as with prescription. (Weinerman, 1968, p. 1429)

Weinerman concluded that only if such ideological changes take place, along with the organizational and financial ones, will prepaid group practice be successful. We concur and add that one might apply his prescription to American medicine as a whole.

Neighborhood Health Centers

The "Neighborhood Health Center" (NHC) movement of the late 1960s and early 1970s saw the development of a particular kind of ambulatory health care facility, based on the concepts of full-time, salaried physician staffing, multidisciplinary team health care practice, and community involvement in both policy-making and facility operations (Zwick). The movement was strongly stimulated by the federal Office of Economic Opportunity (OEO), which was a principal factor in the so-called "War on Poverty" conducted by President Lyndon Johnson's administration in the period 1964–68. The "Neighborhood Health Centers" discussed here are generally limited to those developed with federal government support. Other institutions with similar features also came into being, sponsored by volunteer groups (Schwartz, 1971; *Medical World News,* 1971) and other governmental jurisdictions. However, information available on them is very sketchy, and by and large their impact was negligible. In any case, the NHCs discussed herein were prototypical.

The NHC does not represent an entirely new concept in the United States. The nineteenth-century dispensary, discussed above, performed some similar functions, although it was organized differently. Health department ambulatory care programs developed during the last quarter of the nineteenth century had some elements that would appear later in NHCs, such as districting, but were almost entirely categorical and therefore not comprehensive. The period 1910–1919 was marked by the development of several health centers in different parts of the country; they truly attempted to offer comprehensive services to designated areas from a freestanding, not hospital-based institution (Rosen). C.-E.A. Winslow noted in 1919: "The most striking and typical development of the public health movement of the present day is the health center" (Rosen). However, he was overoptimistic. Herman Biggs, M.D., then Commissioner of Health of New York State, tried vigorously, but quite unsuccessfully, to get the state and local health departments away from the categorical disease approach and into the business of delivering comprehensive health services during the period 1920–23 (Winslow, ch. 17).

With the resurgence of political conservatism in the United States following World War I and the concomitant change in policy of the American Medical Association (it came to oppose any health care delivery mode not based on private practice, except for delivery to the very poor), the NHC movement of that period disappeared (Rosen).

The experience with PPGP in the thirties, forties, and fifties influenced the development of NHC movement of the sixties and seventies. An ambulatory care service developed at the municipal Gouverneur Hospital on New York City's Lower East Side was significant. It was intended by the city administration to provide comprehensive care on the model described by the Committee on the Costs of Medical Care. Its first director, the late Dr. Howard Brown, came from one of the prototypical PPGPs, the Health Insurance Plan of Greater New York, with many concepts new to municipal health services. Indeed, a comprehensive ambulatory care program was installed in Gouverneur (Light and Brown). It was very influential in the early development of OEO NHCs around the United States because it was already fully operational by the time the OEO program got underway and served as a model that many persons who were establishing NHCs came to observe.

Another early model OEO NHC was Montefiore's Neighborhood Medical Care Demonstration project in the Bronx, New York (Lloyd and Wise; Montefiore), which became the Martin Luther King Neighborhood Health Center. In a way, this NHC too had its links with the past, since one of the largest and most successful Health Insurance Plan groups in New York City was based at Montefiore. In other parts of the country as well, individuals who became involved with NHC development had had experience with prepaid group practice. Thus, although NHCs had many new features, they definitely fit into an historical continuum. Indeed, the major medical (although not social, administrative, or political) program elements of the contemporary NHC were proposed in an American Public Health Association policy statement on community health services adopted in 1963 (American Public Health Association).

NHCs appeared in many different shapes and sizes, had a variety of different starting points, various sources of funding, and a variety of program variations (Schwartz, 1970; Abrams and Snyder; Collins; C. D. Gibson, 1968; Lashof; Curry; Kovner and Seacat; Davis and Tranquada). However, they do share

certain common features. NHCs were usually situated in medically underserved minority-occupied urban areas. They generally
attempted—with varying degrees of vigor and success—to institute the concept of multidisciplinary group practice, utilizing
nurses, social workers, neighborhood health workers (often people from the area served, especially trained by the NHC, usually
with a combination of basic nursing and social service skills),
and sometimes lawyers, in a health care team to deal with patients and their problems. Physicians were on salary or paid
by the session. Ultimately the NHCs aimed to institute one-
stop shopping for ambulatory care, to provide a comprehensive
range of preventive and rehabilitative as well as treatment services which were acceptable, affordable, and of high quality,
and to intervene in the cycle of poverty.

Starting an NHC was an expensive proposition. Capital costs
were high, staffing to meet multiple health problems was heavy
and expensive, and many potential patients had no means of
paying for care, either self or third-party. NHCs were funded by
a combination of starting-up grants, usually from OEO or HEW
(the latter under provisions of the Comprehensive Health Planning Amendments to the Public Health Law, P.L.89–749, and
from various programs of the Children's Bureau), and third-
party payments, usually Medicaid and Medicare. NHCs were
related in one way or another to a "back-up hospital," which is
intended to supply inpatient services, specialist consultation,
sophisticated laboratory and x-ray services, and supervision, if
not the direct employment, of the medical staff.

The original OEO legislation mandated "maximum feasible
participation" in the operation and administration of the NHCs
(as well as all other OEO programs) by those persons they
served. "Maximum feasible participation" was never precisely
defined. However, its existence as an OEO requirement led to
many a conflict between the hospitals and medical schools originally involved to a greater or lesser extent in operating programs, and the representatives of the served communities over
the question: "Who's in charge here?" (Goldberg et al.; Torrens).

"Community Advisory Boards" were mandated by OEO. Board
members usually came from underserved areas that had often
received what little care they did get from the hospital that now
had the grant, a hospital that, on the basis of its past performance, was perceived by residents of the service area as being

unsympathetic, to say the least. Community boards therefore wanted the final say on major policy questions. The hospitals, on the other hand, had the responsibility for the program, particularly its medical quality, and were reluctant to give up any significant degree of authority. This situation, exacerbated at times by linguistic and cultural barriers, often led to tense and painful experiences for both sides. Later, fiscal responsibility for operation of some NHCs was turned over to nonprofit corporations representing the served communities, a long-range requirement of the original OEO program guidelines. These bodies then contracted with the back-up hospitals to provide needed services, retaining primary control for themselves.

Additional problems were created by the OEO view that at least as significant a role for the NHCs as the provision of health care was the provision of job opportunities to residents from the NHC service area. This created two important areas of conflict. NHCs usually served severely depressed minority-group urban areas where it is most difficult to find persons with requisite health care skills and training, particularly in the professional and semi-professional job categories. Furthermore, control of job positions for which neighborhood residents might be eligible became a plum, for both positive and negative reasons.

Funding has been a problem for many centers. There always seemed to be a great deal of red tape involved in spending committed funds. The annual grant reapplications for the next year's appropriation produced almost unending difficulties. In recent years especially, the actual amounts of money available have become increasingly inadequate. With the demise of OEO in the seventies, the federal role in the NHC program was moved over to DHEW. Federal grant funding was cut back (Geiger). As this happened, NHCs were forced to rely more and more on Medicaid/Medicare third-party funding and a means-tested, sliding fee scale. This often meant severe program cuts, job losses, and sometimes closure.

Office of Economic Opportunity and other NHCs have been evaluated extensively on a national scale. There have been general program evaluations (Resource Management Corporation; Sparer and Johnson), evaluations of quality of care (Morehead, 1970; Morehead et al., 1970; Morehead and Donaldson), and analyses of costs (Sparer and Anderson). By most accounts, in the mid-1970s NHCs seemed to be doing reasonably well in terms of quality. Many noted deficiencies can be traced back to the lack of resources discussed above. However, serious questions are raised by expecting small-scale, underfinanced health organizations like NHCs to alleviate poverty in isolation from the macroeconomic, political, and social system. Many participants were disillusioned by the failure to achieve this formidable goal. Moreover, the health centers' emphasis on the poverty population created a curious dilemma: in attempting to develop an organization to enhance the health of the poor, the NHC was at the same time perpetuating a separate and distinct system of health care for the poor. Ideally, health care for the poor should be integrated into the mainstream of medical care.

At peak development in the early 1970s, it was estimated that there were nationally at one time or another about 200 NHCs (Health-PAC Bulletin). By 1974, that number had fallen to around 150 (Roemer, 1975a). At most, the NHCs provided 0.5% of the total volume of ambulatory visits nationally, a small fraction. Nevertheless, despite these limitations, they have been very important in demonstrating the feasibility of new approaches to the provision of health care. NHCs, however, require large front-end investments. They operate in areas where most patients simply cannot afford the costs of their own care. With the coming of national health insurance, a major question is, will the private practice sector, which can operate in most lower-working-class neighborhoods under a liberal government-financed fee-for-service reimbursement system (Bernstein) allow the NHC movement a new lease on life and a new period of growth and development?

Organized Home Care

One of the oldest and yet most neglected sites of ambulatory care is the home. In 1972, 2% of the noninstitutionalized population over 65 were bedfast, 6% were homebound, and another 6% could only go outside with difficulty (Nielson et al.). For many persons with chronic diseases in which "cure" is not possible, proper management can make a great deal of difference in their lives. For many patients who are not acutely ill, but need to spend a great deal of time in bed, the home may be a more comfortable, less isolating, lower-cost alternative to the hospital.

The AHA defines home care as the provision of health care to the patient in his/her place of residence (American Hospital Association, 1972). The AHA notes that for some people, care by a family member under the guidance of a doctor is enough, whereas other patients may require care from nurses or occupational and physical therapists. *Coordinated* home care, according to the USDHEW, is a program "that is centrally administered and through coordinated planning, evaluation and follow-up procedures, provides for physician-directed, nursing, social work and related services to selected patients at home" (Allen et al.).

Historically, there have been two streams of development in home care (Kasten). A hospital may extend some of its services in the community to provide care in the home under medical direction, or a community agency such as a Visiting Nurse Service or a Public Health Department may build upon an existing program of services in collaboration with one or more hospitals to provide coordinated care (Richter and Gonnerman, 1972, 1974). There are many combinations of service that appear in different home care programs. The prototypical hospital-based program was established at the Montefiore Hospital in the Bronx in the late 1940s (Bluestone). That program provided medical, social, nursing, housekeeping, transportation, medication, occupational therapy, physical therapy, and diagnostic services in the home on a virtually as-needed basis (Cherkasky). The basis of the concept was a "hospital without walls" (Richter and Gonnerman, 1972). Essential to a comprehensive home care program for the chronically ill is guaranteed readmission to the hospital, whether for medical reasons or for "social" reasons, such as "giving the family a rest" in instances when caring for the sick relative is physically and/or emotionally demanding.

Stimulated by financial support through Medicare and Medicaid, the number of home health agencies grew from 250 in 1963 to over 1,400 in 1966 (Lenzer and Donabedian; Scutchfield and Freeborn). The complexity of insurance regulations has hindered the development of home health care (Van Dyke and Brown). For instance, Medicare Part A requires that home health care follow a period of inpatient hospitalization; Part B, while not requiring hospitalization, imposes coinsurance and deductibles, which may be a severe burden for the patient. Services reimbursed when provided in the hospital—such as maintaining a hygienic environment and preparing a diet—are not reimbursed when provided at home. Reimbursement inadequacies are particularly disturbing when one considers that continuity of health care could mean the difference between prolonging the ambulatory status of the patient and increasing the risk of hospitalization (Trager).

Lenzer and Donabedian (1967) catalogued the pros and cons of home care. As advantages they cited: the company of one's family; a freer, more cheerful atmosphere; comfort; the support and understanding of a visiting nurse; more personal freedom and dignity than in the hospital. And, of course, the patient who is enjoying these advantages is not occupying a costly hospital bed. In addition, patients treated at home may make more progress in the activities of daily living and experience less deterioration in indices of socioeconomic functioning (Katz). Home care may decrease the number of hospital admissions and nursing home placements (Nielson et al.) and may also decrease the length of stay for patients treated at home but subsequently admitted to a hospital. The home may be a more effective site for patient learning and motivational activities (Stone et al.), and it may engender a higher level of patient satisfaction than institutionalized care. It may also be less expensive to patient and health care systems (Hurtado et al.). But, for home care to be appropriately and effectively utilized, it is essential that physicians be knowledgeable about and in favor of home health services. This is often not the case.

Home care is not without disadvantages. Successful home care requires the deep involvement of family members and may disrupt family functioning at the same time that it permits the family to remain technically intact. The indirect costs may be high, when, for example, cost of family member's time is considered. There may be lack of coordination between physician, home health agency, family, and patient. In addition, we need to know much more about the quality of care delivered in the home before reliable judgments can be made. Nevertheless, if quality can be assured, it can be assumed that home care is an important dimension of a coordinated health care system.

Primary Care

"Primary Care" is a popular subject in the health care literature today (Dorsey, 1970; Magraw; Hansen; Last and White; Schonfeld et al.; Tudor Hart, 1973, 1974; Mechanic; Janeway). Primary care has been variously defined (White, 1967, 1973a; Haggerty; Rogatz et al.). A working definition states that primary care is:

medical attention to the great majority of ills, provided continuously over a significant period of time by the same appropriately

trained individual (or team), who is sympathetic, understanding,
knowledgeable, and equipped, who is as capable of keeping people
well as he is of returning them to health when they fall ill.
(Jonas, 1973, p. 177)

This can be contrasted with definitions of secondary and tertiary
care, the set in which the term "primary care" usually appears.
According to Roemer (1975b, p. 263) :

Secondary care consists only of curative services . . . ordinarily
obtained on referral from the primary care level. . . . [It] includes
the services of specialists [beyond the primary-type internist or
pediatrician], whether the patient is ambulatory, or hospitalized
. . . in a peripheral or district general hospital. . . . Likewise, long-
term care of chronic illness . . . is a part of secondary care. . . .

Tertiary care includes the services of the 'super-specialists' for
rare disorders or the care of serious long-term conditions of relatively low frequency . . . [usually] at a regional medical center. . . .

One of the reasons for including a brief discussion of primary
care in this chapter is to point out precisely that primary care is
not limited to ambulatory care. The list of the functions of a primary care system as developed by the Committee on Medical
Schools and the Association of American Medical Colleges (the
Pellegrino Committee) makes this quite clear:

1. Assessment of total [patient] needs before these are categorized
by specialty. 2. Elaboration of a plan for meeting those needs in
the order of their importance. 3. Determination of who shall meet
the defined needs—physicians, general or specialist; non-physi-
cian members of the health team; or social agencies. 4. Follow-up
to see that needs are met. 5. [Provision of such care] in a continuous, coordinated and comprehensive manner. 6. Attention at each
step . . . to the personal, social and family dimensions of the
patient's problem. 7. [The provision of] health maintenance and
disease prevention [at the same level of importance as the provision of] cure and rehabilitation. (Committee on Medical Schools,
p. 753)

Of course, the ever-increasing specialization and subspeciali-
zation of American medicine in this century has made primary
care increasingly difficult to find (Freymann, p. 152). Various
levels of government have recognized this fact and increasingly,
government financial aid, particularly to medical education, has

been tied to improving training in primary care. Several major battles have resulted from this emphasis. One major battle is whether the basic primary care doctor is to be a Family Physician or an Internist-Pediatrician combination (McWhinney; Petersdorf; Hudson and Nourse; Coordinating Council on Medical Education). Another is what other specialties, if any, have a legitimate claim to a piece of the pie (Alpert and Charney, p. 2; Rubin et al.). If the pie turns out to be a rather small one, of course, the interest in and concern with the problem will drop rapidly.

One of the possible outcomes of these struggles may be simply a change of label without touching what is inside the jar, a favorite American solution to problems. Of course, many other categories of health care provider are necessary to the provision of primary care, but the centrality of the physician in the American health care delivery system makes the position of physicians of central concern. In a medical education system that trains specialists and biomedical researchers (Stevens, ch. 16), and does not focus on the broad needs of the population at large (Freymann, chs. 6, 26), providing for the education of physicians in primary care presents serious difficulties (Alpert and Charney). As White (1973a, p. 362) says: "One wants to avoid the confusion inherent in the encounter between the patient who says to the doctor, 'I hope you treat what I've got' and the physician who says, 'I hope you've got what I treat'." Simply tinkering with the curriculum will not do. As the description of the *functions* of the primary care physician developed by the Pellegrino Committee shows, physician primary care is above all not a collection of services, but a state of mind:

[The primary-care physician] must be capable of establishing a profile of the total needs of the patient and his family. This evaluation should include social, economic, and psychologic details as well as the more strictly "medical" aspects. He must know what resources are available for meeting those needs. He should then define a plan of care, deciding which parts are to be carried out by himself and which by others. The plan should have a long-range dimension. It should be understandable to the patient and his family, and it should include a follow-up on whether indicated measures have been undertaken and whether they have been effective. (Committee on Medical Schools, p. 754)

Which brings us back to ambulatory care.

Although primary care is not limited to ambulatory care, ambulatory care is central to primary care. If primary care is to become a major function for physicians, ambulatory care—service, teaching, and research—will have to become a major function of the institutions that train them.

References

Abrams, H. K., and Snyder, R. A. "Health Center Seeks to Bridge the Gap between Hospital and Neighborhood." *Modern Hospital*, May, 1968, p. 96.

Albin, S. L. et al. "Evaluation of Emergency Room Triage Performed by Nurses." *American Journal of Public Health, 65,* 1063, 1975.

Allen, D. et al. "Agencies' Perceptions of Factors Affecting Home Care Referral." *Medical Care, 12,* 828, 1974.

Alpert, J. J., and Charney, F. *The Education of Physicians for Primary Care.* Washington, D.C.: USDHEW Publication No. (HRA) 74–3113, Autumn, 1973.

American Hospital Association. *The Hospital and the Home Care Program.* Chicago, Ill.: 1972.

American Hospital Association. *Hospital Statistics. 1974 Edition.* Chicago, Ill.: 1974.

American Medical News. "Can the HMO Puzzle Ever Be Put Together?" August, 1972.

American Public Health Association. "The Development of Community Health Service Centers—Present and Future: Policy Statement." *American Journal of Public Health, 54,* 140, 1964.

Auger, R. C., and Goldberg, V. P. "Prepaid Health Plans and Moral Hazard." *Public Policy, 22,* 353, 1974.

Axelrod, J. "Group Practice of Medicine and Surgery." *Resident Physician, 2,* September, 1956.

Baehr, G. "Pre-paid Group Practice: Its Strength and Weaknesses, and Its Future." *American Journal of Public Health, 56,* 1898, 1966.

Bates, L. E. "Health Insurance Plan of Greater New York." *Hospitals, J.A.H.A.,* March 16, 1971.

Beloff, J. S. "Adopting the Hospital Emergency Service Organization to Patient Needs." *Hospitals, J.A.H.A.,* April 16, 1968.

Bernstein, G. *An Analysis of Private Physician Participation in the New York City Medicaid Program.* New York: Health Services Administration, 1968. Process.

Blake, E., and Carnoy, J. "The Vanguard of the Rearguard." *Health-PAC Bulletin,* February, 1973, p. 2.

Bluestone, E. M. "Home Care: An Extra-Mural Hospital Function." *Survey Midmonthly, 84,* 99, 133, April, 1948. Reprinted in: Committee on Medical Care Teaching of the Association of Teachers of Preventive Medicine, *Readings in Medical Care,* p. 408. Chapel Hill, N.C.: University of North Carolina Press, 1958.

Brian, E. "Foundation for Medical Care Control of Hospital Utilization: CHAP—A PSRO Prototype." *New England Journal of Medicine, 288,* 878, 1973.

Brindle, J. *The Health Insurance Plan of Greater New York Program.* Presented at National Forum on Hospital and Health Affairs, May 21, 1971, Duke University.

Carnoy, J. et al. "The Kaiser Plan." *Health-PAC Bulletin,* November, 1973.

Cashman, J. *What Thirteen Local Health Departments are Doing in Medical Care.* Washington, D.C.: Public Health Services, USDHEW, 1967.

Center for Health Administration Studies. *Health Maintenance Organization: A Reconfiguration of the Health Services System.* Proceedings of the Thirteenth Annual Symposium on Hospital Affairs. Graduate School of Business, University of Chicago, 1971.

Cherkasky, M. "The Montefiore Hospital Home Care Program." *American Journal of Public Health, 39,* 29, 1949.

Collins, B. "Denver Builds Citywide Health Network." *Modern Hospital,* May, 1968, p. 102.

Committee on the Costs of Medical Care. *Medical Care for the American People.* Chicago, Ill.: University of Chicago Press, 1932. Reprinted, USDHEW, 1970.

Committee on Medical Schools and the AAMC in Relation to Training for Family Practice. "Planning for Comprehensive and Continuing Care of Patients through Education." *Journal of Medical Education, 43,* 751, 1968.

Comptroller General of the United States. *Study of Health Facilities Construction Costs.* Washington, D.C.: Government Printing Office, 1972.

Comptroller General of the United States. *Better Controls Needed for Health Maintenance Organizations Under Medicaid in California.* Washington, D.C.: Report to the Committee on Finance, U.S. Senate, September 10, 1974.

Consumer Reports. "HMO's: Are They the Answer to Your Medical Needs?" October, 1974, p. 756.

Coordinating Council on Medical Education. "Physician Manpower and Distribution: The Primary Care Physician." *Journal of the American Medical Association, 233,* 880, 1975.

Curry, W. "Small Health Group Builds Big Success in the Southwest." *Hospitals, J.A.H.A.,* July, 1969, p. 95.

Danchik, K. M. "Physician Visits. Volume and Interval Since Last Visit —1971." *Vital and Health Statistics,* Series 10, Number 97. Data from the National Health Survey. Washington, D.C.: Health Resources Administration, USDHEW, March, 1975.

Davis, M. S., and Tranquada, R. E. "A Sociological Evaluation of the Watts Neighborhood Health Center." *Medical Care, 7,* 105, 1969.

Dorsey, J. L. "Manpower Problems in the Delivery of Primary Medical Care." *New England Journal of Medicine, 282,* 871, 1970.

Dorsey, J. L. "The Health Maintenance Organization Act of 1973 (P.L. 93-222) and Prepaid Group Practice Plans." *Medical Care, 13,* 7, 1975.

Egdahl, R. H. "Foundations for Medical Care." *New England Journal of Medicine, 288,* 491, 1973.

Ellwood, P. M. et al. "Health Maintenance Strategy." *Medical Care, 9,* 291, 1971.

Emergency Medical Services Systems Act of 1973. P. L. 93–154.

Falk, I. S. "Group Practice Is the Pattern of the Future." *Modern Hospital,* September, 1963.

Fleming, S. "Kaiser Foundation—Permanente Program." *Hospitals, J.A.H.A.,* March 16, 1971.

Flexner, A. *Medical Education in the United States and Canada.* New York: The Carnegie Foundation, 1910. Reprinted, Washington, D.C.: Science and Health Publications, 1960.

Freymann, J. G. *The American Health Care System: Its Genesis and Trajectory.* New York: Medcom Press, 1974.

Geiger, H. J. "New Health Careers and the Illusion of Change." *Social Policy, 6,* 30, 1975.

Gersonde, R. J. "Two Approaches to Providing Physician Coverage in E. R." *Hospital Topics, 49,* 50, February, 1971.

Gibson, C. D. "The Neighborhood Health Center: The Primary Unit of Health Care." *American Journal of Public Health, 58,* 1188, 1968.

Gibson, G. "Status of Urban Services." Parts I and II. *Hospitals J.A.H.A.,* December 1, December 16, 1971.

Gibson, G. "Evaluative Criteria for Emergency Ambulance Services." *Social Science and Medicine, 7,* 425, 1973.

Gibson, G. "Guidelines for Research and Evaluation of Emergency Medical Services." *Health Services Reports, 89,* 99, 1974.

Goldberg, G. A. et al. "Issues in the Development of Neighborhood Health Centers." *Inquiry, 6,* 37, 1969.

Goodrich, C. H. et al. *Proposal for Bellevue Ambulatory Care Program.* New York: Department of Medicine, New York University Medical Center, 1965. Mimeo.

Goodrich, C. H., Olendzki, M. C., and Crocetti, A. F. "Hospital-based Comprehensive Care: Is It a Failure?" *Medical Care, 10,* 363, 1972.

Grupenhoff, J. T. *Health Maintenance Organization Legislation in 1972.*
    Vol. 1, The Health Legislation Report Series. Washington, D.C.:
    Science and Health Publications, Inc., 1973.
Haggerty, R. J. "The University and Primary Medical Care." *New
    England Journal of Medicine, 281,* 416, 1969.
Hanlon, John. "Emergency Medical Care as a Comprehensive System."
    Health Services Reports, 88, 579, 1973.
Hannas, R. R. "Emergency Medicine—A Survey." *Southern Medical
    Bulletin,* December, 1971, p. 11.
Hannas, R. R. "Spreading the Specialty Spectrum." *Harvard Medical
    Alumni Bulletin,* July/August, 1975, p. 23.
Hansen, M. F. "An Educational Program for Primary Care." *Journal
    of Medical Education, 45,* 1001, 1970.
Harrington, D. C. "San Joaquin Foundation for Medical Care." *Hospi-
    tals, J.A.H.A.,* March 16, 1971.
Harvard Law Review. "The Role of Prepaid Group Practice in Reliev-
    ing the Medical Care Crisis." *84,* 887, 1971.
Harvey, J. C. "The Emergency Medical Services Systems Act of 1973."
    New England Journal of Medicine, 292, 529, 1975.
"Health Maintenance Act of 1973." P. L. 93-222.
Health PAC Bulletin. "NENA: Community Control in a Bind." June,
    1972.
Hudson, J. I., and Nourse, E. S. "Perspectives in Primary Care Educa-
    tion." *Journal of Medical Education, 50,* December, 1975, Part 2.
Hurtado, A. et al. "The Utilization and Cost of Home Care and
    Extended Care Facility Services in a Comprehensive Prepaid
    Group Practice Program." *Medical Care, 10,* 8, 1972.
Janeway, C. A. "Family Medicine—Fad or for Real?" *New England
    Journal of Medicine, 291,* 337, 1974.
Jonas, S. *A Review of the Ambulatory Care Services of Mount Sinai
    Hospital, Chicago, Illinois.* Prepared for E. D. Rosenfeld Asso-
    ciates, Inc., New York, 1968. Process.
Jonas, S. *Some Thoughts on the Development of Methodist Hospital of
    Brooklyn, N.Y.* Prepared for WHK Associates, Inc., New York,
    1971. Process.
Jonas, S. "Some Thoughts on Primary Care: Problems in Implementa-
    tion." *International Journal of Health Services, 3,* 177, 1973.
Jonas, S. *Organized Ambulatory Services and the Enforcement of
    Health Care Quality Standards in New York State.* Report to the
    Task Force on the Impact of National Health Insurance on the
    State of New York. New York: New York Metropolitan Regional
    Medical Program, 1975. Process.
Jonas, S. et al. "Monitoring Utilization of a Municipal Hospital Emer-
    gency Department." *Hospital Topics, 54,* 43, 1976.
Kasten, J. "The Case for Standards in Home Care Programs." *The
    Gerontologist, 3,* 14, 1963.

Katz, S. "Comprehensive Outpatient Care in Rheumatoid Arthritis." *Journal of the American Medical Association, 206,* November 4, 1968.

Knowles, J. H. "The Role of the Hospital: The Ambulatory Clinic." *Bulletin of the New York Academy of Medicine, 41,* 2nd Series, January, 1965, p. 68.

Kovner, A. R., and Seacat, M. S. "Continuity of Care Maintained in Family-centered Outpatient Unit." *Hospitals, J.A.H.A.,* July 1, 1969, p. 89.

Lashof, J. C. "Chicago Project Provides Health Care and Career Opportunities." *Hospitals, J.A.H.A.,* July 1, 1969, p. 105.

Last, J. M., and White, K. L. "The Content of Medical Care in Primary Practice." *Medical Care, 7,* 41, 1969.

Lenzer, A., and Donabedian, A. "A Needed Research in Home Care." *Nursing Outlook, 18,* October, 1967.

Levy, H., and Fein, O. "Crippled HIP." *Health-PAC Bulletin,* October 1972, p. 15.

Light, H. L., and Brown, H. J. "The Gouverneur Health Services Program: An Historical View. *Milbank Memorial Fund Quarterly, 45,* 375, 1967.

Lloyd, W. B., and Wise, H. B. "The Montefiore Experience." *Bulletin of the New York Academy of Medicine, 44,* 1353, 1968.

MacColl, W. A. *Group Practice and Prepayment of Medical Care.* Washington, D.C.: Public Affairs Press, 1966.

Magraw, R. M. "Trends in Medical Education and Health Services." *New England Journal of Medicine, 285,* 1407, 1971.

McWhinney, I. R. "Family Medicine in Perspective." *New England Journal of Medicine, 293,* 175, 1975. (Letters in response. *NEJM, 293,* 781, 1975.)

Mechanic, D. "General Medical Practice." *Medical Care, 10,* 402, 1972.

Medical World News. "The Crisis in Emergency Care." December 4, 1970.

————. "Storefront Clinics." September 3, 1971.

————. "A Bid for Independence." October 20, 1972, p. 47.

————. "AMA Gives Ground but Fights On." December, 1972, p. 18.

————. "The Emergency Physician." February 1, 1974.

"Montefiore Neighborhood Medical Demonstration: The Early Experience." A series of articles by several authors. *Milbank Memorial Fund Quarterly, 45,* July, 1968.

Morehead, M. A. "Evaluating Quality of Care in the Neighborhood Health Center Program of OEO." *Medical Care, 2,* 118, 1970.

Morehead, M. A., and Donaldson, R. "Quality of Clinical Mangement of Disease in Comprehensive Neighborhood Health Centers." *Medical Care, 12,* 301, 1974.

Morehead, M. A. et al. "Comparisons Between OEO Neighborhood Health Centers and Other Health Care Providers of Ratings of the

Quality of Health Care." Presented at Medical Care Section, American Public Health Association, 1970, Houston, Texas.

Murray, R. H. "The Use of Technology in Ambulatory Health Care." *Bulletin of the New York Academy of Medicine, 48,* 955, 1972.

Myers, B. A. "Health Maintenance Organizations: Objectives and Issues." *HSMHA Health Reports, 86,* 585, 1971.

Myers, B. A. et al. "The Medical Care Activities of Local Health Units." *Public Health Reports, 83,* 757, 1968.

National Ambulatory Medical Care Survey. *Monthly Vital Statistics Report,* Vol. 24, No. 4, Supplement (2), July 14, 1975.

Newport, J., and Roemer, M. I. "Comparative Perinatal Mortality under Medical Care Foundations and Other Delivery Models." *Inquiry, 12,* 10, 1975.

Nielson, M. et al. "Older Persons after Hospitalization: A Controlled Study of Home Health Aide Service." *American Journal of Public Health, 62,* 1094, 1972.

Petersdorf, R. G. "Internal Medicine and Family Practice." *New England Journal of Medicine, 293,* 326, 1975.

Prager, S. "Doctor of Primary Medicine." *Journal of the American Medical Association, 220,* 410, 1972. (Letters in response, *JAMA, 221,* 192–194, 1972.)

Prussin, J. A. *Health Maintenance Organization Legislation in 1973-74, 2,* The Health Legislation Report Series. Washington, D. C.: Science and Health Publications, Inc., 1974.

Reidel, D. C. et al. *Federal Employees Health Benefits Program.* Washington, D.C.: Health Resources Administration, USDHEW, 1975.

Resource Management Corporation. *Evaluations of the War on Poverty: Health Programs.* Washington, D.C.: General Accounting Office, Contract No. GA-654, 1969.

Richter, L., and Gonnerman, A. "Hospital Administered Home Care Programs." *Hospitals, J.A.H.A.,* May 1, 1972, p. 41.

Richter, L., and Gonnerman, A. "Home Health Services and Hospitals." *Hospitals, J.A.H.A.,* May 16, 1974, p. 113.

Roemer, M. I. "Organized Ambulatory Health Service in International Perspective." *International Journal of Health Services, 1,* 18, 1971.

Roemer, M. I. "From Poor Beginnings, the Growth of Primary Care." *Hospitals, J.A.H.A.,* March 1, 1975, p. 38. (a)

Roemer, M. I. "A Realistic System: Health Maintenance Organizations in a Regionalized Framework." In Roemer, R. et al., *Planning Urban Health Services.* New York: Springer Publishing Co., 1975. (b)

Roemer, M.I., and Shonick, W. "HMO Performance: The Recent Evidence." *Health and Society, 51,* 271, 1973.

Roemer, M. I., et al. "The Ecology of Group Medical Practice in the United States." *Medical Care, 12,* 627, 1974.

Rogatz, P. et al. *Organization and Quality of Health Services.* Health Services Working Conference One, Fairleigh-Dickinson University, January 15, 1970, p. 28.

Rorem, C. R. *Private Group Clinics.* Publication No. 8, The Committee on the Costs of Medical Care. Chicago, Ill.: University of Chicago Press, 1931. Reprinted, New York, Milbank Memorial Fund, 1971.

Rosen, G. "The First Neighborhood Health Center Movement—Its Rise and Fall." *American Journal of Public Health, 61,* 1620, 1971.

Rosenberg, C. E. "Social Class and Medical Care in Nineteenth-Century America: The Rise and Fall of the Dispensary." *Journal of the History of Medicine and Allied Sciences, 29,* 32, 1974.

Rubin, A. A. et al. "Effective Primary Care by the Subspecialty Center." *New England Journal of Medicine, 293,* 607, 1975.

Satin, D. G., and Duhl, F. J. "Help?: The Hospital Emergency Unit as Community Physician." *Medical Care, 10,* 248, 1972.

Saward, E. W. "The Relevance of Prepaid Group Practice to the Effective Delivery of Health Services." Presented at the 18th Annual Group Health Institute, Sault Ste. Marie, Ontario, Canada, June 18, 1969. Reprinted, USDHEW, n.d.

Schlenker, R. E. et al. *HMO's in 1973: A National Survey.* Minneapolis, Minn.: InterStudy, 1974.

Schonfeld, H. K. et al. "Number of Physicians Required for Primary Care." *New England Journal of Medicine, 286,* 571, 1972.

Schwartz, J. L. *The National Free Clinic Survey.* Berkeley, Calif.: University of California Institute of Business and Economic Research. Reprint No. 9, 1971.

Schwartz, J. L. "Early Histories of Selected Neighborhood Health Centers." *Inquiry, 7,* 3, 1970.

Scutchfield, D., and Freeborn, D. "Estimation of Need Utilization and Costs of Personal Care Homes and Home with Services." *HSMHA Health Reports, 85,* April 1971.

Sheps, C. G. "Conference Summary and the Road Ahead." *Bulletin of the New York Academy of Medicine,* Vol. 41, No. 1, 2nd Series, January, 1965, p. 146.

Shortell, S. M. "Determinants of Physician Referral Rates: An Exchange Theory Approach." *Medical Care, 12,* 13, 1974.

Silver, G. A. "Group Practice—What It Is." *Medical Care, 1,* 94, 1963.

Silver, G. A. et al. "An Experience with Group Practice: The Montefiore Medical Group, 1948–1956." *New England Journal of Medicine, 256,* 785, 1957.

Sparer, G., and Anderson, A. *Cost of Services at Neighborhood Health Centers: A Comparative Analysis.* Washington, D.C.: Program Planning and Evaluation Division, Office of Health Affairs, Office of Economic Opportunity, 1972.

Sparer, G., and Johnson, J. "Evaluation of OEO Neighborhood Cen-

ters." Presented before the Medical Care Section, American
Public Health Association, 1970, Houston, Texas.

Spencer, J.H. *The Hospital Emergency Department.* Springfield, Ill.:
Charles C. Thomas, 1972.

Starr, P. "The New Medicine." *The New Republic,* April 19, 1975, p.
15.

Stevens, R. *American Medicine and the Public Interest.* New Haven,
Conn.: Yale University Press, 1971.

Stone, J. et al. "The Effectiveness of Home Care for General Hospital
Patients." *Journal of the American Medical Association, 205,* July
19, 1968.

Strickland, S. P. "Politics, Science and Dread Disease." Cambridge,
Mass.: Harvard University Press, 1972.

Terris, M. "Crisis and Change in America's Health System." *American
Journal of Public Health, 63,* 313, 1973.

Terris, M., Conference Chairman. "Group Practice: Problems and
Perspectives." The 1968 Health Conference. The New York Academy of Medicine. *Bulletin of the New York Academy of Medicine,
44,* November, 1968, pp. 1277–1434.

Torrens, P. "Administrative Problems of Neighborhood Health Centers." *Medical Care, 9,* 487, 1971.

Torrens, P., and Yedvab, D. "Variations among Emergency Room Populations: A Comparison of Four Hospitals in New York City."
Medical Care, 8, 60, 1970.

Trager, B. "Home Health Services and Health Insurance." *Medical
Care, 9,* 88, 1971.

Tudor Hart, J. "Relation of Primary Care to Undergraduate Education." *The Lancet,* October 6, 1973, p. 778.

Tudor Hart, J. "The Marriage of Primary Care and Epidemiology."
Journal of the Royal College of Physicians, London, 8, 299, 1974.

USDHEW. *Health Maintenance Organizations: The Concept and Structure.* Washington, D. C.: 1971.

Van Dyke, F., and Brown, V. "Organized Home Care." *Inquiry, 9,* 3,
1967.

Warner, J., and Aherne, P. *Profile of Medical Practice. '74.* Chicago,
Ill.: Center for Health Services Research and Development, American Medical Association, 1974.

Webb, S. B., and Lawrence, R. W. "Emergency Services: Physician
Staffing and Reimbursement Trends." *Hospitals, J.A.H.A.,* October 1, 1972, p. 69.

Weinerman, E. R. "Anchor Points Underlying the Planning for Tomorrow's Health Care." *Bulletin of the New York Academy of Medicine,* 2nd Series, *41,* 1213, 1965.

Weinerman, E. R. "Problems and Perspectives of Group Practice." *Bulletin of the New York Academy of Medicine,* 2nd Series, *44,* 1423,
1968.

Weinerman, E. R. et al. "Yale Studies in Ambulatory Medical Care v. Determinants of Use of Hospital Emergency Services." *American Journal of Public Health, 56*, 1037, 1966.

Weinerman, E. R., and Edwards, H. R. "Yale Studies in Ambulatory Medical Care I. Changing Patterns in Hospital Emergency Service." *Hospitals, J.A.H.A.*, November 16, 1964.

Wetherille, R. L., and Nordby, J. M. *A Census of HMO's: July 1975.* Minneapolis, Minn.: Interstudy, 1975.

Wetherille, R. L., and Quale, J.N. *A Census of HMO's: July 1974.* Minneapolis, Minn.: Interstudy, 1974.

White, K. L. "Primary Medical Care for Families—Organization and Evaluation." *New England Journal of Medicine, 277*, 847, 1967.

White, K. L. "Organization and Delivery of Personal Health Services—Public Policy Issues." *Milbank Memorial Fund Quarterly*, January, 1968. Reprinted, McKinlay, J. B., Ed., *Politics and Law in Health Care Policy.* New York: Prodist, 1973. (a)

White, K. L. "Life and Death and Medicine." *Scientific American, 229*, September, 1973, p. 23. (b)

White, K. L. "Health and Health Care: Personal and Public Issues." The 1974 Michael M. Davis Lecture. The Center for Health Administration Studies, Graduate School of Business, The University of Chicago, 1974.

Wilder, C. S. "Volume of Physician Visits, United States, July 1966—June 1967." *Vital and Health Statistics*, Series 10, No. 49. Rockville, Md.: National Center for Health Statistics, USDHEW, 1968.

Williams, G. "Kaiser." *Modern Hospital*, February, 1971, p. 67.

Winslow, C.-E.A. *The Life of Herman M. Biggs.* Philadelphia, Pa.: Lea and Febiger, 1929.

Wolfe, S., and Badgley, R. F. "The Family Doctor." *The Milbank Memorial Fund Quarterly, 50*, April 1972, Part 2.

Yolles, T. K. "Emergency Medical Service Systems: A Concept Whose Time Has Come." *Journal of Emergency Nursing, 1*, 31, 1975.

Zwick, D. I. "Some Accomplishments and Findings of Neighborhood Health Centers." *Milbank Memorial Fund Quarterly*, October, 1972. Reprinted in Zola, I. K., and McKinlay, J.B., Eds., *Organizational Issues in the Delivery of Health Services*, p. 331. New York: Prodist, 1974.

7

Hospitals

Michael Enright and Steven Jonas

Introduction

The hospital is the institutional center of the health care delivery system. Because of its complexity, the hospital has been described as a city whose major enterprise is the restoration of its citizens' health; and indeed, all the major services, resources, and social forces of a city have parallels in a hospital.

Like our cities, the hospital has changed dramatically in character in the past century. While in the nineteenth century a person entering a hospital had less than a 50% chance of leaving it alive, today a patient can expect to benefit from his hospital stay. The hospital has evolved from a place of refuge where a person went to spare his family the anguish of watching him die, to a multiservice institution providing interdisciplinary medical care to ambulatory as well as bed patients. Moreover, the present day hospital has other functions aside from delivering health and medical services. It is the center of most clinical training, both graduate and undergraduate, and is the principal locus of continuing education, formal and informal, for most physicians. It also trains other health providers and conducts health and medical research. It is the workplace for most United States physicians (in addition to their office practices) and the only place where they are likely to be subject to peer review at the present time. And the hospital has symbolic importance: being the most visible component of the health care delivery system, the hospital *is* that system in the minds of many laymen; its increasingly complex and sometimes bewildering structures and methods have come to represent the growing complexity of the delivery system as a whole.

In this chapter we will deal primarily with the most common type of hospital—the short-term, general, acute-care institution under private or nonfederal public ownership. The second largest category—mental hospitals—is covered in Chapter 8, while federal hospitals are dealt with in Chapter 10. Certain aspects of rising hospital costs are covered in Chapter 9, while hospital licensing, regulation, and quality control are discussed in Chapters 12 and 13.

Historical Development

The historical development of hospitals has been related to provision of care for poor persons (Stern, chs. 2, 6; Freymann, pp. 28–29) and to provision of medical care for the acutely ill (Freymann, pp. 21–29, ch. 4). Hospitals (the name shares a Latin root with hostels and hotels) began in the Middle Ages as places of refuge for the sick, the weary, and the poor. Most were church-sponsored. Beginning in the seventeenth century, several Western European countries, notably England, began to attempt to deal with the problem of the poor at the local level (de Schweinitz, chs. 3–5). Under the original Elizabethan Poor Laws, much of the relief provided was given to persons living in their own dwelling-places. However, local governments were also given the authority, and in some cases the responsibility, to build or provide institutions to house the poor. The poor comprised those who were unemployed owing to lack of jobs, skills, or education; orphans or children whose parents could not care for them; the dependent elderly; and the mentally retarded, as well as the ill. From the first appearance of such institutions—generally called poorhouses or almshouses—until well into the twentieth century, some or all of these categories were housed together in certain jurisdictions in England and the United States.

In the American colonies, the earliest hospitals were actually infirmaries in poorhouses: at Henricopolis in Virginia (1612); Blockley in Philadelphia (1732); Charity Hospital in New Orleans (1736); and in the Public Workhouse and House of Correction in New York City (1736) (Stern, ch. 6). The first public institution designed solely for the care of the sick was the "pesthouse" built on the same grounds as the New York workhouse. It was not until 1848 that the administrations of the two institutions were formally separated and an independent hospital created (Freymann, pp. 28–29).

Private, voluntary hospitals in the United States go back to the eighteenth century (Freymann, pp. 22–24). These institutions also cared for the poor: since hospitals could do little for their patients, there was no reason for the self-supporting sick to go to them. The first voluntary hospital in the American colonies was the Pennsylvania Hospital in Philadelphia (1751). The New York Hospital was founded in 1769, followed by the Massachusetts General in Boston in 1811 (Freymann, pp. 22–24). However, by 1873, there were only an estimated 178 hospitals in the United States (Stevens, p. 52).

Not until the turn of the twentieth century did a patient admitted to a general hospital have a better than even chance of getting out alive. That milestone was achieved largely by the development of general hospital hygiene and surgical anesthesia and asepsis.

By 1909, there were more than 4,359 hospitals with more than 421,000 beds (Stevens, p. 52). The rapid advance of medical science accounted for the expansion of the hospital, which began to assume its role as the center of the medical care system (MacEachern, pp. 21–27). Medical care had become too complex for the physician to carry his entire armamentarium in his black bag; special equipment and consultation with other medical specialists became essential.

The types of patients in the hospitals have changed with each medical discovery. In 1923, the discovery of insulin drastically changed the character of diabetes as a hospital disease; liver extract reduced the incidence of pernicious anemia in 1929; sulfonamides began to reduce pneumonia and some other infectious diseases in 1935, a trend which accelerated with the widespread use of antibiotics beginning in 1943, and the continuing development of immunization techniques. The development of rehabilitation services began to bring more disabled patients to the hospital. The 1950s saw chronic illness becoming progressively more important as a hospital problem. As noted in Chapters 2 and 3, infectious diseases have generally been conquered, leaving hospitals to cope with the pathology of the degenerative and neoplastic diseases, and trauma (Letourneau, 1964, p. 548). In the first half of the twentieth century there was a striking development of specialty hospitals—for example, general surgical, orthopedic, and eye and ear—largely as a result of benefactors' responses to the initiative of individual physicians (Ginzberg, p. 328). Fiscal exigencies, considerations of efficiency, and medical advances have sharply curtailed this development in recent years, and many former specialty hospitals now have closed or admit a full range of patients. Currently, most new specialty hospitals formed are parts of larger medical centers.

Classification of Hospitals*

The AHA principally classifies hospitals by size, type, mode of ownership, and length of patient stay. There are also cross-tabulations by geographic location, medical school affiliation, and an all-inclusive descriptor combining several of the principal characteristics: the "community hospital," which is defined as "all non-federal, short-term general or other special hospitals, excluding hospital units of institutions [such as prisons and universities], whose facilities and services are available to the public" (*Hospital Statistics, 1975 Ed.*, p. xvii). Hospital size is determined by number of beds, excluding bassinets for newborns (*Hospital Statistics, 1975 Ed.*, p. xxiv). There are four types of hospital: mental, tuberculosis, other special, and general. "Other special" hospitals comprise the following categories: narcotic addiction; maternity; eye, ear, nose, and throat; rehabilitation; orthopedic; chronic disease; mental retardation; alcoholism; or "other"—that is, a special hospital other than a mental or tuberculosis hospital. A general hospital—one which is none of the above—is the category that includes the majority of hospitals in the United States.

There are two principal modes of ownership: private and public. Private hospitals are categorized by the use to which they put their surplus income. They may be investor-owned for-profit (proprietary), or not-for-profit (voluntary). Public hospitals are categorized by the level of government jurisdiction that owns and operates them: federal, state, or local. Length-of-stay categories

---

* *Sources of data*: There are two major agencies that count and classify hospitals in the United States—the American Hospital Association (AHA) and the National Center for Health Statistics of the USDHEW. The AHA annually publishes the Guide Issue of its journal *Hospitals*, followed by a companion publication, *Hospital Statistics* (which until 1972 was published as part of the *Guide Issue*). These publications list each hospital registered by the AHA, giving its basic characteristics, as well as much summary data. *Hospitals* also includes "Hospital Indicators," monthly compilations of data on trends in hospital use and financing. The NCHS publishes *Health Resources Statistics* on an annual or biennial basis, as well as results of the Hospital Discharge Survey, which appear periodically in *Monthly Vital Statistics Report* and *Health and Vital Statistics*. In 1976, a publication somewhat similar to *Health Resources Statistics*, called *Health: United States, 1975*, appeared. It may either supplement or supplant the former. (All of these publications are discussed in Appendix I.) The NCHS defines its terms and counts slightly differently from the AHA. This chapter uses AHA definitions and data except as specifically noted.

are long and short; in the former the average length of stay is 30 days or more, whereas in the latter the average length of stay is less than 30 days.

Types of Hospitals: Data

Table 7.1 provides some statistics on the various types of hospitals, showing number of hospitals, beds, average daily census, and occupancy rate by type, ownership, and length of stay. The voluntary general short-term hospital is the most common type, followed by the local government general short-term hospital. The other principal groups are the federal short-term hospitals, the state mental hospitals, and the proprietary short-term hospitals. In terms of beds, the two major groups are the short-term general hospitals (average size 160 beds), and the long-term (average size 900 beds). Altogether in 1974, there were 1.5 million beds in 7,174 hospitals, with an average daily census of 1.2 million patients and an overall occupancy rate of 77% (*Hospital Statistics, 1975 Ed.*, Table 7.1).

Table 7.2 shows selected characteristics of community hospitals for 1964, 1973, and 1974. Although the number of hospitals is increasing only gradually, the number of beds increased by more than 25% between 1964 and 1974. During that decade the number of hospitals with fewer than 24 beds decreased by 47%; the number of hospitals with between 25 and 49 beds decreased by 21%; while the number of hospitals with more than 400 beds increased by more than 80% (*Hospital Statistics, 1975 Ed.*, p. ix).

The wide variation in the size of community hospitals is related to a variety of factors: community size, availability of manpower, number of hospitals serving a given community, and availability of funds for construction and operation.

In the period 1964–74, total admissions to community hospitals increased by 26%, while the average daily census increased by 27%. During the same time, the population increased by slightly more than 10%, so increased admissions and average daily census reflect a real increase in hospital utilization. Average length of stay has been less stable than would appear from the figures in Table 7.2 because they do not show the peak of 8.4 days in 1968 when the impact of Medicare on length of stay reached its peak.

Teaching Hospitals

The term "teaching hospital" generally refers to hospitals in which undergraduate and/or graduate teaching of medical stu-

Table 7.1

Short- and Long-term Hospitals Registered with the American Hospital Association

TYPE AND CATEGORY	SHORT-TERM				LONG-TERM			
	No.	Beds (× 1,000)	Average Daily Census (× 1,000)	Occupancy Rate	No.	Beds (× 1,000)	Average Daily Census (× 1,000)	Occupancy Rate
General								
Nongovernmental not-for-profit	3,304	643	501	78%	4	0.4	0.3	75%
Investor owned (for profit)	743	68	46	68	2	0.4	0.3	87
Local government	1,656	179	127	71	4	1.1	1.0	90
State government	150	30	20	68	11	2.5	2.0	85
Federal government	334	88	69	78	23	16.6	14.0	85
Total	6,187	1,009	763	76	44	21.0	18.0	85
Psychiatric								
Nongovernmental not-for-profit	44	3	2	69	44	5.6	4.5	81
Investor owned (for profit)	66	4	3	65	49	4.6	3.5	77
Local government	4	0.6	0.4	56	16	9.7	7.4	78
State government	23	4	3	71	297	352.0	283.0	80
Federal government	0	0	0	0	27	29.0	25.0	87
Total	137	11.6	8.4	69	433	401.0	324.0	81
TB and other respiratory disease								
Nongovernmental not-for-profit	1	0.07	0.04	59	3	0.2	0.1	49
Local government					11	1.3	0.8	60
State government					31	6.6	4.3	65
Total	1	0.07	0.04	59	45	8.1	5.1	63
Other special								
Nongovernmental not-for-profit	77	7	5	70	100	14	12	85
Investor owned (for profit)	32	1	0.8	63	8	0.8	0.7	83
Local government	8	0.9	0.6	69	53	22	18	82
State government	7	1.1	0.9	74	39	13	10	80
Federal government	1	0.5	0.3	61	2	1.1	0.9	82
Total	125	10.7	7.4	69	202	51	42	82
Total	6,450	1,032	778	75	724	481	389	81

Source: Hospital Statistics, 1975 Ed., Tables 2A and 2B. (See Appendix I, A10.)

Table 7.2

**Selected Characteristics of Community Hospitals Registered
with the American Hospital Association, 1964, 1973, 1974**

	1964	1973	1974
Number of hospitals	5,712	5,789	5,875
Number of beds (thousands)	721	898	926
Average number of beds per hospital	126	155	158
Total admissions	26,000	32,000	33,000
Average daily census (thousands)	550	680	700
Average length of stay (days)	7.7	7.8	7.8
Occupancy, percent	76.3	75.7	75.6
Total expenditures (billions)	. . .ᵃ	28.3	32.6
Expenses per patient day (dollars)	. . .ᵃ	102.44	113.55
Assets per bed (dollars)	. . .ᵃ	41,758	45,013
Outpatient visits (millions)	91	173	189

Source: *Hospital Statistics, 1975 Ed.,* pp. vii–xvi. (See Appendix I, A10.)
ᵃ Comparable figures not available.

dents and/or house staff (interns, residents, and specialty fellows) takes place. The term is not applied to hospitals with teaching programs for nurses, technicians, therapists, and other allied health workers, but not physicians. The AHA publishes information on hospitals affiliated with medical schools, which account for most teaching hospitals (*Hospital Statistics, 1975 Ed.,* Table 8). In 1974, there were 662 (9% of all hospitals), with 298 thousand beds (20% of all beds). Their average size, excluding mental hospitals, was around 400 beds, while the average size for all hospitals, excluding mental hospitals, was around 160 beds. They provided 10.2 million admissions (29% of the total), and on the average day cared for 31% of all hospitalized patients. They provided one-third of all out-patient visits. Their occupancy rate was 80.5% and the average length of stay was 8.6 days (for definitions see next section below). Thus, teaching hospitals have an importance in the hospital system quite out of proportion to their number.

Hospital Utilization

There are several measures of hospital utilization, which are for the most part self-explanatory: admissions, average daily census (average number of patients in the hospital), occupancy rate (percentage of beds occupied), average length of stay, total patient days (the product of average daily census by number of days in time-period considered), and discharges. These data can be modified and compared in various cross-tabulations: by geography (region, state), by hospital characteristics (bed-size, type, category of ownership), and by patient age, sex, and demographic modifiers. Analyses of hospital utilization data are vast; we will cover only a small portion of it.*

In 1974, there were 35.5 million admissions to hospitals in the United States (*Hospital Statistics, 1975 Ed.*, Table 1). Of the admissions, 98% were to short-term hospitals (although only two-thirds of the patient-days of care were in short-term hospitals) (*Hospital Statistics, 1975 Ed.*, Table 2). Two-thirds of these admissions were to voluntary general hospitals, 18% to local government hospitals. Although only 1.8% of admissions were to short and long-term psychiatric hospitals, these accounted for 28% of the patient days of care.

There are many determinants of hospital admission. Being separated or divorced, having comprehensive insurance, and having a long traveling time to a regular source of medical care all increase an individual's chance of being hospitalized (Andersen, p. 13). The length of stay in a hospital is most closely associated with degree of anxiety about health, but is also related to a person's age, family structure, beliefs about health care, and availability of hospital services (Andersen, p. 13).

Women are more likely to be hospitalized than men. When obstetrical admissions are eliminated, the average length of all admissions is about the same for males and females (Reidel et al., p. 22). Length of stay in a hospital decreases with patients' level of education and with higher income, and increases with age (Phelps, p. 112). By January 1976, the average length of stay was 7.5 days, down from 7.8 in 1974 ("Hospital Indicators").

Persons over age 65 account for nearly one-fourth of all patients ("Hospital Indicators"). Length of stay has been declining with medical progress. In 1947 pneumonia patients stayed 16 days in hospital; in 1972, they stayed 6.8 days. An appendec-

---

* As mentioned elsewhere, hospital utilization data are available from several recurrent sources. The AHA's *Guide Issue* and "Hospital Indicators" are very useful in giving provider-perspective information. Patient-perspective information for short-term hospitals is collected in the *Hospital Discharge Survey*. The data are published periodically in *Monthly Vital Statistics Report* (until 1972 in *Vital and Health Statistics*, Series 13), in three categories: Utilization of Short-Stay Hospitals —Summary of Nonmedical Statistics; Utilization of Short-Stay Hospitals, by Diagnosis; and Surgery in Short-Stay Hospitals.

tomy once required 14 days of hospitalization; by 1972 it required 6.6 days. A maternity stay in 1947 was 10 days; by 1972 it was down to 3.6 days (Commission on Professional and Hospital Activities).

The 10 leading discharge diagnoses from short-stay hospitals are: complications of pregnancy, childbirth, and the puerperium; malignant neoplasms, ischemic heart disease; mental disorders; diseases of the urinary system; fractures; hypertrophy of tonsils and adenoids; other heart and hypertensive disease; infective and parasitic diseases; and benign neoplasms and neoplasms of unspecified nature (National Center for Health Statistics, June 10, 1975, Table 1).

The average length of stay (ALOS) in community hospitals in 1975 was 7.4 days ("Hospital Indicators"). It has remained unchanged for three years. There is wide variation by age. Patients 65 and over stayed an average of about 11.4 days while those 65 and under stayed about 6.3 days. There is also variation by region and hospital bed-size. For example, for persons 65 and over, in January 1976 the ALOS in community hospitals ranged from 8.7 days in the Pacific states to 14.3 days in the mid-Atlantic states, and from 8.7 days in hospitals of 25–49 beds to 13.2 days in hospitals with 500 or more beds. Variation in ALOS by hospital size may be explained in part by variation in severity of disease, but regional differences are difficult to explain on medical bases alone. By type of short-term hospital, the ALOS is shortest in the proprietaries (6.7 days), longest in the voluntaries (7.9 days), with local government hospitals falling in between (7.5 days) (*Hospital Statistics, 1975 Ed.*, Table 2A).

Other Institutional Beds

In 1974 there were approximately 16,100 nursing homes* in the United States (National Center for Health Statistics, Sept. 5, 1974) ; 73% were operated under proprietary auspices while 27% were nonprofit. The preponderance of private, profit-making

---

* We have not covered nursing homes and other nonhospital health care facilities in any detail, although they are, of course, important components of the health care delivery system. We thus provide just the briefest sketch of the situation. A short bibliography on nursing homes will be found in Appendix II. Ongoing data on nursing homes and their patients can be found in *Vital and Health Statistics*, Series 12 and 13, and in the "Nursing Home Survey" published periodically in *Monthly Vital Statistics Report*.

ownership is the most important characteristic of U.S. residential facilities for the aged. It is the principal factor behind the scandals over wretched care, wretched conditions, and financial fraud which periodically wrack the industry (Thomas; Subcommittee on Long-term Care; Moreland Act Commission; Temporary State Commission).

In 1974, nursing homes provided care for about 1.1 million persons, approximately 5% of the U.S. population aged 65 and over. The number of beds in nursing homes more than doubled between 1963 and 1973, from 569,000 to 1,328,000. This increase was due in part to the coverage of the charges for certain types of nursing home care under the Medicare and Medicaid programs, as well as to changes in family living arrangements and advances in medical technology. Some of the growth in nursing home use appears to be the result of placement in nursing homes of older patients who in earlier years would have been resident in state and county mental hospitals. There are wide differences in the nursing home bed-population ratios among the different regions of the country.

In addition to the 1,513,000 beds in hospitals and the 1,328,000 in nursing homes, in 1971 there were about 448,000 beds in other residential health and health-related facilities. These included facilities for the mentally retarded (214,000 beds), orphans and dependent children (61,000 beds), unwed mothers (6,500 beds), alcohol and drug abusers (13,000 beds), the deaf and blind (24,000 beds), the physically handicapped (8,000 beds), and "other" (sheltered care homes, boarding homes, juvenile correctional facilities, and the like), which had 121,000 beds. These beds accommodate a total of 383,000 persons (National Center for Health Statistics, 1974).

Distribution and Relative Bed Supply
Introduction

In 1948 there were approximately 3.4 nonfederal general medical and surgical hospital beds per 1,000 civilian resident population, with a geographical range from a low of 2 beds per 1,000 population in the south to a high of 6 beds per 1,000 population in the industrial north and far west. By 1973, the community hospital bed-population ratio was approximately 4.3 per 1,000. There was some variation around the mean, ranging from 3.1 per 1,000 in New Mexico to 6.5 per 1,000 in North Dakota, among the contiguous states, and from 2.1 per 1,000 in Alaska to 7.2 in the District of Columbia (National Center for Health Statistics, 1976, Table B. II. 2). The ratio in a majority of states lies within ± 0.5 beds per 1,000 of the mean. Nevertheless, there are no known variations in health status, positive or negative, which can explain the variations that do exist.

Although improvements in bed distribution and increase in bed supply since World War II have been regarded as an achievement in providing access to hospitals for people in rural areas, the overall number of hospital beds in America has come to be regarded as excessive. This is difficult to quantify because a generally accepted definition of an excess bed cannot be found (Sattler and Bennett, p. 30). The number of beds required for a given geographic region is a function of the number of patient-days of hospital care required by the population (expressed as average daily census) and the occupancy level deemed appropriate for the hospitals of a given area (Sattler and Bennett, p. 30). However, beds have not been built in accordance with such a rational formula but rather because of medical need, local wealth, civic pride, and competition.

Once built, the availability of hospital beds promotes their use (Klarman, p. 139). The popular formulation of this relationship is known as Roemer's Law (Roemer) abbreviated as "a built bed is a filled bed." Thus, adding beds can cost the system money even if the beds are all used, because they may be filled with unnecessary admissions.

A relatively high proportion of hospital costs are either fixed, or varied with difficulty in the face of short-term changes in utilization. Personnel costs accounted for about 53% of community hospital costs in 1975 ("Hospital Indicators," April 16, 1976, Table 1). Of the balance, capital costs for plant already purchased do not vary and utility costs can be reduced only slightly. Only expenditures for food and consumable supplies do not have to be made when a bed is empty. For these reasons, it can be estimated that on a short-term basis an empty bed costs about 70% as much to maintain as does a filled one (Blue Cross/Blue Shield). High occupancy provides a stimulus to shorten length of stay and pressure for maximum use of diagnostic and therapeutic facilities. However, increased occupancy raises hospital costs only modestly, while raising hospital income dramatically, assuming that the patient has a payment source. Thus, the incentive for hospitals is to admit patients. The only way to really save money in the hospital sector is to close beds and eliminate those high fixed costs. Simply holding down admissions will not solve the problem: it saves third-party insurers money in the short-run, but does not reduce total health expenditures much in the long run.

Overbedding

A great deal of controversy has been generated in recent years over the related, but different, questions of overbedding and overutilization of beds. Overbedding means an excessive bed supply, resulting in unused beds. Researchers at the University of Michigan's Program and Bureau of Hospital Administration have determined that a general hospital of 300 beds or more can easily operate in the 85–95% occupancy range (Sattler and Bennett, pp. 36–39). In 1975, the community hospital adult bed occupancy rate for hospitals of all sizes was around 75% nationally ("Hospital Indicators," April 16, 1976, Table 1). Although in 1974, the President of the AHA said, "We've already got more beds than we need" (*Medical World News*, Nov. 8, 1974, p. 114), in 1975 the AHA officially took the position that the 75% occupancy figure does not necessarily mean that there are too many beds: the ideal bed/population ratio has not been determined, flexibility is needed to meet emergency situations, there are variations in occupancy rate by region and medical service which are not reflected in national figures (American Hospital Association, April 1, 1975).

Nevertheless, in 1976, as part of an effort to control hospital costs, the American Hospital Association took an official position against building new hospitals or expanding existing ones, but did not argue against replacing dilapidated ones or recommend closing existing ones. The President of the AHA warned the membership against allowing costs to continue to increase and provided an 11-point antiinflation package (American Hospital Association, Annual Report, 1975). The USDHEW regarded this sign of leadership from the private sector as encouraging and essential if that sector expects to continue its dominant role in the health care delivery system (*Medical World News*, Nov. 8, 1974).

However, a simple end-to-expansion policy may not be sufficient. A moratorium on the construction of additional hospital beds has been proposed (Rogatz, Aug., Oct., 1974). Legally acceptable means of closing beds down must be devised. Financial resources to provide support for geographically necessary but underutilized hospitals must be generated so that these hospitals will be able to survive. In dealing with the question of unnecessary hospitalization, Rogatz said that alternatives to inpatient care, such as Health Maintenance Organizations, and ambulatory surgical facilities, which will reduce the need for hospital beds, should be promoted. Physicians, he said, must be given an incentive to avoid unnecessary hospitalization.

In the study cited above, Sattler and Bennett concluded that for 1975 the estimated national community hospital bed excess was about 70,000 (1975, pp. 40–42). They assumed that although larger hospitals could safely operate with a 90% occupancy rate, smaller ones could not: enough beds to allow for emergencies must be provided. They suggested that a weighted national average occupancy rate of 81% for hospitals of all sizes would be optimal. Estimating the average cost of carrying an excess bed to be $18,250, the authors found that the 81% rule would produce an annual saving of over $1 billion (p. 46).

The Comptroller of the United States has pointed out that excess beds are accompanied by sophisticated equipment, often purchased with little assurance of use sufficient to justify cost (p. 98). Because of this "overequipping" an estimated 25% of the population receives hospital care in facilities with expensive equipment that inflates costs, but that is not necessary for patient care.

In 1975, the Health Research Group (HRG) of Public Citizen, the Ralph Nader organization, issued a report called *The $8 Billion Hospital Bed Overrun: A Consumer's Guide to Stopping Wasteful Construction* (Ensminger). The writer used 85% as his optimum community hospital occupancy rate, rather than 81%, and thus arrived at a figure of 100,000 excess beds. Using a conservative construction cost figure of $50,000 per bed, he estimated the cost of building these beds at $5 billion; the annual maintenance cost he estimated to be $2 billion. The "$8 Billion Overrun" refers only to annual operating costs: the $2 billion for maintaining excess beds, plus $6 billion for claimed unnecessary admissions, a subject to which we shall turn shortly.

The American Hospital Association issued a sharply worded critique of the report (July, 1975), concentrating on alleged HRG methodological errors and defending the hospital industry's efforts to control bed-supply, utilization, and costs. Six months later HRG issued a point-by-point rebuttal of the AHA critique (Health Research Group). Readers will have to judge the validity of each side's position for themselves. However, one point is striking. The AHA never claims that there are *no* extra beds, or *no* unnecessary hospitalizations; but they seem more interested in defending the status quo than in determining the true overbedding figures. It would be wise for the industry to take action before sanctions are imposed by law or by administrative fiat on the part of regulatory authorities.

Overutilization

Overutilization means that a significant proportion of hospital admissions are unnecessary. If they were not made, the occupancy rates would be even lower than they already are, and the excess bed figure would be even higher. There is significant evidence to support this position.*

The analysis of possible overutilization of hospitals has focused particularly closely on surgery. John Bunker, comparing the frequency of surgery in England and Wales with that in the United States, said: "There are twice as many surgeons in proportion to the population in the United States as in England and Wales, and they perform twice as many operations. . . . Indications for surgery are not sufficiently precise to allow determination of whether American surgeons operate too often or the British too infrequently . . ." (p. 135). It appeared from this study that there might be a Roemer's Law for surgeons too: when surgeons are present, they will operate.

The controversy flared into the national press in 1975 when

---

* In Chapter 6, we cited a lengthy review of the performance of Health Maintenance Organizations by Roemer and Shonick (1973). They cited a series of studies over many years showing that prepaid group practice subscribers have hospitalization rates that average 40% below those of Blue Cross/Blue Shield and other item-of-service reimbursement plans (1973, pp. 281–291). Ensminger cited a short series of studies making the same point (1975, pp. 26–28). A 1976 study reported on the utilization experience of persons covered by Medicaid in 10 Health Maintenance Organizations with a combined enrollment of almost 1.3 million people, of whom about 225,000 were on Medicaid (Gaus et al.). The Medicaid group-practice subscribers were compared with matched controls. The experimental group used less than one-half of the hospital services used by the control group, measured both by admissions and days of care (Gaus et al., Table 4). In none of these studies is there any evidence that the health status of one group is different from that of another.

congressional hearings were held by Representative John Moss. The congressmen examined a New York City study in which second opinions were required before surgery could be authorized; the study concluded that 17.6% of operations are unnecessary (McCarthy and Widmer). They also reviewed evidence that the surgery rate for Medicaid recipients in the U.S. is almost 2½ times that for the general population ("Getting Ready," July 18). Ensminger, citing the McCarthy-Widmer study, as well as a study by Lewis (1969) and a book by a pseudonymous Dr. Williams (1971), estimated that the national excess surgery rate is 20% (pp. 17–19). He estimated the dollar cost of that surgery at $3 billion. (Added to the $2 billion for excess beds and an estimated $3 billion for overlong hospital stays, Ensminger arrived at his $8 billion overrun total.) Ensminger also raised the issue of unnecessary death as the ultimate side-effect of unnecessary surgery. He estimated that if there are 3 million unnecessary surgical operations each year, there must be about 15,000 unnecessary deaths (assuming normal surgical and anesthetic mortality) resulting from the unnecessary operations (p. 18). This dispute blossomed further when in early 1976 *The New York Times* projected McCarthy and Widmer's figures nationally. Their estimates were somewhat lower than Ensminger's, but still substantial: 2.4 million unnecessary operations and almost 12,000 needless deaths (*New York Times*, Jan. 27, 1976).

The response of organized medicine to these charges was as sharp as the AHA's response to the overbedding instigations. Dr. Francis D. Moore, chief of surgery at the Peter Bent Brigham Hospital in Boston said: "Fraudulent operations are extremely rare and it's irresponsible to suggest otherwise. . . . The person who wrote that story in *The New York Times* ought to be horsewhipped" (*Medical World News*, May 3, 1976, p. 50). *The American Medical News*, the AMA newspaper, criticized *The Times* "for exaggeration, for distortion of admittedly true facts, for extrapolating sound data beyond reasonable limits" (*American Medical News* p. 4). A former AMA President, Malcolm Todd said: "These figures are outrageously exaggerated" (*American Medical News*, p. 15).

Few surgical voices called for vigorous investigation of problems in surgery, George Zuidema of Johns Hopkins (*Medical World News*, p. 92) being one exception. However, it is an issue with a long history. *Medical World News* compiled a lengthy bibliography with citations going back to 1946 (1976, p. 66). As with overbedding, the question is not whether unnecessary surgery and overutilization occur, but to what extent they prevail. It is up to the hospital industry and the medical profession to determine the true state of affairs and then to take action to save dollars and lives.

Hospital Structure
The Operating Divisions of a Hospital*

The principal hospital operating divisions are medical, nursing, other diagnostic and therapeutic support, financial, personnel, hotel, and community relations. Most hospitals provide services both to inpatients (who are admitted to the hospital and assigned a bed) and to outpatients (who come to an emergency department, an outpatient clinic, or to a diagnostic or therapeutic service for a procedure not requiring admissions).

Medical. The medical division is generally organized along the lines of the medical specialities. The larger the hospital and the more specialized the medical services, the more medical departments are found, particularly in teaching hospitals. There is no universal logic to the way in which medical departments are categorized. Some are separated from the others by type of skill involved, some by the age or sex of their main patient group, and some by the organ or organ system which is their primary purview.

The principal departments are *internal medicine* (diagnosis and therapeusis for adults, in general with problems involving one or more internal organs or the skin, in which the principal tools do not involve a physical alteration of the patient's body by the physician); *surgery* (diagnosis and therapeusis in which the principal tools involve a physical alteration of the patient's body by the physician); *pediatrics* (diagnosis and therapeusis for children, primarily but not entirely with nonsurgical techniques); *obstetrics/gynecology* (diagnosis and therapeusis for women, relating to the sexual/reproductive system, which uses both surgical and nonsurgical techniques); and *psychiatry* (diagnosis and therapeusis for people of all ages with mental and emotional

* We are here considering primarily community hospitals, as defined above. Although some of the broad generalizations and principles apply to other kinds of hospitals, many of the details do not. For more specific information on state mental hospitals and federal government hospitals, see Chapters 8 and 10 respectively.

problems, using primarily nonsurgical techniques). A sixth important medical department in many hospitals is *general/family medicine* (diagnosis and therapeusis for people of all ages with all conditions, using nonsurgical and surgical techniques, although the practice of the latter in general/family medicine has been declining in recent years).

Other medical departments, when they exist, tend to be organized around organs and organ-systems: ophthalmology (eye); otolaryngology (ear, nose, and throat); urology (male sexual/reproductive system, and the renal system for both males and females); orthopedics (bones and joints); and so on. Radiology (the use of X-ray and other radiation sources) is a medical department with a primarily diagnostic function, although radiotherapy is also important. Pathology, in medical practice, serves only a diagnostic function, both before and after treatment. Anesthesiology is principally concerned with preparing patients so that they may be surgically operated upon with no pain or discomfort during the procedure.

Other health services. The functional divisions of the nursing service follow the pattern discussed in Chapter 5. The diagnostic and therapeutic services (which may or may not be attached to one of the medical departments) include: laboratory (usually under the direction of the department of pathology); electrocardiography (usually a part of internal medicine); electroencephalography (part of neurology); radiography (part of radiology); pharmacy; social service; inhalation therapy (often part of anesthesiology or pulmonary medicine); nutrition as therapeusis; physical, occupational, and speech therapy (often attached to the department of rehabilitation medicine, if there is one); and medical records.

Administrative functions. Financial, personnel, and hotel service are the major operating functions of the hospital administration. The hotel services include maintenance of plant and equipment, housekeeping, laundry, and dietary (cooking and delivery of meals). Other primarily administrative functions include community/public relations, organizing volunteer services, operating the medical library, and long-range planning.

Administration

Health administration encompasses planning, organizing, directing, controlling, and coordinating the resources and procedures by which needs and demands for health and medical care and a healthful environment are fulfilled, by provision of specific services to individual clients, organizations, and communities (Austin, p. 139). The hospital's chief administrator is the direct representative of the Board of Trustees or other governing authority in the management of the hospital, and is responsible to the governing authority alone for the performance of his or her duties. The administrator is responsible for seeing that all policies approved by the board, including medical staff by-laws, are implemented.

Hospital management is primarily concerned with efficiency in terms of controlling expenditures and effectiveness in terms of assuring benefits. The hospital has a major incentive to contain costs in order to increase its ability to provide a broader range of services to as many of the sick as possible. Opportunities to contain hospital costs exist in four areas: planning of facilities and services, scheduling of patients and patient services, medical control of facilities utilization and quality of service, and administrative control of manpower and expenditures (Phillips).

Financial aspects of administration are complemented by other administrative skills such as planning the evolution of the hospital role; defining and redefining corporate objectives; and developing policies with appropriate strategies to assure their implementation. Areas in which these skills are utilized are medical staff and board of trustees relations; maintenance of the physical plant and equipment; maintaining awareness and responsiveness to the legal environment; and fostering educational programs, medical and health care delivery research, and cooperation with other hospitals and health agencies (Davis and Henshaw, pp. 5–7).

Community relationships in administration. Hospital administrators, in addition to dealing with professional medical concerns, have a social role in filling community demands for health care. Some hospitals are regarded as detached from their communities, and demands are being made that they change their institution-centric (Freymann, Section V) mode of functioning and share control of decision-making processes with community groups. Social roles in which hospitals which choose to can become involved include eliminating unemployment and underemployment in their communities, improving inadequate educational services, and combatting personal and institutional racism (Dornblaser, p. 811).

In developing its role in relation to its community, the hospital must also consider other health agencies and community health programs. In some communities, it may be quite logical to have health services centralized in the hospital, while in others it may be appropriate to decentralize some services to a neighborhood health center or other agency, which may be either independent of the hospital or contractually related (see Chapter 6).

Providing outpatient care, which is either preventive or else treats a problem that might previously have necessitated hospital admission, lowers the cost of medical care, but may increase demand for inpatient services by referrals. At any rate, it will probably increase the average cost per admission because of the higher proportion of more seriously ill patients admitted.

From the mid-sixties to the early seventies, there was plentiful federal support for experimental or demonstration community health care programs (see Chapter 6), but in the mid-seventies, many programs begun in the previous 10 years were curtailed for lack of adequate support. As more people are deprived of health services, the resulting political pressures may lead to a return to more federal support for such programs.

In order for hospitals to make appropriate decisions, some consumer advocates feel that the medical mystique must be cast aside and consumers must be given a share of responsibility for their own health care (Belsky and Gross, p. 229). According to this view, those who control the system must develop and implement a mechanism for consumers to influence decisions affecting the community. Hospitals must develop the additional resources to respond to consumer requests for improved services.

However, in a time of increasingly scarce resources, it is not clear whether hospitals will expand or contract their community role. The relationship between consumer expectations and hospital financial problems is certainly an area of potential conflict.

Sharing strategies. Administrators make efforts to see that the services that their hospitals do provide are accessible to the community and appropriate to its health needs. The range of services must be broad enough to leave no critical needs unmet, but not so broad as to require wasteful investment of community resources in high-cost, low-utility technology if it can be made available to the community through cooperation with some other agency. Administrators also attempt to see that the services provided are continuous rather than episodic and that hospital services interface through appropriate referral mechanisms with other health services in the community; or through sharing services with other agencies.

Since institutions have historical relationships with a patient population, and are reluctant for political and social reasons to appear to be reducing services, a sharing strategy among hospitals is sometimes used to reduce the burden of a given service. For example, one hospital may be responsible for emergency medical care with back-up services being provided by one or several others.

The sharing strategy is also being implemented by administrators on a larger scale in the consolidation of hospitals through various forms of mergers (Brown and Money, 1975). Further, management of some hospitals is being provided under contract by other hospitals or management firms. The result is the development of multiple hospital chains under centralized management. These conglomerates can attract expensive management expertise and can organize on a regional basis in order to share this management and medical expertise. Many of these chains are proprietary operations which will be subject to the same forces that have made many small proprietary hospitals become voluntary: the pressures of public expectations that a wide range of services be provided (Brown and Money, 1975).

This seems to offer a major opportunity for voluntary, not-for-profit institutions to expand their services and influence, without new capital, and to acquire and use the range of talent essential in modern hospital operations. The end result may be a hospital market that can buy and sell specific services and programs to meet the changing health needs of the public (Brown and Money, 1975).

Personnel. Since over 50% of a hospital budget is spent on personnel services, appropriate use of personnel resources is a major concern among administrators. The number of personnel required to provide patient care is increasing constantly. In 1950 there were 1.78 full-time equivalent employees per patient in non-federal short-term hospitals; by 1973 the number had increased to 3.15 (*Hospital Statistics, 1975 Ed.*, p. xii).

New medical technology, which is being developed continuously, has a direct effect on hospital personnel costs. For every new piece of equipment purchased for the hospital, additional persons, who may require extensive training, are required to perform tasks created by the machine. Further, as medical care becomes more complex, many duties formerly carried out by physicians or nurses are delegated to other persons who are specifically trained to provide a broad range of related services.

Personnel costs contribute to hospital inflation not only because there are more employees but also because they now earn more than ever before. Increases in the minimum wage, the infusion of funds that followed the implementation of Medicare, unionization, and the greater skills demanded of those who work with complex medical technology have all resulted in increased wages (Raske, p. 68).

Hospital employees are now covered under the Federal Wage and Hour Standards Act. The right of collective bargaining through hospital unions is protected by law and may be enforced by state labor agencies.* Three factors which have influenced the impact of unionization on hospital wages are (a) the percent of hospital employees covered; (b) laws requiring nonprofit hospitals to recognize collective bargaining agents, and (c) spreading union coverage for workers in general (Sloan, p. 36). It has been argued that these measures serve the public interest because the state should assure decent wages for all persons working in its jurisdiction, while hospitals must be able to maintain a qualified and stable labor force which must be sought in the competitive labor market (Shain and Roemer).

Hospital Governance

The majority of hospitals, in 1975, were voluntary. The voluntary principle is historically associated with charity, emphasis on good quality of care, concern for the public interest, and involvement in education and training. These elements are found also to various degrees in all types of hospitals, often deriving from the example of the private nonprofit hospital.

Profit and nonprofit hospitals differ in that economic criteria are most important in decision-making in for-profit hospitals, whereas a wider variety of criteria influence decision making in nonprofit hospitals (Rushing). These differences influence the way that the hospital operates. Specifically, not-for-profit hos-

---

* A useful series of papers which can introduce the reader to the subject of unionization, collective bargaining, and strikes in the health care field is contained in the *International Journal of Health Services*, 5, 5, 1975.

pitals with higher occupancy rates have a higher ratio of personnel to patients than do for-profit hospitals with the same occupancy levels. Also, average daily charges of for-profit hospitals are positively associated with community wealth; for non-profit hospitals there is no evidence of such a relationship (Rushing, pp. 474, 477).

The typical private community hospital is organized according to a constitution and by-laws, investing in a board of trustees the responsibility for all aspects of the operation of the hospital, including ultimate responsibility for the medical care delivered in that institution. That responsibility is then delegated to a medical staff, which has its own set of by-laws, approved by the board of trustees (Letourneau, 1964, p. 92).

Hospitals receive authority to operate from the government of the state in which they are located. The agency with hospital licensing powers varies from state to state. Boards of voluntary hospitals are given the legal authority to operate the hospital, set policy, and make all major decisions. Day-to-day decisions are made by administrative and professional personnel who manage the hospital. New York State law, for example, specifies that the board shall appoint the hospital administrator, shall appoint members of the medical staff, and shall approve the by-laws and regulations of the medical staff (Somers, 1969, p. 108).

Voluntary hospitals. Boards of trustees for voluntary hospitals were formed originally out of a sense of obligation felt by the upper class in America to provide for the welfare of the sick poor in the cities. This was done by financing the building and operation of hospitals. Hospital trusteeship has since become legally formalized in all states.

Making and soliciting philanthropic contributions is not now a major activity of hospital trustees (Stephenson, p. 38). Although the amount of dollars contributed to hospitals has remained relatively constant, the increases in national medical care expenditures have made such contributions relatively less significant. In 1974, philanthropic contributions amounted to 3.9 billion, covering around 10% of total hospital expenditures. This was a 2.6 percent gain over 1973 (Garber), but at the same time hospital expenses increased by 12.2%. Many voluntary hospitals still want to continue their charity role, providing care free to patients who have no source of payment, both as a moral and social commitment. Although some administrators and boards consider this stance inconsistent with economic efficiency, hospitals having the resources and management skills to generate support for their commitment will continue to provide charity care.

Before the 1940s and 1950s, when hospital administration had not yet emerged as a career, hospitals actually needed trustees to deal with the administrative problems that the nurse superintendent—at that time the senior administrator—was not trained to handle. As hospitals moved from caring for the sick/poor to caring for the community at large, medical matters became more important to trustees. Their role changed from providing minimal charity services to guaranteeing that each patient is maximally safe when he enters the hospital (Stephenson, p. 40).

The board of trustees is the legally responsible body for the financial mantenance of hospital services. It acts as an organ of review, appraisal, and appeal in a judicial manner. It assures the physical integrity of the hospital. It must be cognizant of the appointments and privileges granted to each physician and be assured that all services provided in the hospital are of adequate professional caliber and it must review the medical staff constitution and by-laws (Stephenson, pp. 40-41). It also reviews the short- and long-range objectives of the hospital, and reviews and approves the various budgets.

Some characteristics of hospital trustees were identified in a survey conducted by the American Hospital Association Bureau of Research Services (Kessler, pp. 21–26). It reported that 39% of the respondents had annual incomes of more than $40,000. More than one-half of the trustees surveyed indicated no limit on the number of years they could serve without interruption. In general, boards of trustees cannot be considered to be broadly representative of the communities their hospitals serve. In Detroit in 1971, 76% of board members were business or professional people (*Health Perspectives,* Nov. 73–Jan. 74, Table II (a)). In 1973, among the memberships of the boards of trustees of hospitals in Manhattan, New York, with 300 or more beds, 87% were male, 67% were business people or non-health professionals, and another 3% were health professionals (*Health Perspectives,* Nov. 73–Jan. 74, Table II (b)).*

---

* Given that trustees are often businesspeople and that they substantially influence hospital expenditures, conflicts of interest can arise when hospitals do business with firms with which their trustees are associated (*New York Times,* Dec. 26, 1975, April 18, 1976; *Newsday,* Feb. 27, 1976, March 15, 1976).

According to the survey, trustees perceive recovery of operating costs as the most crucial problem hospitals face (Kessler, pp. 21–26). Only 4% of the trustees surveyed received monetary compensation, although three times that number thought compensation for trustees desirable. Areas of major interest identified by respondents included legal definition of trustee responsibilities, the quality of hospital care, qualifications of an effective trustee, medical staff relations, financing national health care, and ethical concerns.

Some changes are imminent in the membership of hospital boards. A professional trustee may develop in the future, with expertise in a specific area and with experience on boards of several hospitals (Stephenson, p. 80). *Ex officio* members who represent other agencies will be given seats on hospital boards; in exchange for their information, they will acquire an informal base for political action outside the traditional structures. These changes are not occurring universally, but can be expected as the necessity for community cooperation, interagency sharing, and trustee expertise becomes apparent to even the most traditional boards (Mott and Chalk).

One reorganization of hospital boards which is occurring and does reduce the control of trustees over administration is adoption of the corporate model, integrating the board of trustees and the administration of the hospital. The new board will have full-time presidents and salaried vice-presidents covering the specialties of management (*Modern Hospital*, 1970).

Another imminent change is the addition of community representatives to hospital boards. Those who argue for broader representation on boards say that the wishes and value systems of the vast majority of persons in the community are represented only to the extent that upper- and middle-class board members understand those wishes and value systems, and choose to pay attention to them (Mott and Chalk). (Not only the poor, but the lower middle class are underrepresented on most hospital boards. In fact, nonrepresentation of major sectors of society is almost universal, and the wealthy are not even any longer providing significant financial support.) It is possible that broadening the makeup of the governing board will bring improvements, or at least a system that the majority of people want. If members of the community were recruited, the board's broadened power base might yield greater community support; the likelihood of relevant decision making would increase; and legitimate testing ground for new ideas would be provided.

Public hospitals. There are a variety of governance forms for public hospitals. At the federal level, the Department of Defense, the Veterans' Administration, and the Public Health Service operate their hospitals without boards of trustees or their equivalent. The hospital directors are directly accountable to their administrative superiors, and indirectly to the President and the Congress. State hospitals are also run directly by government departments, usually Mental Health or Hygiene for psychiatric facilities, and Health for the remaining tuberculosis sanatoria. These hospitals usually do not have boards of trustees, although the government department may be in part responsible to a Board of Mental Hygiene, or Health, which may exert some board of trustee-like influence on individual hospitals. As at the federal level, state hospital directors are mainly accountable to their administrative superiors, and indirectly to the Governor and the state legislature.

At the local level, governance becomes more complex. For example, until 1969 in New York City, the 18 municipally owned hospitals were operated by a Department of Hospitals. Hospital directors were directly accountable to the commissioner, and indirectly accountable to the mayor and the city council. (A similar situation currently prevails in Los Angeles, San Francisco, Boston and Philadelphia.) Hospital boards, where they existed, were mere window-dressing.

In 1969, New York City adopted the public corporation approach. A semi-independent Health and Hospitals Corporation was established. Public officials sit on the Board but do not have a majority of its seats. All appointments are made by elected officials, and the chairman is the Commissioner of Health. The chief operating officer is the Corporation's president, elected by the Board, usually on recommendation from the mayor. However, the president is under the mayor's control only through the latter's control of part of the Corporation finances; there is no formal administrative line from the Corporation president to the mayor. The hospital directors report directly to the Corporation president, and the Corporation Board functions like a board of trustees of a voluntary hospital. There are "community advisory boards" for each municipal hospital but they have little power as yet. Cook County Hospital in Illinois has a similar structure, except that it has a governing commission and an executive director. In that case, however, the mayor appoints all of the Commission's members.

County hospitals in semiurban, suburban, and rural areas may be run directly by a department of the county government, or may have a board of managers, as is the case in Nassau County, New York. These boards are usually appointed by the chief executive officer of the county, and/or the county legislative body. The pursestrings are usually controlled by the county government. But in certain jurisdictions, county hospital boards are independent authorities with the power to levy their own taxes and sell their own bonds for capital construction.

The concern of community residents about hospital services is also directed toward local government hospitals, many of which have historically been regarded as second-class institutions. Some are now being upgraded, however, and are seeking to provide a single standard of care to all members of the population. To do so they must be operated not as charity hospitals but as institutions open to all patients and all physicians in the city. To assume this role, they must have operating autonomy including adequate financing (Brown, 1970). However, it may be too late to bring these changes about.

If public hospitals do not adopt new financing mechanisms, they may have to shut down. Declining occupancy figures, and the closing of county hospitals in California (Blake and Bodenheimer) and municipal hospitals in New York are regarded by some as a harbinger of similar events in other states. They point out that Medicare and Medicaid gives the patient free choice of physician and hospital, and the private sector is increasingly being chosen. In California, 30% of all patients requiring hospitalization did switch from the public to the private sector between 1966 and 1974. Other observers are more optimistic as to the future of public hospitals. With public funding, the hospitals are upgrading their facilities so that they now have special treatment units and semiprivate rooms, like voluntary hospitals (Beyers). Haughton believes that if the dual system is ever to be replaced by one which would guarantee the benefits of American health care technology to all of our people fairly and equitably, the initiative would have to come from the public sector (1975).

However, this is a difficult and strongly debated policy question. The United States has had two classes of community hospital since the end of the nineteenth century, when scientific, technological, and medical advances fueled the explosion in hospital construction. First there were the voluntary hospitals, which in the earlier days had cared for a class of patients, among the acutely ill at least, similar to those found in public hospitals. In modern times, however, they increasingly came to admit more patients who could pay or had hospitalization insurance. Second were the local government hospitals which, where they existed, cared for those who could not gain admission to the voluntaries.

It is difficult to determine whether the two classes of institutions provided different levels of medical care. Where municipal hospitals are principal teaching institutions of medical schools— New York's Bellevue, the Boston City, the Philadelphia General, and Los Angeles General—the technical medical quality is probably superior to that of the average community hospital. However, in general surroundings, amenities, overall staffing, buildings, equipment, and budgeting, many local government hospitals are distinctly inferior.

There are periodic scandals involving New York City hospitals which go back over decades, usually as a result of journalistic or political exposés. The findings are always the same: staff shortages, antiquated buildings, broken equipment, dirt, insects, poor food, unattended patients, and so on. Outpatients have suffered particularly hard from long waits, hard benches, understaffing, poor record keeping, and inefficient organization. The results of the investigations were usually the same too: negligible. To its credit, New York City embarked on a major hospital construction program after the last major exposé in the mid-sixties, replacing some of its most antiquated buildings. Ironically, these came on line in the mid-seventies, just at a time when the city was facing its worse financial squeeze. The Health and Hospitals Corporation was then forced to close some of its facilities, including one new building, stop its construction program, and curtail services at all of its institutions. The care in a new building with staff shortages cannot be much better than that in an old building with staff shortages, and could be worse (*New York Times*, July 30, 1976).

With some kind of universal financial entitlement to health services for all Americans in the offing (see Chapter 15), the question of what to do with local government hospitals becomes pressing. Should they be improved and strengthened? Should advantage be taken of universal coverage to put them on a sound financial basis, since it should be possible for them to exist almost entirely on third-party reimbursement for services rendered? Should they be opened to private patients, as some already are? Or should it be assumed that the poor-law heritage and the pauper stigma, civil service rules, and detrimental local party political influence have injured them beyond repair?

If so, public hospitals should be closed or turned over to nonprofit corporations. Some fear that this would amount to the people's "losing their hospitals." But the public receives little benefit from having poor quality hospitals. Maintaining local government hospitals in an era of universal financial entitlement might well perpetuate the two-class system. Moreover, voluntary hospitals that were significantly accountable to public authorities might actually be more attuned to the communities than public hospitals have been in the past.

Medical Staff

The physician is traditionally described as a guest in the hospital and as its primary customer. Except when a physician chooses to run a hospital for profit, he has no personal responsibility to see that the hospital is available to provide care for his patients. The physician uses the hospital as his workshop, as noted above. In exchange for this privilege, he is obligated to participate in governance of the medical staff and hospital. Further, he is obligated to participate in care given in areas of the hospital for which the medical staff accepts collective responsibility, such as the emergency room or outpatient clinic (Letourneau, 1964, pp. 20–26).

When a physician admits a patient to the hospital, he is free to order whatever tests or treatments he deems necessary. Thus he basically determines the amount of services used and consequent costs of individual patients' care. He also influences the growth and expansion of the institution. Physicians have every reason to want the best possible institutional setting in which to practice medicine, especially when it is provided at no personal cost to them.

Although the doctor is technically a guest in the hospital, it is responsible for the care its staff renders his patients on the physician's orders. Until relatively recently, hospitals could not be held liable for the wrongful conduct of a physician, but this principle is being significantly changed by a series of judicial decisions (Health Law Center, pp. 31–34). Changing legal doctrines of negligence and corporate liability of hospitals have recently established that hospitals are legally and, to the extent that they cause a tort to a patient, financially responsible for the care provided by their entire professional staff, including physicians (Somers 1969, pp. 32–36).

The medical staff by-laws specify procedures for election of medical staff officers by the membership. The officers are given authority under the by-laws to enforce rules and regulations. The officers delineate privileges and recommend disciplinary action when necessary through the committee structure. They enforce the by-laws and must oversee the committee structure and submit reports of medical staff activities to the board of trustees.

There are numerous medical staff committees. The executive committee coordinates all activity, sets general policies for the medical staff, and accepts and acts upon recommendations from the other medical staff committees. The joint conference committee acts as liaison between the medical staff and the governing board in deliberations over matters involving both medical and nonmedical considerations. The credentials committee reviews applications by physicians to join the medical staff, and considers the qualifications of education, experience, and interests before making recommendations to the executive committee, which will then make recommendations for appointment to the board of trustees.

The infections control committee is responsible for preventing infections in the hospital through routine preventive surveillance, tracking down of outbreaks of infection, and education of hospital personnel. The pharmacy and therapeutics committee reviews pharmacologic agents for inclusion in the list of drugs approved for use in the hospital. The tissue committee is responsible for insuring quality control of surgery, principally by examining and evaluating bodily tissues removed during operations.

The medical records committee is responsible for certifying complete and clinically accurate documentation of the care given to patients. The committee also acts as a judge of clinical care based on the written record.

The utilization review committee evaluates the appropriateness of admissions and length of stay in the hospital, and may review use of services and facilities for patients whose hospital care is being paid for by Medicare. Utilization review never worked very well, for reasons that are not entirely clear. In the mid-70s, it was allied with the Professional Standards Review Organization (PSRO) system (see Chapter 13).

The tissue, medical audit, and utilization review committees and the PSRO provide for review of physician's professional work by other physicians (see Chapter 13). As the hospital has become more complicated and more critical of medical practice, the medical staff has been subjected to more scrutiny. In the hospital, the medical chain of authority exists side by side with an administrative chain. There are many areas of confused jurisdiction and overlapping or conflicting powers. Hospital-physician cooperative efforts attempt to integrate these hierarchies. Thus physicians have become more involved in hospital governing boards; boards of trustees review the methods used to appoint physicians to hospital staffs; and more full-time salaried physicians have been hired, resulting in direct physician-hospital reporting lines (R. N. Wilson, p. 179).

Because of the vested interests of various medical departments in a hospital, and latent or open conflict with trustees or administration, the method of selecting a full-time or part-time chief of the medical staff or of medical departments is potentially explosive. To avoid controversy, in some hospitals appointments are made for a specified period of time rather than for indefinite or lifetime periods of tenure. As full-time chiefs of service become more common, many functions now handled by volunteer committees—such as utilization review, medical records, and continuing medical education—may gradually be taken over by full-time paid employees (McGill).

Many hospitals are now hiring salaried medical care directors and utilization review teams. As hospitals are made more accountable for alleged misconduct of attending physicians, they seek to have their own agents—rather than the voluntary medical staff—responsible for the quality of medical care (*Medical World News*, Oct. 1974).

As more salaried physicians are being hired by hospitals, private physicians are beginning to fear their impact. The American Medical Association reports that the number of hospital salaried physicians other than house staff doubled from 10,000 in 1963 to 20,000 in 1973. They are employed in the hospital to supervise medical care in intensive care units, outpatient departments, and medical education. Nonsalaried physicians fear competition for patients, the possibility of a closed medical staff, additional supervision of their medical care, a change in traditional patient care orientation to more emphasis on teaching and research, and reduced availability of beds (*Medical World News*, Oct. 1974).

The Economics of Hospital Operations

The hospital is the largest consumer of the health care dollar (see Chapter 9). The flow of resources into the hospital industry is subject to several constraints and is likely to be altered considerably in the future under any national health insurance program, and by increased regulation. Currently funds come from commercial and government insurance, philanthropy, private payment from a small number of patients, and various other sources of grant and contract funding for demonstrations and experiments.

Hospital costs are defined as the expenses hospitals incur in the treatment of patients.* Hospitals experience financial difficulties as a result of one or a combination of the following: (a) a decrease in volume of services sold; (b) an inability to increase charges because of constraints imposed by third-party payors; (c) poor financial planning; (d) bad management planning and control; (e) lack of coordination and cooperation between medical and administrative staffs; (f) the notion that quality is a function of cost; (g) too tight control by the board of directors, who lack adequate training or experience over the operation of the institution (Sattler and Bennett, p. 59).

If there are too many beds in a community, it is obviously impossible to have high occupancy and controlled use of hospital resources. Strategies to maximize revenues, payrolls, or prestige run counter to a general movement toward cost containment. More careful cost budgeting, consistent occupancy goals, better reporting of exceptional expenditures, and cost benefit justifica-

* It is hard to describe hospital costs further because at present there is no unit of measurement of the outcome of hospital services except in terms of patient/days. However, patient/days are not a unit of output, only a time frame in which hospital services are provided. When hospital expenses are expressed in terms of a patient/day, the result is average cost per day. Comparing the cost per patient/day in 1967 ($53.14) and in 1972 ($96.70), we find an apparent increase of 82.1%, but real hospital costs rose by about only one-half of that figure. The rest was due to inflation. The real increase results from the fact that a patient/day in 1972 involved more tests, more personnel, more education, and more diagnostic and therapeutic services than in 1967 (Raske, p. 67).

The USDHEW, after analyzing the rise in hospital unit costs over a 20-year period from 1952 to 1972, concluded that approximately half of the average annual increase in hospital unit cost was attributable to hospitals increasing the number and the quality of their labor and non-labor inputs (Raske, p. 68). In a slightly more recent study of the period 1950–1973, Worthington similarly concluded that the single most important factor in rising hospital costs is technological change, as reflected in increased real inputs (1975).

tion are all necessary for adequate financial control (Griffith, pp. 33–34).

Voluntary hospitals have traditionally acknowledged that part of their responsibility is to provide care to the medically indigent. Funds for this purpose were generated by pricing certain hospital services higher than the cost of providing them, to those who could afford to pay, so that a number of medically indigent patients could receive those services for free. Traditionally, laboratory and radiology services have been used to generate this excess revenue. Now, with 85% of patients having their hospital bills paid by a third party, which is willing to pay only the actual costs of services received, this source of revenue is rapidly disappearing. Although Medicare and Medicaid programs have reduced to some extent the number of persons seeking free care, in many states large numbers of the poor still have no source of payment. Medicaid eligibility levels are changed sporadically by state governments, and the future of the program is problematic. Thus the sources of funds used by hospitals to care for the poor are not constant. Few hospitals have endowments sufficient to finance this care; few can generate excess revenue and, for those which can, there are many other competing uses for it.

Lowering hospital costs. In this environment, there are many incentives to reduce costs. Ironically, many efforts to reduce the cost of medical care to the community increase the cost of providing medical care in the hospital. Providing care on an ambulatory basis, when possible, to avoid hospitalization, or making efforts to shorten the length of stay for hospitalized patients, increases the cost of a day of hospital care, for several reasons. Patients who do occupy hospital beds will be sicker and require more services per day. A reduction in occupancy means less expenditure by the third-party payors, which reimburse hospitals on an item-of-service basis, but it also means less revenue for the hospitals, which still have their relatively high fixed expenses. Shortening length of stay also lowers third-party expenditures, but it increases cost per patient day because more technical services have to be provided each day, on the average. As pointed out above, the only long-term way to lower costs is to reduce the capital investment and operating expenses by not building additional beds or adding new equipment, and by closing existing beds. Reimbursing hospitals for providing days of hospital care rewards them for admitting patients, not for providing a spectrum of health services which might, or might not, include hospitalization for any particular patient.

This is a complex social problem that could be partially solved by altering the financial structure used to pay for care. Decisions made would have to take into account the effect of the procedure on the patient, the cost, the patient's ability to pay, and the recommendation of his physicians. The appropriate use of high-cost technology is a central issue in providing hospital services. The number of hospitals offering special, expensive services has increased over the past decade. Facilities for open-heart surgery, radioisotope diagnosis and therapy, cobalt therapy, renal dialysis units, and computerized axial tomography have proliferated. Regional planning for the distribution of specialized, expensive hospital services has been a subject of much talk, but little action.

The Health Planning and Resources Development Act of 1974 (see Chapter 12), which could restrict payment by federal third-party payors for services rendered in nonapproved facilities and programs, may discourage implementation of technological advances that have not been proven necessary or effective. It may encourage regional planning among hospitals for the distribution of new equipment, procedures, and services on a rational basis, rather than the present all-too-common competitive approach. However, in the past, such controls have been relatively ineffective. If a hospital could justify sufficient use of such equipment to make it pay for itself, or even generate a profit, it was possible to justify it to planning agencies on the basis of adequate demand. The extent to which this demand was manufactured by the novelty of the diagnostic effort was not considered. Another approach that may have some effect is the refusal of certain private third-party payors to reimburse hospitals for the performance of expensive specialized services like open-heart surgery, if their volume of service doesn't meet minimum levels. This should encourage the closing of marginal, underutilized services with high fixed costs.

In some cases new technology does not lead to increased costs. The hospital laboratory and the accounting and materials management functions can reduce the numbers of people required to carry out work, because the materials with which the new equipment comes in contact are not living patients, but specimens or information. However, while there has been extensive automation in laboratories in the last 10 years, the absolute number of personnel has not declined: costs per test are dropping, but the total number of tests performed is increasing. Thus, the cost benefits of few productivity increases are being passed on to consumers, while the health benefits of many of them remain to be evaluated.

Obsolete facilities also add to costs. The capital needs of hospitals currently exceed $1.5 billion per year. The increased need for funds results from obsolescence of costly equipment owing to the rapid rate of technological change, the growth in demand for health care services caused by the expansion of private health insurance programs and government assistance programs, and the historic long-term growth trend in the U. S. population (M. K. Deets).

Capital costs. Capital expenditures are limited by the reimbursement formulas of Blue Cross, Medicare, and Medicaid. Capital projects must, therefore, be funded by such external sources as private grants, government grants, and long-term commercial borrowing. Of the total expenditure for hospital construction in 1973, $820 million came from government grants, philanthropy, and internal operations, while $1.35 billion came from borrowing, a ratio of 1 to 1.6 (Sattler and Bennett, p. 51). The price of capital for hospitals has been increasing, seemingly faster than prices of capital for other industries. Yet, payment of depreciation and interest costs by third parties may enable a hospital to cover the cost of expansion whether it was justified or not. Therefore, it is essential that planning agencies continue to attempt to exercise controls, including approval of capital expenditures; in the past, being subject to political pressure from health care providers, they have not been able to fulfill this responsibility (Lave and Lave, p. 63). (See also discussions of certification of need in Chapters 12 and 13.) According to an official in the New York State Health Department, real control over capital formation in the hospital industry is the single most important step in cost-control (Fleck).

Additional cost increases may be generated by universal entitlement to health care through a national health insurance program; expansion of community health services regardless of established need; patient safety and security in health facilities; adjustments or shortages in health manpower; extension of the human life span; and continuing medical innovation (Phillips, p. 75). All of these demands tend to diminish the ability of hospitals to provide the maximal range of services to all who want them. In the future hospital services could become so expensive that they will be unavailable except in absolutely life-threatening situations.

Conclusion
Problems of Hospitals

If the first problem hospitals face is costliness, the second is the imbalance in the hospital sector between acute and long-term care.

This imbalance has by no means developed accidentally:

> The mold from which today's health care system was cast took its shape around 1850. There were still relatively few general hospitals or health facilities of any type in Britain [our most important medical *organizational* forebear] and the fledgling United States, but the institutional organization of health care was already firmly established. Separate administration and staffing of the curative services—for acute, chronic, and psychiatric illnesses —became such a strong precedent that it continues even when all three components have a common source of support, as they do now in Britain. . . .
>
> As the four disparate fragments of our system for delivering care developed [acute, long-term, psychiatric, and preventive services], the voluntary hospital component was the only one whose primary institutional objective was *always* treatment of disease. Voluntary hospitals were able to cater to patients selected for certain illnesses, generally acute ones, because donors were entitled to prescribe the scope of their charity, and because a medical staff that contributed its time without remuneration could reasonably dictate the nature of its worth. Both the philanthropic trustees and the medical staffs agreed on leaving to the state the prevention of disease and the intractable problems of mental illness and chronic infirmity. . . .
>
> The contrast between the history of voluntary hospitals and that of the other three fragments of the health care system is striking. A common thread runs through the chronicle of the last three—entanglement with overwhelming numbers of people and with complex social, economic, and political problems. . . . Voluntary hospitals have been able to limit their involvement for almost 200 years, while the other three components sequestered the problems which were destined to become the main health concerns of the late 20th century (Freymann, pp. 47–48).

The third major problem concerns the mode by which most

physicians taking care of patients in hospitals are paid, and the influence which physicians have over hospital operations. The physician makes most of the decisions regarding the commitment and use of hospital resources, yet, because he is usually paid directly by the patient or his insurer, he has no direct financial relationship to the hospital, nor any responsibility for its financial status. It is as if modern school boards provided everything necessary for education except payment of the teachers, who would proceed to collect fees directly from the students, as indeed they did before the educational reforms of the mid-nineteenth century.

Fourth, hospitals have problems with vertically organized administrative structures which are not well integrated horizontally at the service levels. In many hospitals the operating divisions to which we referred earlier fall roughly into three separate vertical organizational groupings: medical staff, nursing, and support/hotel services. Within each of these structures there can be further fragmentation, e.g. the different medical services, internal medicine, surgery, pediatrics, etc., may function quite separately from each other. The vertical lines of authority may meet in the office of the director; sometimes they never meet. This kind of separation can make it very difficult to provide integrated programs of patient care in which unitary direction is needed at the functional level in order to best meet patient needs. For example, in outpatient services, it is very difficult to provide comprehensive patient-centered care when there is no coordinated leadership at the functional level of service for the medical, nursing, social work, and clerical personnel who are all essential to providing that care (Jonas, 1973).

A fifth problem is the isolation of many hospitals from the real health and medical needs of their communities. This does not apply solely to short-term general hospitals. In health terms, Freymann describes the present era as the Age of Darwin and Freud, since "most of our woes now stem from two causes: either our genetic heritage or the buffeting of our environment or both" (1974, p. 74). However, he says many health care institutions, not just short-term hospitals, are still armed primarily to fight the wars of the era immediately past, the Age of Pasteur, when "infection was the main foe of medicine" (1974, p. 13). This orientation, of course, arises not only from institutional rigidity but also from the character of medical practice, which is still largely stuck in the Age of Pasteur as well.

In most hospitals, outpatient services have a distinctly second-class status, preventive medicine is practiced to a minimal extent, home care and rehabilitation services are treated as luxuries. Community-based chronic disease control programs are not undertaken. Mental hospitals have little to do with community mental health. Proprietary nursing homes have not the least interest in dealing with the complications of aging in a positive way, since they want patients *in*, not *out*. Hospitals, and other health care institutions, with certain impressive and encouraging exceptions, to be sure, resolutely turn inwards, wishing that everyone would just go away and leave them to do their job as they see it: taking care of sick people in bed.

Solutions

Complex problems do not have simple solutions, and we do not pretend to offer panaceas. But in the context of a program of universal financial entitlement to health services, an approach to hospital reform is available. We turn once again to Freymann, who has developed the concept of the "Mission-Oriented Hospital" (1974, ch. 18).

The Mission-Oriented Hospital has two principal attributes: "(1) Each hospital has a mission defined and continuously modified by the specific needs of the community it serves. (2) Individuality and flexibility are secured by ongoing use of a rational planning process" (1974, p. 248).

The concept is based on four "theorems":

1. The need for medical *cure* that dominated men's minds from the dawn of time to the end of the Age of Pasteur will wane, but the need for total health *care* will remain.

2. Health care must be a continuum because a healthy life is a continuum from conception to death—not a vacuum punctuated by episodes of illness.

3. Since the needs of each individual vary widely, an organization meeting these needs cannot be frozen into classification by organ, by diagnosis, or by medical specialty.

4. Since the mission of the health care system is to maintain health, the system should interfere as little as possible with the functional capacity of those it serves. Ambulatory or home care are ideals; confinement to an institution must be dictated only by biologic necessity. (pp. 247–248)

Freymann recognizes that "the word 'hospital' itself presents a problem, for today it connotes a building that houses patients. I think 'hospital' could be used in a different sense—to signify a dynamic complex of facilities and skilled personnel organized to provide all types of health services" (p. 247). He points out that:

> . . . while general hospitals were originally intended only for the acutely sick, history has dictated that they become the centers about which the American health care system revolves. To consider creating new centers for the care of the well and limiting 6,000 general hospitals to their 18th Century function is to fly in the face of reality. But [to meet their new functions] they must be designed [physically and programmatically] not as enclaves but as open accessible places where the scattered fragments of the health care system can at least be brought together. (p. 212)

To accomplish this goal, we must end the "tyranny of the bed" (pp. 197–223, 249). In this "tyranny," as we have seen in this chapter, the principal measures of what a hospital is, and does, are related to beds—that is, admissions, length of stay, occupancy, average daily census, and bed-days of care, rather than to any measures of illness or health.

The mission-oriented approach would in fact make the hospital into a *health* center rather than an *illness* center. The hospital would relate to the needs of its community in a rational, planned, dynamic manner. By definition, the acute/chronic/preventive distinctions would become things of the past. Cost problems would be dealt with directly because we already know from group practice experience that in reasonably comprehensive ambulatory care, even without special prevention programs, where there is no special incentive for physicians to hospitalize patients, hospitalization rates are significantly lowered.

The present-day administrative problems would not be automatically resolved by a mission-oriented approach. However, they would have to be solved in order to accomplish mission-orientation. Mission-orientation demands an administrative structure that is functionally decentralized to operate integrated programs requiring staff teams at the patient-care level, not one which has vertically organized reporting lines separating health care providers into independent hierarchies.

The challenge of implementing mission-orientation lies in finding the doctors who can do it. To change hospitals to mission-orientation will require "mission-oriented" physicians who can understand health and illness in populations as well as in individuals, and can see patients in their socioeconomic context. But the bulk of medical training takes place in our present-day, inward-directed hospitals. How to break out of this vicious circle is a separate discussion (Jonas, in press). But the future is bright; solutions and resources are available. All we need is to summon the will.

References

American Hospital Association. *Annual Report.* May, 1975.
————. "Are There Too Many Hospital Beds?" *Hospitals, J.A.H.A.,* April 1, 1975, p. 17.
————. *A Critique of the Public Citizen Health Research Group Report $8 Billion Hospital Bed Overrun.* Chicago, Ill.: Bureau of Research Services, July 1975.
American Medical News. "Unnecessary Surgery." February 9, 1976.
Andersen, R., et al. *Equity in Health Services: Empirical Analyses in Social Policy.* Cambridge, Mass.: Ballinger Publishing Co., 1975.
Austin, C. J. "Emerging Roles and Responsibilities in Health Adminis-tration." In *Education for Health Administration,* Vol. 1, pp. 137–151. Ann Arbor, Mich.: Health Administration Press, 1975.
Beaudry, M. L., Sr. "Broadening the Institution's Health Care Base." *Hospital Progress,* March, 1975, pp. 66–69.
Belsky, M., and Gross, L. *Beyond the Medical Mystique: How to Choose and Use Your Doctor.* New York: Arbor House, 1975.
Berki, E. *Hospital Economics.* Lexington, Mass.: D. C. Heath, 1972.
Beyers, C. "Are Public Hospitals Headed for the Scrap Heap?" *Prism,* November, 1974, p. 21.
Blake, E., and Bodenheimer, T. *Closing the Doors on the Poor: The Dismantling of California's County Hospitals.* San Francisco, Calif.: Health/PAC, 1975.
Blue Cross/Blue Shield of Greater New York. "Just How Much Hospi-tal Does This City Need?" *New York Times,* August 24, 1976.
Booz, Allen, Hamilton. *Management Memorandum on Hospital Fran-chising.* Chicago: Ill., April, 1973.
Brown, J. H. "Delivery of Personal Health Services and Medical Serv-ices for the Poor." *The Milbank Memorial Fund Quarterly, 46,* 211, 1968.
Brown, M., and Money, W. "The Promise of Multihospital Manage-ment." *Hospital Progress,* August/September, 1975, p. 36.
Brown, R. E. "Forces and Fallacies Affecting the Public Hospital." *Proceedings of the Booz, Allen & Hamilton Seminar on the Public Hospital.* January, 1970.

Bunker, J. P. "Surgical Manpower." *New England Journal of Medicine,* *282,* 135, 1970.

Commission on Professional and Hospital Activities. *Length of Stay in PAS Hospitals U.S., 1972.* Ann Arbor, Mich., 1973.

Comptroller General of the United States. *Study of Health Facilities Construction Costs.* Washington, D.C.: Government Printing Office, 1972.

Davis, S., and Henshaw, S. *Decision Analysis in Hospital Administration.* Washington, D. C.: Association of University Programs in Health Administration, 1974.

Deets, M. K. "The Financial Gap: The Concept of Leverage in Hospital Building Program." *Hospital Progress,* May, 1972, p. 62.

de Schweinitz, K. *England's Road to Social Security.* New York: 1943. Reprinted, A. S. Barnes and Co. Perpetual Edition, 1961.

Dobkin, J. "Health Care in the 1980's: What Should Hospitals Do Today?" *The Hospital Medical Staff,* December, 1975, pp. 30–36.

Donabedian, A. "An Evaluation of Prepaid Group Practice." *Inquiry, 6,* 1969.

Donabedian, A. *Aspects of Medical Care Administration.* Cambridge, Mass.: Harvard University Press, 1973.

Doody, M. "Guidelines for Implementing Cooperative Programs/A Review." *Hospitals, J.A.H.A.,* June 1, 1974, p. 55.

Dornblaser, B. M. "The Social Responsibility of General Hospitals." *Hospital Administration,* Spring, 1970, p. 6.

Duff, S., and Hollingshead, A. *Sickness and Society.* New York: Harper and Row, 1968.

Emanuel, W. J. "Hospital Policy: Professional Associations as Unions." *Hospital Progress,* January, 1976, p. 51.

Ensminger, B. *The $8 Billion Hospital Bed Overrun.* Washington, D.C.: Public Citizen's Health Research Group, 1975.

Fabro, J. A. "Full-Time Physicians in Hospitals." *Medical World News,* October 4, 1974, p. 41.

Fleck, A. Personal communication. March 7, 1975.

Freymann, J. G. *The American Health Care System: Its Genesis and Trajectory.* New York: Medcom Press, 1974.

Garber, S. "Development: Annual Administrative Review." *Hospitals, J.A.H.A.,* April 1, 1975, p. 61.

Gaus, C. R. et al. "Contrasts in HMO and Fee-for-Service Performance." *Social Security Bulletin,* May, 1976, p. 3.

Georgeopoulos, B. *The Community General Hospital.* New York: Macmillan, 1962.

Georgeopoulos, B., ed. *Organization Research on Health Institutions.* Ann Arbor, Mich.: University of Michigan Press, 1971.

"Getting Ready for National Health Insurance: Unnecessary Surgery." Hearings before the Subcommittee on Oversight and Investigations of the Committee on Interstate and Foreign Commerce,

House of Representatives. Washington, D. C.: July 15, 17, 18 and September 3, 1975.

Ginzberg, E. *A Pattern for Hospital Care.* New York: Columbia University Press, 1949.

Griffith, J., Hancock, W. M., and Munson, F. C. "Practical Ways to Contain Hospital Costs." *Hospital Financial Management*, January, 1975, p. 46.

Haughton, J. C. "Role of the Public General Hospital in Community Health." *American Journal of Public Health, 65*, 21, 1975.

Health Law Center. *Problems in Hospital Law.* Rockville, Md.: Aspen Systems Corporation, 1974.

Health Perspectives. "Profile of Governing Bodies of New York City Voluntary Hospitals." Nov. 73–Jan. 74.

"Health Philanthrophy Registers a 2.6 Percent Gain in 1974." *Hospitals, J.A.H.A.*, March 16, 1976, p. 29.

Health Research Group-Public Citizen. *Consumer Health Action Network*, January, 1976, p. 7.

Hellinger, F. J. "Hospital Charges and Medicare Reimbursement." *Inquiry, 12*, 313, 1975.

"Hospital Indicators." *Hospitals, J. A. H. A.*, April 16, 1976, p.45.

"Health Care in the 1980's: What Should Hospitals Do Today?" *The Hospital Medical Staff*, December, 1975, p. 30.

Hospital Statistics, 1975 Edition. Chicago, Ill.: American Hospital Association, 1975.

Jonas, S. "Some Thoughts on Primary Care: Problems in Implementation." *International Journal of Health Services, 3*, 177, 1973.

Jonas, S. *The Health-Oriented Physician: The Future of Medical Education in the United States.* New York: W. W. Norton, in press.

Kernaghan, S. G., and Manzano, A. "The Complex Face of Charity." *Hospitals, J.A.H.A.*, June 1, 1975, p. 47.

Kessler, R. "A Profile of the Hospital Trustee." *Trustee*, January, 1975, p. 21.

Klarman, H. E. *The Economics of Health.* New York: Columbia University Press, 1965.

Lave, R., and Lave, L. *The Hospital Construction Act.* Washington, D. C.: American Enterprise Institute for Public Policy Research, 1974.

Letourneau, C. U. "A History of Hospitals." *Journal of the International College of Surgeons, 35*, 527, 1961.

Letourneau, C. U. *The Hospital Medical Staff.* Chicago, Ill.: Starling Publications, 1964.

Lewis, C. E. "Variations in the Incidence of Surgery." *New England Journal of Medicine, 281*, 880, 1969.

McCarthy, E. G., and Widmer, G. W. "Effects of Screening by Consultants on Recommended Elective Surgical Procedures." *New England Journal of Medicine, 291*, 1331, 1974.

MacEachern, M. T. *Hospital Organization and Management.* Berwyn, Ill.: Physician's Record Co., 1962.

McGill, C. S. "A Look Into the Hospital of the Future." *Trustee,* December, 1974, p. 14.

McMahon, J. A. "How Much Care Can We Afford?" *Prism,* October, 1974, p. 17.

Medical World News. "Full-Time Physicians in Hospitals." Oct. 4, 1974, p. 41.

————. " 'More Beds than We Need,' AHA Admits." November 8, 1974, p. 114.

————. "How Much Unnecessary Surgery?" May 3, 1976, p. 50.

Modern Hospital. "Power to the Coalitions: Experts See New Balance of Health Care Forces." April, 1970, p. 39.

Moreland Act Commission. *Regulating Nursing Home Care: The Paper Tigers.* Albany, N.Y., October, 1975.

Mott, A., and Chalk, A. "The Board Structure Has to Change!" *Trustee,* January, 1975, p. 28.

National Center for Health Statistics. *Health Resources Statistics: Health Manpower and Health Facilities, 1974.* Rockville, Md.: USDHEW, 1974.

————. "1973–74 Nursing Home Survey—Provisional Data." *Monthly Vital Statistics Report,* September 5, 1974.

————. "Utilization of Short-Stay Hospitals, by Diagnosis: United States, 1973." *Monthly Vital Statistics Report,* Vol. 24, No. 3, Supp. (2), June 10, 1975.

————. *Health, United States, 1975.* USDHEW Pub. No. (HRA) 76–1232. Washington, D. C.: Government Printing Office, 1976.

Newsday. "Poll Shows LI Hospital Conflicts." February 27, 1976.

————. "60 Doing Business as Hospital Trustees." March 15, 1976.

New York Times. "Hospitals Lax on Conflict of Interest Data." December 26, 1975.

————. "Incompetent Surgery Is Not Found Isolated." January 27, 1976.

————. "Hospitals Resist a Trustee Conflict-of-Interest Bill." April 18, 1976.

————. "Care at Lincoln Hospital Scored." July 30, 1976.

Phelps, Charles E. "Effects of Insurance on Demand for Medical Care." In *Equity in Health Services.* Anderson, R., Kravits, J., and Anderson, O., Eds. Cambridge, Mass.: Ballinger Publishing Co., 1975.

Phillips, D. F. "American Hospitals: A Look Ahead." *Hospitals, J.A.H.A.,* January 1, 1976, p. 73.

Pointer, D. D. "How the 1974 Taft-Hartley Amendments Will Affect Health Care Facilities." *Hospital Progress,* October, 1974, p. 68.

Raske, K. E. "The Components of Inflation." *Hospitals, J.A.H.A.,* July 1, 1974, p. 34.

Reidel, D. C. et al. *Federal Employees Health Benefits Program Utilization Study.* USDHEW Pub. No. (HRA) 75–3125. Washington, D.C.: Government Printing Office, 1975.

"Rising Hospital Costs . . . A Look at the Causes." *The Volunteer Leader,* March, 1973, p. 4.

Roemer, M. "Bed Supply and Hospital Utilization: A Natural Experiment." *Hospitals, J.A.H.A.,* November, 1961.

Roemer, M, and Shonick, R. "HMO Performance: The Recent Evidence." *Health and Society, 51,* 271, 1973.

Rogatz, P. M. "Excessive Hospitalization Can Be Cut Back." *Journal of the American Hospital Association,* August 1, 1974, p. 51.

Rogatz, P. M. "Let's Get Rid of those Surplus Hospital Beds." *Prism,* October, 1974, p. 13.

Rushing, W. "Differences in Profit and Nonprofit Organizations: A Study in Effectiveness and Efficiency in General Short-Stay Hospitals." *Administrative Science Quarterly, 19,* 474, 1974.

Sattler, F. L. "A Rational Look at the Hospital and Debt Financing." *Hospital Topics,* Jan./Feb., 1975, p. 18.

Sattler, F. L., and Bennett, M. D. *A Statistical Profile of Short-Term Hospitals in the United States as of 1973.* Minneapolis, Minn.: Interstudy, 1975.

Shain, M., and Roemer, M. I. "Hospitals and the Public Interest." *Public Health Reports, 76,* 401, 1961.

Sloan, F. A. *Determinants of Hospital Wage Inflation.* Washington, D. C.: National Center for Health Services Research, 1974.

Snoke, A. W. "A Blueprint for Change." *Hospitals, J.A.H.A.,* July 1, 1974, p. 61.

Somers, A. *Hospital Regulation: The Dilemma of Public Policy.* Princeton, N.J.: Princeton University Press, 1969.

Somers, H. M., and Somers, A. *Medicare and the Hospital.* Washington, D. C.: The Brookings Institution. 1967.

Stephenson, H. R. "Hospital Trusteeship." *Hospitals, J.A.H.A.,* December 16, 1963, p. 38.

Stern, B. J. *Medical Services by Government.* New York: The Commonwealth Fund, 1946.

Stevens, R. *American Medicine and the Public Interest.* New Haven, Conn.: Yale University Press, 1971.

Stine, O. C., and Pickard, R. "Regional Perinatal Centers in Maryland." *Maryland State Medical Jounral, 23,* 46, 1974.

Subcommittee on Long-Term Care. *Nursing Home Care in the United States: Failure in Public Policy.* Special Committee on Aging, U. S. Senate, November, 1974.

Temporary State Commission on Living Costs and the Economy. *Report on Nursing Homes and Health Related Facilities in New York State.* Albany, N.Y., April, 1975.

Thomas, W. C. *Nursing Homes and Public Policy: Drift and Decision in New York State.* Ithaca, N.Y.: Cornell University Press, 1969.

Wasyluka, R. G. "New Blood for Tired Hospitals." *Harvard Business Review,* September-October, 1970, p. 65.

Welham, W. F., and Judnich, F. A. *A Comparison of Patient Length of Stay: Military versus Civilian Health Care Delivery Abstract.* In *Government Reports Announcement, 74,* 45, 1974.

Williams, L. *How to Avoid Unnecessary Surgery.* Nash Publishing, 1971.

Wilson, J. Q. "Innovation in Organization: Notes Toward a Theory." In Thompson, J., Ed., *Approaches to Organizational Design.* Pittsburgh, Pa.: University of Pittsburgh Press, 1966.

Wilson, R. N. "The Physician's Changing Hospital Roles." *Human Organization,* Winter, 1959–60, p. 179.

Worthington, N. L. "Expenditures for Hospital Care and Physicians' Services: Factors Affecting Annual Changes." *Social Security Bulletin,* November, 1975, p. 3.

8

Mental Health Services

Lorrin M. Koran

Introduction

Despite great progress in the past quarter century, the delivery of mental health care, like the delivery of general health care, is beset by many difficulties. The pluralistic nature of the service delivery system creates certain problems: inequitable access based on geography, class, and diagnosis; inadequate coordination of different phases of care; fragmented planning, evaluation, and regulation; and insufficient coordination with such other human services as general medicine, education, and welfare. Other difficulties stem from our inability to cure many mental disorders, from limited manpower, and from inadequate community-based treatment facilities. The social stigma attached to mental patients, public apathy toward them and resistance to placing services in "good" neighborhoods also hamper care. Finally, many mental health professionals are dealing with extraordinarily complex problems, especially when working with groups affected by poverty and racism.

The challenge of the 1970s and 1980s is to find ways to resolve these difficulties. To help the reader participate in the search, this chapter will discuss the forms of mental disorder; the kinds of mental health care; the history of that care in the United States, the prevalence of mental disorders; mental health manpower; the delivery of services; insurance coverage; and legal issues.

The Forms of Mental Disorder

The Diagnostic and Statistical Manual of Mental Disorders of the American Psychiatric Association (DSM-II, 1968) includes over 140 different "mental disorders" grouped in the following 10 categories.

1. mental retardation (subnormal general intellectual func-

tioning associated with impaired learning ability and/or impaired social maturation)
2. organic brain syndromes (disorders caused by or associated with impairment of brain tissue function, e.g., dementia)
3. psychoses with no known physical pathology (characterized by disordered perception, thinking, emotions, and/or behavior, e.g., schizophrenia)
4. neuroses (characterized by anxiety and psychological defenses against anxiety, e.g., obsessive-compulsive neurosis)
5. personality disorders, including sexual deviations, alcoholism, and drug dependence (characterized by deeply ingrained patterns of maladaptive behavior, e.g., paranoid personality)
6. psychophysiologic disorders (characterized by physical symptoms caused by emotional factors, e.g., peptic ulcer)
7. special symptoms, e.g., sleep disorders
8. transient situational disturbances (acute reactions to overwhelming environmental stress in people without apparent underlying mental disorder)
9. behavior disorders of childhood and adolescence
10. conditions without manifest psychiatric disorder, e.g., marital maladjustments.

Some of these conditions may be deviant behaviors rather than illness. For example, the American Psychiatric Association removed homosexuality from its manual of mental disorders in 1975. Indeed, a few mental health professionals believe all mental disorders are social myths (Szasz), but the reasoning and evidence to the contrary are powerfully convincing (Murphy; Kendall).

"Mental health care" encompasses diverse preventive, therapeutic, and rehabilitative activities. Preventive mental health care aims to promote mental health and prevent specific mental disorders. The first objective is difficult to attain because it is vague—few people agree on exactly what "mental health" is. The second has met with some success; such disorders as syphilitic dementia and pellagrinous psychoses, for example, are now widely prevented. The effectiveness of efforts to prevent functional mental disorders such as neuroses and alcoholism through school programs and other means remains unproven (Zusman).

Therapeutic mental health services include individual, family, and group psychotherapies; hypnosis; psychodrama; milieu therapy; medications; electroconvulsive therapy; and psycho-surgery. *Psychotherapies* rely primarily on structured conversation to change patients' attitudes, feelings, beliefs, defenses, personality, and/or behavior. The therapist's procedures vary with his school of psychotherapy and with the nature of the patient's problem: a situational crisis is handled differently from a long-standing problem in interpersonal relations. Psychoanalysis, for example, employs techniques such as dream interpretation, free association, and interpretations based on psychoanalytic theory to bring about personality restructuring. Most forms of psychotherapy, however, have much in common (Frank). Psychotherapy, *hypnosis* and *psychodrama* are generally used to treat mental disorders other than psychoses and organic brain syndromes. *Milieu therapy* involves arranging the physical setting and social organization of an inpatient ward to encourage socially acceptable and responsible behavior. Most *drugs* effective in treating mental disorders have been available for only 10 to 20 years. These include phenothiazines and other drugs for schizophrenia; tricyclic and monoamine oxidase inhibitors (MAOI) for treating depression; lithium for manic-depressive psychosis; and benzodiazepines for anxiety states. Amphetamine has been used to treat hyperactive children since the 1930s. *Electroconvulsive therapy*, which is effective in treating certain forms of depression, schizophrenia, and mania, was introduced in 1938 (Kalinowsky and Hippius, p. 3). *Psychosurgery* (neurosurgical operations for mental disorders) was widely used to treat schizophrenia in the late 1940s and early 1950s, but is rarely used today, and then usually as a treatment of last resort (Sweet; Bernstein et al.)

Rehabilitative mental health care includes occupational therapy and re-education to help the patient return to normal living patterns. It may begin in an inpatient setting with patient government and social activities, and can progress through transitional settings such as halfway houses, group homes, or supervised apartments. Rehabilitative care is usually required only for patients with psychoses, drug addiction, or alcoholism.

Brief History of Mental Health Care in the United States

The mentally disordered in colonial America were slightly better treated than their European counterparts: fewer were tortured, burned, hanged, or drowned as witches. The Salem witch trials of 1691–92, during which 250 persons were tried and 19 executed, were an exception, not the rule. Throughout the colonial period most mentally ill people were kept at home or wandered from town to town where they were lodged in jails or almshouses (workhouses). This remained the pattern until the 1840s (Shryock).

As early as 1756, however, mentally ill patients were admitted to the newly established Pennsylvania Hospital, and in 1773 the first American mental asylum was established under government auspices in Williamsburg, Virginia. These two institutions marked the beginnings of humanitarian treatment of mentally disordered patients in America, although some treatments administered within their walls until the early 1800s seem barbaric—bloodletting, purges, and emetics.

In the early 1800s, the Quakers and American physicians exposed to European psychiatry encouraged the view that mental illness could be treated and espoused kind and sympathetic methods. Partly as a result, a few mental hospitals were opened where "moral treatment" (combining work, recreation, education, and kind but firm management) was predominant (Bockoven). Violent patients, however, were segregated in separate wards, and in most of the country mentally disordered paupers and blacks were sent to workhouses and jails (Mora). In 1841 Dorothea Dix began her successful 30-year crusade to encourage states to build hospitals specifically for the care of the mentally ill. Many mental hospitals were built, usually in rural areas since the countryside was believed to provide refuge from noxious urban and familial influences. Despite Dix's successes, the quality of care in state mental hospitals rapidly declined. Outright neglect and custodial care were fostered by the overcrowding of the hospitals with criminals, alcoholics, vagrants, and state paupers, by a tendency to build larger institutions to keep expenditures down, and by an increasing pessimism regarding the curability of mental disorders. Since mental hospitals were located away from population centers, the dismal conditions within them were easily ignored for a time. In the 1870s and 1880s a wave of reform began, with criticisms of commitment procedures, the use of restraints, and the low level of staff training (Deutsch). Between 1890 and 1900 New York State reformed its institutions for mental patients, but its example was not widely followed.

In 1908 Clifford Beers, a former mental patient, exposed the cruel conditions in public and private asylums with his autobiography, *A Mind That Found Itself.* Together with William

James, Adolf Meyer, and others, Beers helped launch the
National Committee for Mental Hygiene, which lobbied on behalf
of the mentally disordered and carried out a national census of
institutionalized mental patients until the Bureau of the Census
took over in 1923. During World War I, the Surgeon General's
Office asked the National Committee to organize the psychiatric
branch of the Army Medical Corps. For many years the Committee surveyed conditions in mental hospitals. (Inspection and
accreditation of mental hospitals was not undertaken by the Joint
Committee on Accreditation of Hospitals, the accrediting body
for general hospitals, until 1958.)

At the beginning of this century, mental health care was primarily hospital-based and biologically oriented regarding etiology
and treatment. During World War I, however, the contributions
of psychological and social influences to etiology and treatment
were forcibly brought home to professionals and the public alike.
Thousands of men were rejected for service because of psycho-
neuroses. War neuroses ("shell shock") accounted for a large
proportion of psychiatric casualties. Psychiatrists saw that situational stress could precipitate a mental disorder in "normal" individuals as well as in those with "psychopathic constitutions."
Psychological and social influences techniques were soon widely
employed by military psychiatrists to treat war neuroses and
return soldiers to the front (Strecker). Early intervention prevented chronic disability. These lessons were lost on the military
until World War II, but psychiatrists carried them back into
civilian life.

In the 1920s the mental hygiene movement, nurtured by the
National Committee for Mental Hygiene and strengthened by the
psychological theories of Freud and experience gained in World
War I, captured the popular imagination. As Deutsch writes,

> Enthusiasm for mental hygiene swept the social work field. . . .
> [There was an] accelerated trend toward organizing mental
> hygiene clinics in the community. Most of them were connected
> with mental hospitals; some were attached to outpatient depart-
> ments of general hospitals or to social agencies, courts, and
> correctional institutions; some were independently created. . . .
> the movement was oversold by overenthusiastic converts who
> advanced mental hygiene as a sure cure for practically every ill
> that beset the world. . . . (pp. 362–363)

In the 1930s the mental hygiene movement slowed under the
weight of the Depression, the limited scientific knowledge regard-

ing prevention of mental disorders, and conflicts among various schools of psychiatric theory.

Between 1910 and World War II, psychoanalysis gradually came to dominate psychiatric training, outpatient care, and popular views of the nature of man. It did little, however, for severely disturbed individuals who, for the most part, remained in poorly funded, sparsely staffed, biologically oriented, custodial state institutions. In the 1930s, new hope for these severely disturbed patients was raised by the discovery of new biological treatments —insulin coma, cardiazol convulsive treatments, electroconvulsive therapy, and psychosurgery. The Public Works Administration added more than 60,000 beds to state and local mental institutions.

World War II again focused public attention on mental disorders: 1.75 million men were rejected for service because of mental or emotional disturbances and a large number of veterans returned with emotional problems. In 1946 Congress passed the National Mental Health Act, which established the National Institute of Mental Health (NIMH) and gave new federal support for mental health services, training, and research. The Veterans' Administration established psychiatric hospitals and outpatient clinics. Most inpatient treatment, however, still took place in state institutions whose deplorable conditions were graphically described by two journalists, Mike Gorman and Albert Deutsch. Partly to compensate for limited professional manpower, institutions and outpatient clinics began to use group psychotherapy which allowed one professional to treat many patients at once.

By the mid-1950s, the number of persons hospitalized in state and county mental hospitals reached its peak, 558,900. At the same time, however, effective drugs for treating schizophrenia and mania were discovered (reserpine and chlorpromazine). These drugs replaced insulin coma and psychosurgery and allowed many patients to behave more acceptably in institutions, to leave them, or to avoid hospitalization entirely. Effective drug treatment stimulated the introduction of milieu therapy, halfway houses, and aftercare.

In 1955 Congress established the Joint Commission on Mental Illness and Health, representing 36 organizations, to examine American mental health care. The Commission's 1961 report, *Action for Mental Health,* concluded that half the patients in the state mental hospitals were not receiving active treatment. The Commission's recommendations set the stage for the emphasis on community mental health that marked the 1960s. The Commission recommended establishing one fully staffed community mental health clinic per 50,000 citizens, limiting the bed complement of psychiatric hospitals to a maximum 1,000, and employing only brief and local inpatient care.

Many of the Commission's recommendations were incorporated in a 1963 Message to Congress by President John F. Kennedy, the first presidential message Congress had ever received on behalf of the mentally ill and the mentally retarded. Congress responded with the Mental Retardation Facilities and Community Mental Health Centers Construction Act, which, in part, created federal support for community-based mental health services delivered by community mental health centers. The 1960s also saw the introduction of additional effective drug treatments for mental disorders—benzodiazepines for anxiety, tricyclic and MAO-inhibiting drugs for certain depressions, and lithium for manic-depressive psychosis. Behavior therapy became popular for treating certain neuroses and behavior disorders, and research to identify the effective elements in various psychotherapies blossomed. Congress continued to expand the NIMH financial support for psychiatric and behavioral science research, psychiatric education in medical schools, residency training of psychiatrists, and community mental health centers.

Currently, mental health professionals have evidence that some forms of psychotherapy are effective for specific mental disorders (Bergin; Malan; Weissman et al.). Effective drugs are available for treating many mental disorders (Davis and Cole; Cole and Davis 1975a and b; Fieve). The number of patients in state mental hospitals today is less than 40 percent of the number in 1955, and mental health care is widely available in many different organized care settings. Learning theory and public health concepts as well as psychoanalytic and biological theories are guiding mental health care planning. Unfortunately, however, patients still in need of care are being discharged from state hospitals, for fiscal reasons, into communities that are ill prepared to provide them with the supportive services they require.

The Prevalence of Mental Disorders

Epidemiological studies of the prevalence of mental disorders have encountered the same problems as epidemiologic studies of somatic diseases—deciding what constitutes a "case," establishing operational diagnostic criteria, choosing a method of case-finding.

For these reasons, prevalence estimates for mental disorders have varied widely. A review of community surveys of mental disorder carried out before 1960 found one-day prevalence rates ranging from 3,640 to 33,300 per 100,000 population (Plunkett and Gordon, p. 90). A later review found estimates of psychiatric morbidity in North American and European studies ranging from about 1% to 64% of the population (Dohrenwend and Dohrenwend, p. 10). Estimates of the prevalence of psychoses like schizophrenia vary less widely, perhaps because the diagnostic criteria, though variable, are considerably less variable than those for "mental disorder" in general. Estimates of the prevalence of schizophrenia in a variety of populations range from 0.7 to 7.0 per 1,000 population, with most estimates much nearer the 0.7 figure (Gruenberg and Turns).

Instead of estimating the prevalence of mental disorder, one can estimate the proportion of the population disabled by mental disorder. The National Center for Health Statistics (NCHS) estimated (based on household survey data) that 0.2% of the ambulatory population over age 18 in 1969 were severely disabled by mental illness. But the survey questionnaire promoted under-reporting and interviewees were apparently reluctant to admit to having received psychiatric care (NIMH, 1976, Series B, No. 7, p. 14). By correcting for these sources of under-reporting, a recent study estimated that the prevalence of any degree of disability arising from mental disorder in the NCHS survey population was 2.5%, and the prevalence of severe disability was 0.92% (NIMH, 1976, Series B, No. 7).

Mental Health Manpower

Health professionals serving the mentally disordered include psychiatrists, nonpsychiatric physicians, psychologists, social workers, and registered nurses. In addition, services are provided by vocational rehabilitation counselors, occupational therapists, teachers, and by other health workers such as licensed practical nurses. In January 1972, an NIMH survey identified 420,000 filled staff positions in 3,200 mental health facilities in the United States (NIMH, 1973, Series B, No. 6). The distribution of mental health professionals working in these facilities is shown by profession in Table 8.1. About a third were professional patient-care staff, a third other patient-care staff, and a third nonpatient-care staff. Combining part-time and full-time staff into full-time equivalent (FTE) staff, about 83% of FTE staff were

Table 8.1

**Distribution of Staff Positions by Discipline and Status,
U.S. Mental Health Facilities, January 1972**

Discipline	All Staff	Full-time	Part-time	Trainee
Psychiatrists	16.3%	8.1%	30.8%	31.5%
Nonpsychiatric physicians	4.8	3.3	7.4	8.0
Psychologists	10.7	8.4	13.2	18.2
Social workers	17.2	18.4	12.9	18.6
Registered nurses	27.9	33.6	18.9	15.0
Other mental health prof.	16.0	19.5	10.7	7.9
Physical health professionals	7.1	8.7	6.1	0.8
Total prof. patient care staff	100.0%	100.0%	100.0%	100.0%

Source: NIMH, *Staffing of Mental Health Facilities—United States 1972* (Mental Health Statistics, Series B, No. 6), Table D.

employed in public facilities and 17% in private facilities. State and county mental hospitals accounted for almost 60% of FTE staff.

Psychiatrists

Psychiatrists are physicians with postgraduate training, usually a year's medical or other internship followed by three years of psychiatric residency training. Psychoanalytic psychiatrists (analysts) undergo additional years of part-time didactic education, a personal psychoanalysis, and supervision of their analytic treatment cases before being certified by a psychoanalytic institute. About 10% of psychiatrists are psychoanalysts. About 50% have passed examinations entitling them to be certified in psychiatry by the American Board of Psychiatry and Neurology.

By 1973 about 19,000 psychiatrists had completed training in adult psychiatry and an additional 2,268 were trained in child psychiatry (National Center for Health Statistics, 1974, p. 178). The primary professional activity of about half of psychiatrists was office-based practice, with the other half devoting most of their time to full-time hospital work, or to a mixture or teaching, research, and administration. The distribution of psychiatrist and other professional positions in mental health facilities is shown in Table 8.2. Of full-time psychiatrist positions in 1971, almost half were in state and county mental hospitals.

Like other physicians, psychiatrists are geographically maldistributed, ranging from one psychiatrist per 4,400 people in New York and one per 5,100 in Massachusetts to one per 40,500 in Alabama and one per 45,100 in South Dakota (in 1973)

Table 8.2

**Distribution of All Positions by Discipline and Type of Facility,
U.S. Mental Health Facilities, January 1972**

FACILITY	Psychiatrist	Psychologist	Social Worker	Registered Nurse	"Other Professional"
			POSITION		
State & county mental hospitals	25.3%	20.6%	25.6%	39.8%	38.8%
Private mental hospitals	7.6	2.9	2.4	9.1	4.9
VA psychiatric services	5.1	8.6	5.9	14.5	15.0
General Hospital psychiatric services	29.4	13.0	12.3	23.7	9.3
Outpatient psychiatric services	17.8	33.7	27.8	2.4	6.2
CHMCs	12.2	17.1	16.9	9.6	11.4
Residential treatment centers	2.6	4.1	9.1	0.9	14.4
All facilities	100.0%	100.0%	100.0%	100.0%	100.0%

Source: NIMH, *Staffing of Mental Health Facilities—United States 1972* (Mental Health Statistics, Series B, No. 6).

(Marmor, p. xiv). Within states, psychiatrists are more concentrated in urban areas than the general population. They are somewhat more maldistributed across the 50 states than pediatricians, internists, and surgeons (Marmor, p. xiv).

Psychologists

Psychologists are nonmedical professionals who may have either a master's or a doctorate degree in one of several kinds of psychology—experimental, social, general, or clinical (Shakow). Only psychologists trained in clinical psychology programs must have supervised clinical experience. Because most states license individuals generically as psychologists, any psychologist, regardless of training, can open a private practice (Meltzer). Private practice has not been the primary professional activity of most clinical psychologists (National Center for Health Statistics, 1974, p. 268). By 1975, however, psychologists were lobbying the federal and state governments for legislation to allow third-party payments to psychologists without requiring physician referral or supervision (Meltzer).

Psychologists working in mental health facilities carry out psychotherapy, research, teaching, and administrative duties, and offer consultation to other human service agencies. Some strain exists between psychiatrists and psychologists regarding the qualifications necessary for practicing psychotherapy. On the one hand, a medical education is not needed to be a skilled psychotherapist or to counsel or treat physically well individuals whose mental disorders do not require medications. But only physicians can prescribe indicated psychotherapeutic drugs, knowledgeably treat the large proportion of psychiatric patients who suffer from both organic illnesses and mental disorder (Herridge; Maguire and Granville-Grossman; Babigian and Odoroff), and be relied upon to recognize organic diseases masquerading behind mental symptoms (Wingfield; Rossman).

Social Workers

Social workers may have a bachelor's, master's or doctorate degree in social work. In 1972, 70% of social workers in psychiatric facilities had a master's or doctorate degree (NIMH, 1973, Series B, No. 6). Social work programs are accredited by the Council on Social Work Education. By 1973 only 11 states, however, licensed social workers (NCHS, 1974, p. 283).

Psychiatric social work received great impetus from the mental hygiene movement and child guidance clinics of the 1920s and 1930s. The social worker obtained diagnostic information concerning the child, his parents, and environment from the child's parents, pooled this information with the psychologist and psychiatrist, and then carried out therapy with the child's parents (Modlin). Today psychiatric social workers bring resources of community health and welfare agencies to bear on their patients' problems; continue in their diagnostic and therapeutic roles; offer consultation to human service agencies; and, to a limited degree, engage in research, teaching, and administration.

Registered Nurses

Some training in psychiatric nursing is part of all general nursing programs. A small percentage of registered nurses pursue specialized training in psychiatric nursing or other fields at the master's or doctorate level. Psychiatric nursing education was stimulated by the availability of federal funds under the 1946 Mental Health Act and by the introduction of psychotherapeutic drugs in the 1950s (O'Toole). By 1972 registered nurses were the largest group providing professional patient care in mental health facilities (NIMH, 1973, Series B, No. 6). Moreover, nurses generally spend more time with patients in inpatient facilities than members of any other mental health discipline.

The roles of psychiatric nurses include supervising patients' interactions on the ward; administering medications; assisting in somatic treatments; assisting patients with activities of daily living; and, in some instances, engaging in individual, group, or family therapy. Psychiatric nurses with advanced training participate in research, teaching, and administration and offer consultation to nurses and others working in medical wards and public health agencies (O'Toole).

Training Mental Health Manpower

In 1947, when the federal government began NIMH funding of mental health manpower training, there were only 3,000 psychiatrists in the United States. By 1973, there were 25,000. In 1970 the Nixon Administration concluded that there were enough mental health professionals of all kinds and announced its intention to phase out federal support. The mental health professions, supported by lay mental health organizations, argued before Congress against this policy decision. Barton (1972) pointed out that if federal support for psychiatry training were withdrawn, almost half the psychiatric residency positions in medical schools would be lost. Psychiatry cannot generate substantial training

funds, as do most other medical specialties, from insurance benefits for care because insurance coverage for psychiatric services
is much more limited. The Ford Administration has continued
attempts to phase out federal support for mental health manpower training. If this occurs or a federal loan proposal is
adopted (Torrey), psychiatry training will be at a severe disad-
vantage, and funds to support training of psychologists, psychiatric social workers, and psychiatric nurses will decline sharply.

Are more mental health professionals needed? Certain observations suggest that they are—the high prevalence of mental disorders, together with estimates of the number of patients a psychiatrist can treat in a year (Sharfstein, et al.) ; the disparity in
patient-care staffing ratios between public and private mental
health facilities (NIMH, 1973, Series B, No. 6) ; the need to rely
on foreign medical graduates to fill 40% of physician positions in
state mental hospitals in New York and Ohio and 90% in West
Virginia (Torrey and Taylor). But assessing medical manpower
needs remains a thorny task: simply increasing the numbers of
mental health professionals will not correct geographic maldistribution and inadequate staffing of public facilities. The current
pattern of financial incentives, prestige, career opportunity
paths, and conditions of work must also be changed. Moreover,
the number and kinds of mental health professionals needed will
be influenced by any governmentally mandated changes in the
health care delivery system. In early 1976 Congress was still
assessing medical manpower and attempting to deal with geographic and specialty maldistribution in ways that were feasible,
equitable, and constitutional (Culliton).

Delivery of Services

Both the public and private sectors of mental health care under-
serve certain groups more than others: children, the mentally
retarded, the brain damaged, alcoholics, drug abusers, the elderly, and individuals in correctional facilities (Talkington). As a
result, services for these groups are receiving increased federal
attention, especially through the CMHC Program discussed
below.

Private Practice

In mid-1973 the American Psychiatric Association performed the
first nationwide study of a random sample of private-practice
psychiatrists (psychiatrists spending 15 hours or more per week

in private practice) (Marmor). The sample, 440 psychiatrists, was skewed toward psychoanalysts. Almost all psychoanalysts are in private practice, whereas nonanalytic psychiatrists may not be. The private-practice psychiatrists saw an average of 32 patients per week, most in individual psychotherapy (including use of medications), but some in group therapy, family therapy, or couple therapy. The average fee was $35 for a 45- to 60-minute visit. Psychoanalysts estimated that 60% of their patients would require 100 or more visits to achieve the goals of therapy, whereas nonanalysts estimated only 16% of their patients would require this many visits.

Who seeks private psychiatric treatment? The APA survey found:

> . . . professional and managerial workers are quite disproportionately represented in the private offices of psychiatrists as compared to blue- and white-collar workers. . . . The percentage of lawyers, physicians, and social workers receiving private psychiatric treatment ranges from 12 to 19 times higher than their actual percentage in the work force. (Marmor, pp. 38–39)

Although most of this differential can be attributed to the expense of private care, psychiatric treatment is socially more acceptable among better-educated groups. (The fact that uninsured and insured patients had the same average number of visits per year shows that expense is not the only determining factor.) Despite common stereotypes to the contrary, more than three-quarters of the psychiatrists' patients were rated moderately or severely functionally impaired; and the proportion of women in private treatment (57%) did not differ significantly from the proportion seen in public treatment settings.

Outpatient Psychiatric Clinics

Over the last two decades use of outpatient psychiatric clinics has greatly increased: clinic outpatient care episodes in 1971 accounted for 57% of all patient care episodes (inpatient, outpatient, and day-care) recorded by NIMH, compared to 23% in 1955. The number of outpatient care episodes in 1971 was six times the number in 1955, a rise traceable to an increase in the number of mental health professionals, in the provision of services to less severely disabled patients, in the emphasis on aftercare, and in the insurance coverage for outpatient care. In clinics that are not affiliated with inpatient facilities, the increased volume of care has meant more care rendered by social workers and psychologists, who constitute most of the staff; in 1972 psychiatrists accounted for only 9% of staff in these clinics (NIMH, 1973, Series B, No. 6). The nearly 2,300 outpatient psychiatric clinics operating in 1971 varied considerably in diagnostic groups served, hours of operation, and treatment modalities offered—for example, some offered only individual psychotherapy (NIMH, 1973, Series A, No. 13).

Although patients seen in outpatient clinics in 1971 resembled in sex distribution those seen in private practice psychiatry, there were striking differences in terms of socioeconomic status and race. Only 4% of patients seen in private psychiatric practice in 1973 were nonwhite, compared to 17% in outpatient psychiatric clinics in 1971 (NIMH, 1974, Statistical Note 79). On the other hand, the cost of a visit to an outpatient clinic was about the same as the cost of a visit to a private psychiatrist (NIMH, 1973, Series A, No. 13; AMA). The difference was in the mixture of government, insurance, philanthropic, and out-of-pocket dollars that paid for the services. Despite the emphasis on organized mental health care settings in many national health insurance bills being considered by Congress in the mid-1970s, no evidence exists that services in these settings are more cost-effective than those delivered in private psychiatric practice. To legislate in favor of organized care settings in the absence of such evidence would be less than rational public policymaking.

State and County Mental Hospitals

Since the mid-1950s state and county mental hospitals have played a progressively smaller role in the total delivery of mental health care. These hospitals accounted for half the patient care episodes recorded by NIMH in 1955 but for only 18% in 1971 (NIMH, 1973, Series B, No. 5, and Statistical Note 23, 1971). The number of resident patients declined by 60% between 1955 and mid-1974 (NIMH, 1975, Statistical Note 114) despite an increase in admission rate every year from 1950 to 1972. As noted above, there are several reasons for the decline: the introduction of antipsychotic drugs in the mid-1950s; the proliferation of nursing and personal care homes to provide custodial care for the mentally disordered elderly; the increased availability of outpatient care and aftercare; the growing efforts to prevent inappropriate admissions; the establishment of community mental health centers; and the reorganization of large mental hospitals into smaller units responsible for particular geographic areas (NIMH, 1974, Statistical Note 77).

State departments of mental health have welcomed the decrease in the resident population since fewer patients mean a higher staff/patient ratio for the same staffing costs, which should facilitate more humane and effective care. Moreover, since antipsychotic drugs were introduced, mental health professionals have come to believe that shorter hospital stays are preferable to longer stays for most patients: longer stays are associated with increased loss of social skills and family and community roles and cost the state more than shorter stays. In general, care in state mental hospitals is more expensive for the state than care in local public outpatient facilities where federal and local funds contribute.

The decline in use of state hospitals has had negative effects, however. Many patients have been discharged into communities ill-prepared to provide the therapeutic and rehabilitative services they need (halfway houses, aftercare clinics, sheltered workshops, rehabilitation centers). The board and care homes to which many patients are discharged may be unlicensed and uninspected. As Greenblatt and Glazier (1975) note, "Without appropriate standards and monitoring procedure, the chronically mentally ill may be prey to incompetent or mercenary caregivers" (p. 1137). This deficiency of local services raises the readmission rate. (Low community and, in some instances, familial tolerance for socially disruptive or ineffective behavior, and the tendency of psychoses to recur despite treatment, also contribute to readmissions.) Aged mentally disordered patients may receive less humane care in nursing and personal care homes—which often use untrained staff—than in state mental hospitals.

Patients with a diagnosis of schizophrenia continue to be the largest group of state hospital admissions (almost 30% in 1972). Patients with alcohol disorders are the next largest group (about 25% in 1972) and, together with drug abuse patients, were a rapidly growing segment of the state and county mental hospital population in the 1960s and early 1970s (NIMH, 1974, Statistical Note 97). Many other mental health facilities refused to treat these patients. Lower-class patients are disproportionately represented in state and county mental hospitals (NIMH, 1971, Statistical Note 34), reflecting the greater prevalence of diagnosed psychosis and alcohol disorders in the lower class, differential societal response based on patients' social class (NIAAA), and lower-class patients' inability to pay for services elsewhere.

Despite the drop in resident population, state and county mental hospitals face a number of problems. First, they have trouble convincing most state legislatures to place a high priority on funds for mental health care: in 1970 the average total expenditure per patient day in private mental hospitals was $50; in state and county mental hospitals it was $13 (NIMH, 1972, Series A, No. 10). Second, they cannot easily attract well-trained staff since they cannot compete with many other facilities or with private practice in terms of location, prestige, working conditions, or income. As a result, state hospitals rely heavily on foreign medical graduates, who are handicapped by limited psychiatric training in their medical schools, by limited educational opportunities in most state hospital psychiatric residency programs, and by language and cultural barriers (Miller et al.). State hospitals have the smallest percentage of professionals (doctors, nurses, psychologists, and social workers) on their staff of any kind of mental health facility (NIMH, 1973, Series B, No. 6).

A third problem is how to use buildings and staff now that the resident population has declined and the emphasis is on community care. One answer is to help urban state and county hospitals provide a range of mental health services designed around community needs. In addition, state and county hospitals can serve patients with special treatment and rehabilitiative needs, e.g., chronic patients with no families, alcoholic patients, and patients dangerous to themselves or others (Demone and Schulberg).

A fourth problem—the difficulty in finding low-cost or publicly supported aftercare services to decrease the need for readmission —is being addressed in part by the federal government's support for community mental health centers, many of which are administratively coordinated with state hospitals.

Community Mental Health Centers

The federal Community Mental Health Centers (CMHC) program was established to improve the delivery of mental health services to the entire U.S. population by eventually creating 1,500 to 2,000 centers. Each center was made responsible for providing services to all residents of a geographic area (catchment area), including a population of from 70,000 to 200,000 people. In addition to providing the requisite services—inpatient care; outpatient care; 24-hour emergency service; partial hospitalization; and consultation and education services to community agencies and professional personnel—centers were encouraged to develop diagnostic, rehabilitative, precare and aftercare services (e.g., home visits and halfway houses), training activities, research and evaluation programs, and an administrative organization fostering continuity of care, accessibility of services, and community participation in planning and operating the center (Koran and Brown).

By mid-1975, 536 federally-funded CMHCs were providing services to catchment areas including about 77 million people. Individual CMHCs vary widely in staffing pattern, financial arrangements, population served, and administrative organization. CMHCs have been organized, for example, as new, independent entities; under the auspices of general hospitals, state mental hospitals, outpatient clinics, or university medical programs; and by means of interagency agreements between two or more cooperating agencies. The catchment areas served range from inner-city ghettos to rural areas and affluent suburbs.

Utilization rates of individual CMHCs also vary widely (NIMH, 1974, Statistical Note 86). Generally, however, the patient population admitted to CMHCs in 1971 contained more low-income, black, and less-educated individuals than the United States population as a whole. Inner-city CMHCs had much higher utilization rates then suburban or rural ones. The difference cannot be attributed to differences in the prevalence of mental disorders, since CMHC utilization rates are also affected by the accessibility of other mental health facilities, patients' ability to pay for private care, community attitudes toward mental health care, and the attractiveness of CMHC facilities (NIMH, 1974, Statistical Note 87).

CMHCs were designed to remedy in mental health care some of the deficiencies long recognized in the U.S. health care delivery system; however, the achievement of this laudable aim has been blocked by various obstacles. Growth of nonfederal sources of funding has been slower than expected, leading Congress in 1970 to extend staffing grants from 51 months to eight years. Part of the difficulty stems from limited coverage for partial hospitalization, outpatient care, and sheltered living arrangements in most insurance policies. Moreover, some CMHCs have had difficulty in obtaining provider status under state Medicaid plans and some states have limited their participation in Medicaid. In addition, local governments often can allocate very little support to CMHCs, particularly in poverty areas. Finally, nongovernmental funds are rarely available to support preventive services like consultation and education. Nonetheless, older CMHCs depend less on federal funds than younger ones (NIMH, 1974, Statistical Note 91).

A basic problem arose from the belief of many federal CMHC program planners and of many CMHC staff that preventive mental health care meant political action to improve the quality of community life. Some CMHCs plunged into local political conflicts about resources allocation and aroused local opposition. Others discovered a CMHC could not miraculously cure social inequities and injustices rooted in economics, politics, and racism (Musto).

The Nixon and Ford Administrations attempted to change the federal commitment to the CMHC Program from a nationwide network of centers to a demonstration program. They argued that the CMHC Program had demonstrated the effectiveness of this service-delivery model, and future costs should therefore be borne by state and local governments, fees, and insurance (Koran et al.).

In the Community Mental Health Centers Amendments of 1975 (Title III of Public Law 94-63), passed over a presidential veto, Congress made clear its commitment to a nationwide network of centers and addressed problems identified in the first decade of the CMHC program's existence (Ochberg). The 1975 Amendments required centers to establish services for children, the elderly, drug addicts, alcoholics, and chronically and severely handicapped patients. Bilingual staff were required if non-English-speaking patients were served. The Amendments also provided grants to support consultation and education services and required centers to create utilization review and other evaluative procedures. Governing bodies of new centers were required to be consumer-dominated and to have power to select a center director and approve the budget.

The experiences of CMHCs with catchment area responsibility, multiagency agreements, continuity of care, consumer participation, and local, state, and federal politics are casebooks that might well be consulted by those interested in planning improvements in general health care service delivery.

General Hospital Psychiatric Inpatient Units

The number of general hospitals with separate psychiatric inpatient services has increased dramatically since World War II, and patient-care episodes in these units have more than doubled between 1955 and 1971. But because of the vast increase in outpatient patient-care episodes, these units account for a slightly smaller percentage of all patient-care episodes in 1971 (17%) than in 1955 (21%) (NIMH, 1971, Statistical Note 23, and 1973, Series B, No. 5).

General hospital psychiatric inpatient units have increased in number for several reasons (NIMH, 1972, Series A, No. 11). Insurance coverage for treatment of mental disorders in general hospitals gradually increased; in the 1960s, limited Medicare and Medicaid coverage for mental illness provided incentives to treat indigent psychiatric patients and to correct the classification of psychiatric patients previously given nonpsychiatric diagnoses so they could qualify for private health insurance reimbursements. In addition, the 1961 report of the Joint Commission on Mental Illness recommended that every general hospital of 100 beds or more have a psychiatric unit; federal Hill-Burton hospital construction funds were released for construction of psychiatric beds; and NIMH training grants greatly increased the number of mental health professionals.

General hospital psychiatric inpatient units offer several advantages over state mental hospitals. The ratio of full-time equivalent staff per 100 average resident patients is much higher (103 vs. 47 in 1972) (NIMH, 1973, Series B, No. 6). Patients are treated close to their homes. Outpatient psychiatric services are frequently available in the same hospital or from private psychiatrists who utilize the inpatient unit. Psychiatric inpatients who have associated or coincidental physical illnesses can readily obtain medical consultation. And psychiatric units provide a base from which psychiatrists can provide consultations for medical and surgical patients with psychiatric disturbances (Lipowski). On the other hand, these units are usually not equipped to meet the vocational rehabilitation and other needs of chronically disabled mental patients.

In psychiatric units of nongovernment general hospitals, patients with depressive disorders are the largest diagnostic group, a reflection both of the treatability of depressive disorders and of these patients' ability to pay. In Veterans' Administration (VA) and public nonfederal general hospitals, patients with schizophrenia are the largest diagnostic group; because schizophrenia is more chronically disabling, these patients are less able to pay for care. In VA hospitals, patients with alcohol disorders are the second-largest diagnostic group (NIMH, 1973, Statistical Note 68). The higher prevalence of alcohol disorders in the armed forces compared to the general population has not stimulated adequate preventive measures (Gunderson and Shuckit).

Private Mental Hospitals

With the rise of general hospital psychiatric inpatient units and other facilities, the contribution of private mental hospitals to mental health care has gradually declined. In 1971 these hospitals accounted for only 2% of all patient-care episodes and 18 states had no private mental hospitals (NIMH, 1973, Series B, No. 5; 1971, Statistical Note 23). This small percentage belies the influence of private mental hospitals on mental health care. Books written by staff psychiatrists in these hospitals— Fromm-Reichman (1950), Sullivan (1953), Stanton and Schwartz (1954), and Menninger (1963)—have strongly influenced psychiatric practice since the early 1950s.

Like psychiatric units in nongovernmental general hospitals, private mental hospitals most frequently admit patients with depressive disorders (about 40% of admissions); schizophrenic patients are the second-largest group (NIMH, 1973, Series B, No. 5).

The ratio of full-time equivalent patient-care staff in private nonprofit mental hospitals is somewhat higher than in psychiatric units in general hospitals, but in private for-profit hospitals it is lower (NIMH, 1973, Series B, No. 6). No studies are available to indicate whether the profit motive is creating care that is more efficient or less complete.

Public Institutions for the Mentally Retarded

Persons with intelligence quotients (I.Q.s) more than two standard deviations from the mean score of 100 on the Revised Stanford-Binet Tests of Intelligence are defined as mentally retarded. Since intelligence scores follow a normal statistical distribution, about 2.5% of the United States population is mentally retarded by this definition. In 1968, the latest year for which data are available, there were 193,000 residents in public institutions for the mentally retarded, about 3 to 4% of all mentally retarded persons in the United States. An additional 34,000 mentally retarded persons were residents in state and county mental hospitals, but the trend was against use of these hospitals for this purpose (NIMH, 1971, Statistical Notes 17 and 18).

Like state mental hospitals, these state institutions for many years sought to provide little more than custodial care. They underwent a profound change in orientation in the 1950s and now aim at treatment and rehabilitation, but have been handicapped by large size and the mixing of patients of all ages and degrees of mental and physical handicap (Cytryn and Lourie). Although it is thought desirable to have small groups living in a home-like atmosphere, it is frequently not practical for financial reasons. Many institutions remain understaffed human warehouses.

Mentally retarded persons receive care in a variety of settings. Of some 123,000 patient-care episodes recorded by NIMH in 1971 involving mentally retarded persons, about one-third took place in the institutions and hospitals mentioned above, about 5% in other inpatient settings, about 20% in the outpatient service of a CMHC, and about 40% in other outpatient settings (NIMH, 1973, Series B, No. 5). Both the federal and state governments, through a variety of agencies, support a large number of programs in addition to mental health care designed to aid the mentally retarded. Among them are special education, vocational training, day care, foster care, and funds for research and training.

Residential Psychiatric Facilities for Children and Adolescents

Residential psychiatric facilities for children and adolescents include residential treatment centers for emotionally disturbed children (RTCs) and psychiatric hospitals for children (CPHs) but not facilities such as training schools for juvenile delinquents (NIMH, 1972, Series A, No. 14). RTCs provide inpatient services primarily to moderately or seriously disturbed children under 18 years of age. The programs and physical facilities are usually designed to meet patients' daily living, schooling, recreational, socialization, and routine medical care needs. Because of the large number and variety of staff needed, costs are high. Treatments include milieu therapy, psychotherapy, behavior modification, psychotropic drugs, and special education (Lewis and Solnit). CPHs differ from RTCs in serving more disturbed children and in relying more heavily on psychiatric and medical treatments. As a result, fewer of their staff are educators and more are mental health professionals.

RTCs and CPHs together accounted for less than a quarter of the inpatient patient-care episodes involving persons under 18 years of age recorded by NIMH in 1971. This suggests most children admitted to psychiatric facilities are admitted to units not specifically designed to meet children's needs. Moreover, RTCs and CPHs do not attempt to treat all serious mental problems of children. For example, three-quarters of RTCs and one-quarter of CPHs will not admit children who are "heavy drug users." The 1970 report of the Joint Commission on Mental Health of Children concluded that there were too few mental health care facilities of all kinds to meet children's needs.

Day Treatment

Day treatment patients spend most of the day at the treatment facility in structured activities but return home in the evenings. Day treatment services—including psychotherapy, pharmacotherapy, and occupational therapy—are used as an alternative to inpatient care, as a transition from inpatient to outpatient care or discharge, or as a locus for rehabilitating or maintaining long-term patients. Most day treatment facilities are affiliated with psychiatric hospitals, psychiatric units in general hospitals, or CMHCs, but some are affiliated with outpatient clinics or other mental health facilities (NIMH, 1974, Statistical Note 96). Day treatment services have grown in number in response to the increased number of patients discharged from mental hospitals improved, even if not fully recovered, on antipsychotic drugs. Between 1962 and 1971, for example, the number of day treatment settings increased sevenfold and the number of persons treated increased fourteenfold (NIMH, 1974, Statistical Note 96).

Despite this impressive growth, expansion of day treatment services has been slowed by the widespread failure of insurance policies to cover day treatment. In rural areas, long travel times also impede the use of day treatment facilities.

Psychiatric Halfway Houses

Psychiatric halfway houses are nonmedical residential facilities that provide room and board in a homelike atmosphere for mentally disturbed individuals who cannot live independently, but who can work or occupy themselves productively during the day if given some support and supervision. Where they exist, halfway houses allow patients a graded transition from the extreme dependency of hospital life to the full responsibility of independent living. Most halfway houses operating in 1971 were less than five years old. Like day treatment services, halfway houses grew in number in the 1950s and 1960s to meet the needs of discharged patients partly recovered on antipsychotic drugs. Two-thirds of patients admitted to halfway houses for adults in 1971 were referred from psychiatric inpatient facilities (NIMH, 1974, Statistical Note 80).

Because patients in halfway houses are not fully recovered, residential neighborhoods usually resist the establishment of a halfway house. Fears about felonious sexual or aggressive behavior of mental patients, for which the empirical evidence is contradictory (Gulevich and Bourne; Rubin), and reasonable fears about the effects of a halfway house on property values make establishing these desirable facilities difficult (Ozarin).

Nursing and Personal-Care Homes

The number of senile or otherwise mentally disordered persons in nursing and personal-care homes increased dramatically between 1963 and 1969, from 222,000 to 427,000. Much of this increase reflected a shift in custodial care for elderly mentally disordered persons from mental hospitals to these homes. Since federal Medicaid covers care in these homes for psychiatric disorders on the same basis as for general medical disorders, but limits coverage of psychiatric care in state mental hospitals, states had a clear financial incentive to transfer patients to nursing and personal-care homes. For example, 75% of persons aged 65 or over, resident in long-term institutions in 1969 with diagnoses of senility or other mental disorders, were in nursing and personal care homes; only 23% were in state and county mental hospitals. Nonetheless, many homes did not accept such patients (NIMH, 1974, Statistical Note 107).

Because staff of nursing and personal care homes usually lack extensive training in the care of mentally disordered persons, many patients do not receive active or appropriate treatment, especially individuals in personal care homes without nursing services. It remains to be demonstrated that these patients would not benefit from treatment, and that these homes offer a socially more economical and humane custodial care than state mental hospitals (Epstein and Simon). A growing body of evidence indicates that many elderly, institutionalized, mentally disordered patients can be returned to their communities if active treatment and supportive community services are available (U.S. Congress, 1971). Recommendations for preventing prolonged institutionalization include more community-based services in CMHCs, halfway houses, and psychiatric clinics; greater availability of home health care services; greater use of active treatments in institutions; and greater cooperation between disparate community agencies that serve the elderly (NIMH, 1974, Statistical Note 107; U.S. Congress, 1971).

Insurance Coverage for Mental Disorders

Insurance coverage for mental disorders is less widespread than for other illnesses. For example, the Social Security Administration estimated that at the end of 1970, 80% of the civilian population had some private health insurance coverage for hospital care of general illnesses; 71% had some coverage for physicians' in-hospital visits; and 45% had some coverage for physician office visits. For mental disorders, the corresponding rates were 63%, 61%, and 38%. Moreover, even when insurance coverage exists for mental disorders, it is usually more limited than for somatic illnesses (Reed et al., p. 162), especially in the case of ambulatory services.

These differences arose in the 1920s and 1930s when hospital insurance began to be written. Hospital treatment for mental disorders then occurred largely in state-funded mental hospitals or in private mental hospitals used primarily by the wealthy. When nonhospital services began to be covered in the 1950s, psychoanalysis was the most common outpatient treatment for mental disorders; it was very costly and was given to individuals functioning well in the community (for example, members of the intelligentsia) as well as to the seriously disturbed. Although treatments and treatment settings have changed, these restrictions have remained because of rising health care costs, the absence of strong consumer demand for mental health coverage, and insurers' continuing fear of the potential cost of this coverage. A recent comprehensive study of utilization experience concluded, however, that broad coverage for mental health services would cost only a few dollars per covered person per year (Reed et al., p. 171). But this study did not adequately consider the effects of benefit limitations and the composition of covered populations (unemployed persons and blue-collar workers were underrepresented) on utilization, or the effects of omitted, uncovered costs (e.g., costs of care in state mental hospitals) (Allison and Volz). Thus, definitive conclusions about the cost of broad coverage for mental health care cannot be drawn. Yet cost should not be the determining consideration: "One does not cover a service because the cost is high or low, but rather, because the service is an essential and desirable one . . ." (Reed, 1974, p. 974). Are people with mental disorders less in need of care than people with somatic illnesses?

Detailed utilization and cost data are available for the interested reader (Reed et al.; Spiro et al.; Reed; Sharfstein and Magnas). For illustrative purposes, information concerning Medicare, Medicaid, and Blue Cross/Blue Shield for federal employees is summarized here.

Medicare

The general benefits and costs to the beneficiary of Medicare, a federal program in which some health care costs of persons 65 and over are covered through the Social Security System, are described in Chapter 9. Under Part A (hospital insurance), benefits for inpatient treatment in a psychiatric hospital are limited to 190 days in a lifetime. Only 150 of these days (90 benefit-period plus 60 lifetime-reserve days) can be used in any one benefit period. Benefits for psychiatric care in a certified general hospital or extended care facility are the same as for any form of medical care. This provision has increased the use of general hospitals to provide psychiatric care for the elderly.

Under Part B (supplementary medical insurance), benefits for physicians' outpatient care for mental illness are limited to 50% of the charges or $250, whichever is less. Benefits for physicians' inpatient care for mental illness are the same as for other illnesses, i.e., not limited. One hundred home visits are also covered and may be provided by mental health agencies.

An American Hospital Association study published in 1973 indicates that "approved claims per 1,000 enrollees, total hospital charges, and the amount reimbursed in psychiatric hospitals were all less than 1 percent of the corresponding figures for all hospitals" (Hall, 1974). This suggests that mental health care accounts for a surprisingly small percentage of Medicare hospital expenditures. Recent utilization statistics for outpatient mental health services under Medicare are not available.

Medicaid

Medicaid, also described in detail in the next chapter, is a combined federal-state program to cover certain health care costs for eligible persons with incomes falling below stated levels. Eligibility standards vary from state to state. However, in no state is care of patients under 65 in mental institutions included; the federal government views this as a responsibility long borne by the states through their own mental hospitals. Although no other restrictions by diagnosis are permitted, states can and have limited the amounts of care they will cover, for example, the number of hospital days.

Few utilization data are available since states are not required to keep records by diagnosis. It has been noted however, that "... a comprehensive program of services for the mentally ill, with emphasis on ambulatory care, is not at present a Medicaid requirement and is not included in the Medicaid plans of a number of states" (Reed et al., p. 144). This deficiency reflects the priority given by both the federal and state governments to the mental health care needs of the poor.

Blue Cross and Blue Shield Plans for Federal Employees

Reed (1974) has provided utilization data for these plans for 1972, when more than 4 million persons were covered under high option benefits. Data for the high option benefits are summarized here because "this option provides relatively comprehensive benefits and virtually equal benefits for mental conditions" (p. 973). Under the high option basic hospital and medical surgical benefits, mental health benefits included 365 days of inpatient care per year in general hospitals or Blue Cross member hospitals, together with in-hospital psychotherapy, electroconvulsive therapy, drugs, X-rays, and laboratory services. Supplemental benefits covered other medically necessary services and supplies in or out of the hospital; the plan covered 80% of the cost of these after a deductible of $100.

Over the decade 1961–1962 to 1972, mental health services took an increasing percentage of benefit payments, rising from 3.9% to 7.1%. This increase supported the belief of some insurance planners that unlimited mental health care benefits would lead to an ever-increasing percentage of benefits being paid out for mental health services. Recent statistics tend to prove this assumption wrong: mental health benefits reached a plateau in 1973 and 1974, when they accounted for 7.3% and

7.2% respectively of benefit payments (Sharfstein and Magnas). The 1962–1971 increase resulted from elimination of benefit restrictions for mental disorders, and probably also reflected a greater willingness to seek psychiatric care and the more widespread availability of services.

Mental Health Care Coverage under National Health Insurance

The broad issues in National Health Insurance are treated in Chapter 15. Insurance coverage of mental health care under NHI can be considered in the following categories: costs, indications for and effectiveness of treatments; services and service providers that should be covered; needs for research; and consumer demand.

Insurance carriers and government officials continue to fear the costs and degree of utilization of mental health care benefits. Previously cited studies (Reed; Reed et al.; Spiro et al.; Sharfstein and Magnas), although not definitive because of benefit and population limitations, suggest that mental health services can be covered at a reasonable cost per subscriber and as a reasonable proportion of benefits paid. Moreover, a few studies suggest that when mental health care is available, utilization of other health care services decreases (Follette and Cummings; Goldberg et al.). Access to costly treatments such as long-term psychoanalysis may or may not need to be limited (Sharfstein and Magnas); any restrictions of this kind should also apply to such costly medical or surgical procedures as long-term renal dialysis. The potential effects of different methods of cost-control should be carefully studied before they are incorporated in large-scale insurance plans (Muller and Schoenberg). Cost-control, if unwisely implemented, can seriously damage the quality of health or mental health care.

Some health insurance experts have questioned mental health coverage on the grounds that the indications for and effectiveness of psychiatric treatments are not well documented and agreement regarding diagnoses and diagnostic criteria is more limited than in other health care fields (Hall). These experts seem unaware that the indications for and effectiveness of medical and surgical treatments are constantly being tested and debated in the medical literature (Ingelfinger et al.; Koran, 1975a; U.S. Congress, 1976). These tests and debates create medical progress. Yet treatments whose benefits are uncertain, such as tonsillectomy, coronary artery bypass surgery (Spodick), certain drug treatments of cancers (Chalmers et al.), and care in coronary care units (Hiatt) have not been denied insurance coverage. If coverage were limited to those medical and surgical treatments for which incontrovertible evidence of effectiveness exists, far fewer treatments would be covered. In any case, the effectiveness of many pharmacological treatments in psychiatry is not in question (Davis and Cole; Cole and Davis 1975a, b; Fieve) and evidence for the effectiveness of psychotherapy is accumulating (Bergin; Malan; Weissman et al.).

Insurers and public policy makers must be helped to understand that "effectiveness" does not mean "cure." Even today, physicians can only hope "to cure sometimes, to relieve often, to comfort always" (Strauss, p. 410). Diabetes, atherosclerosis, multiple sclerosis, and a host of other diseases are treated, not cured. Furthermore, physicians other than psychiatrists often disagree regarding signs and symptoms, diagnostic criteria, and diagnoses (Koran, 1975b). Diagnostic disagreements do not justify limiting insurance coverage of mental disorders or of physical illnesses; they merely reflect the imperfect but progressing state of medical science.

A wide variety of mental health service providers should be covered if high-quality mental health services are to be encouraged. Coverage for ambulatory care services, including newer treatments such as group or family therapy, partial hospitalization, and consultation with another health practitioner or community agency, will need special attention. Covering services of nonphysicians is most important. Questions concerning indications for and duration of treatment by nonphysicians can perhaps be met by requiring physician referral and periodic consultation. Financing the social services often required for adequate mental health care remains a problem (Muller and Schoenberg). Mental health care in facilities such as halfway houses has not been well covered by insurance, though it should be. Although few people would dispute that alcohol and drug abuse frequently create disorders that necessitate physical and mental health care, full insurance coverage of these disorders remains controversial, perhaps because they are often chronic and because they bear a moral stigma.

To plan mental health service coverage most intelligently, we need to study the effects of various cost-control and quality-assurance mechanisms on utilization rates and on the level of mental health in covered populations. Research is also needed on the cost-effectiveness of treatments rendered in different settings—private practice versus public outpatient clinics, for example.

Finally, public demand would be a powerful force for bringing about adequate coverage for mental health services. Continued educational efforts to combat the social stigma and myths surrounding the mentally disordered and the treatments available to them are sorely needed to influence public opinion in this direction (Rabkin; Glasser et al.).

Legal Issues

Laws and their interpretations change with the times, and laws regulating the delivery of mental health services are no exception. In the 1960s and 1970s legal issues receiving attention in the courts have included commitment procedures, the right to treatment, the right to refuse treatment, and confidentiality (Brooks; Stone).

Civil commitment to a mental institution deprives a mentally disordered person of his liberty in exchange for treatment. The grounds for civil commitment vary in different states but include judgments that the person is dangerous to himself or others, unable to care for physical needs, or needs care or treatment. The trend in recent years has been toward restricting the grounds for civil commitment; reducing the length of time a person can be committed by physicians without judical review; abolishing indeterminate stays during which the patient could not initiate discharge or release; and requiring commitment through the courts with due process guarantees for longer-term commitments. In addition, the civil and personal rights of committed and voluntary patients have been given increasing statutory recognition. These rights include the right to communicate with persons outside the institution, to keep clothing and personal effects, to practice religion freely, to receive independent psychiatric examination, to manage or dispose of property, to retain licenses, permits, or privileges established by law, to enter into contracts, to marry, and to sue and be sued (McGarry and Kaplan).

The Mental Health Law Project, sponsored by the American Civil Liberties Union Foundation, the American Orthopsychiatric Association, and the Center for Law and Social Policy, has been engaging in litigation and consulting with legislatures and mental health organizations to help secure these and other patient rights. Because of this attention to procedures and rights, seriously disturbed individuals are being given more humane care. But the conflicts between a patient's right to liberty, his need for care or treatment, and the state's interests in protecting his welfare and in preventing harm to others remain unresolved (Shah).

A constitutional right to treatment for involuntarily committed patients was first recognized by a court in *Wyatt* v *Stickney* (1972). Guardians of involuntarily committed patients sued the Alabama mental health commissioner, charging that inadequate care was rendered in a state mental hospital. The federal district court judge agreed the patients had a right to treatment that included certain standards of care. With the aid of medical and psychiatric consultations, he defined these standards to include individual evaluation, active treatment, minimum staffing ratios, detailed nutritional and physical standards, and compensation for work performed. But the judgment had certain limitations: it did not apply to voluntary patients; it set no penalty for noncompliance. The psychiatrist mental health commissioner, who did not contest the inadequacy of care at the state institutions, was fired and replaced by a finance officer. Although Alabama increased its daily per-patient expenditure, qualified mental health professionals, particularly psychiatrists, have not come forward to work in the state system because of continuing low salaries and poor working conditions.

Still, in time, *Wyatt* v. *Stickney* and similar cases may force state legislatures to allocate more resources to institutional care of the mentally disordered and to community-based care in order to prevent costly admissions and readmissions (Burris). Right-to-treatment cases on behalf of the mentally retarded have had some success in this regard (McGarry and Kaplan). Right-to-treatment litigation does raise the dangerous possibility that lawyers and judges rather than mental health professionals may begin determining the details of hospital administrative practices and the adequacy of individual treatment plans. If courts intrude too far on the decision-making prerogative of mental health professionals working in state institutions and departments of health, even fewer will work there than do now (Robitscher).

The right of committed patients to refuse treatments is not well recognized. Since the committed patient is deprived of his liberty in exchange for treatment presumably in his best interest, to allow him to refuse it would seem contradictory. On the other hand, the state's coercive power must be restrained to prevent capricious application. The committed patient is usually regarded as legally incompetent to decide whether to accept particular treatments, although exceptions are made for electroconvulsive therapy and psychosurgery in a few states, on the grounds that these treatments may harm the patient or change him irrevocably. Psychosurgery is irreversible and its indications and benefits are controversial. Electroconvulsive therapy, however, is much safer than many common surgical procedures, is not known to cause permanent brain damage, and brings about well-documented benefits (Kalinowsky and Hippius). Committed patients' only grounds for refusing medications is religious principle (*Winters* v. *Miller*), which is now recognized by the Supreme Court. With additional litigation and statutory change, reasonable rights to refuse treatments will be ensured in all states, without erecting unnecessary legal barriers to treatment of seriously disturbed individuals.

The confidentiality of patient-psychotherapist communications has important bearings on treatment. If therapists' records or memories can be subpoenaed when a patient introduces a medical or psychiatric condition into a civil litigation (such as a divorce), the public may hesitate to consult psychiatrists or to confide in them. Moreover, the patient may be tempted to exaggerate or prolong his symptoms in therapy to aid his legal case (Dubey). Relying on the evaluation of an independent court-appointed psychiatrist has been suggested to prevent abuse of therapeutic communications, but it has not been widely written into law. Reporting to insurance companies to allow patients to obtain benefits is another area wherein a method for balancing the need for confidentiality against an outside agency's need for information has yet to be satisfactorily devised (Grossman). Protection of confidentiality will be vital in the context of national health insurance.

Conclusion

Mental health care has come a long way in the past 75 years. Asylums and private care have been supplemented by new outpatient clinics, psychiatric wards in general hospitals, day-care programs, halfway houses, and a federally mandated network of community mental health centers. Moreover, many new effective treatments have been discovered. Still, opportunities abound for improving the delivery of mental health care and for increasing our understanding of mental disorders. Issues regarding insurance coverage of mental disorders, legal rights of patients, and legal duties of care-giving institutions remain unresolved. Mental health professionals and members of the general public will still have to participate in politics and government in order to generate government support for mental health services, training, and research. We hope that some readers will wish to take up these challenges that confront us in the last quarter of the twentieth century.

References

Allison, T., and Volz, F. A. "Health Insurance and Psychiatric Care: Utilization and Cost." *Inquiry, 10,* 77, 1973.

American Medical Association. *Profile of Medical Practice—1973.* Chicago, Ill.: American Medical Association, 1973.

American Psychiatric Association. *The Diagnostic and Statistical Manual of Mental Disorders* (DSM-II). Washington, D.C.: American Psychiatric Association, 1968.

Aviram, U., and Segal, S. P. "Exclusion of the Mentally Ill." *Archives of General Psychiatry, 29,* 126, 1973.

Babigian, H. M., and Odoroff, C. L. "The Mortality Experience of a Population with Psychiatric Illness." *American Journal of Psychiatry, 126,* 470, 1969.

Barton, W. "Federal Support of Training of Psychiatrists." *Psychiatric Annals, 2,* 42, 1972.

Beers, C. W. *A Mind That Found Itself.* New York: Doubleday, 1939.

Bergin, A. E. "The Evaluation of Therapeutic Outcomes." In Bergin, A. E. et al., Eds., *Handbook of Psychotherapy and Behavior Change,* Ch. 7. New York: Wiley, 1971.

Bernstein, I. C. et al. "Lobotomy in Private Practice: Long-Term Follow-up." *Archives of General Psychiatry, 32,* 1041, 1975.

Bockoven, J. S. *Moral Treatment in Community Mental Health.* New York: Springer Publishing Co., 1972.

Brooks, A. D. *Law, Psychiatry and the Mental Health System.* Boston, Mass.: Little, Brown and Co., 1974.

Burris, D. S., ed. *The Right to Treatment.* New York: Springer Publishing Co., 1969.

Chalmers, T. C. et al. "Controlled Studies in Clinical Cancer Research." *New England Journal of Medicine, 287,* 75, 1972.

Cole, J. O., and Davis, J. M. "Antidepressant Drugs." In Freedman, A. M. et al., Eds., *Comprehensive Textbook of Psychiatry II,* Ch. 31.2 Baltimore, Md.: Williams and Wilkins, 1975 (a).

Mental Health Services   241

Cole, J. O., and Davis, J. M. "Minor Tranquilizers, Sedatives, and Hypnotics." In Freedman, A. M. et al., Eds., *Comprehensive Textbook of Psychiatry II*, Ch. 31.3. Baltimore, Md.: Williams and Wilkins, 1975 (b).

Culliton, B. J. "Health Manpower: The Feds Are Taking Over." *Science, 191*, 446, 1976.

Cytryn, L., and Lourie, R. S. "Mental Retardation." In Freedman, A. M. et al., Eds., *Comprehensive Textbook of Psychiatry II*, Ch. 20.1, Baltimore, Md.: Williams and Wilkins, 1975.

Davis, J. M., and Cole, J. O. "Antipsychotic Drugs." In Freedman, A. M. et al., Eds., *Comprehensive Textbook of Psychiatry II*, Ch. 31.1. Baltimore, Md.: Williams and Wilkins, 1975.

Demone, H. W., and Schulberg, H. C. "Has the State Mental Hospital a Future as a Human Service Resource?" In Zusman, J., and Bertsch, E. F., Eds., *The Future Role of the State Hospital*, Ch. 1. Lexington, Mass.: Heath, 1975.

Deutsch, A. "The History of Mental Hygiene." In Hall, J. K. et al., Eds., *100 Years of American Psychiatry*, p. 325. New York: Columbia University Press, 1947.

Dohrenwend, B. P., and Dohrenwend, B. S. *Social Status and Psychological Disorder: A Causal Inquiry*. New York: Wiley, 1969.

Dubey, J. "Confidentiality as a Requirement of the Therapist: Technical Necessities for Absolute Privilege in Psychotherapy." *American Journal of Psychiatry, 131*, 1093, 1974.

Epstein, L. J., and Simon, A. "Alternatives to State Hospitalization for the Geriatric Mentally Ill." *American Journal of Psychiatry, 124*, 955, 1968.

Fieve, R. R. "Lithium (Antimanic) Therapy." In Freedman, A. M. et al., Eds., *Comprehensive Textbook of Psychiatry II*, Ch. 31.8. Baltimore, Md.: Williams and Wilkins, 1975.

Follette, W., and Cummings, N.A. "Psychiatric Services and Medical Utilization in a Prepaid Health Plan Setting." *Medical Care, 5*, 25, 1967.

Frank, J. D. "Common Features of Psychotherapy." *Australian and New Zealand Journal of Psychiatry, 6*, 34, 1972.

Frankel, F. H. "Reasoned Discourse of a Holy War: Postscript to a Report on ECT." *American Journal of Psychiatry, 132*, 77, 1975.

Fromm-Reichmann, F. *Principles of Intensive Psychotherapy*. Chicago, Ill.: University of Chicago Press, 1950.

Glasser, M. A. et al. "Obstacles to Utilization of Prepaid Mental Health Care." *American Journal of Psychiatry, 132*, 7, 1975.

Goldberg, J. D. et al. "Effect of a Short-Term Outpatient Psychiatric Therapy Benefit on the Utilization of Medical Services in a Prepaid Group Practice Medical Program." *Medical Care, 8*, 1970.

Greenblatt, M., and Glazier, E. "The Phasing Out of Mental Hospitals in the United States." *American Journal of Psychiatry, 132*, 1135, 1975.

Grossman, M. "Insurance Reports as a Threat to Confidentiality." *American Journal of Psychiatry, 128,* 64, 1971.

Gruenberg, E. M., and Turns, D. M. "Epidemiology." In Freedman, A. M. et al., Eds., *Comprehensive Textbook of Psychiatry II,* Ch. 6.1. Baltimore, Md.: Williams and Wilkins, 1975.

Gulevich, G. D., and Bourne, P. G. "Mental Illness and Violence." In Daniels, D. N. et al., Eds., *Violence and the Struggle for Existence,* Ch. 11. Boston, Mass.: Little, Brown and Co., 1970.

Gunderson, E. K. E., and Schuckit, M. A. "Hospitalization Rates for Alcoholism in the Navy and Marine Corps." *Diseases of the Nervous System, 36,* 681, 1975.

Hall, C. P. "Financing Mental Health Services Through Insurance." *American Journal of Psychiatry, 131,* 1079, 1974.

Herridge, C. F. "Physical Disorders in Psychiatric Illness: A Study of 209 Consecutive Admissions." *Lancet, 2,* 949, 1960.

Hiatt, H. H. "Protecting the Medical Commons: Who is Responsible." *New England Journal of Medicine, 293,* 235, 1975.

Ingelfinger, F. J. et al., Eds. *Controversy in Internal Medicine II.* Philadelphia: W. B. Saunders, 1972.

Joint Commission on the Mental Health of Children. *Crisis in Child Mental Health.* New York: Harper and Row, 1970.

Joint Commission on Mental Illness and Health. *Action for Mental Health.* New York: Basic Books, 1961.

Kalinowsky, L. B., and Hippius, H. *Pharmacology, Convulsive and Other Somatic Treatments in Psychiatry.* New York: Grune & Stratton, 1969.

Kendell, R. E. "The Concept of Disease and Its Implications for Psychiatry." *British Journal of Psychiatry, 127,* 305, 1975.

Koran, L. M. "Controversy in Psychiatry and Medicine." *American Journal of Psychiatry, 132,* 1064, 1975a.

Koran, L. M. "The Reliability of Clinical Methods, Data and Judgments." *New England Journal of Medicine, 239,* 642, 695, 1975b.

Koran, L. M., and Brown, B. S. "The Community Mental Health Center." In Corey, L. et al., Eds., *Medicine in a Changing Society,* Ch. 12. St. Louis, Mo.: C. V. Mosby, 1974.

Koran, L. M., et al. "The Federal Government and Mental Health." In Hamburg, D. A., and Brodie, H. K. H., Eds., *American Handbook of Psychiatry,* Ch. 43. New York: Basic Books, 1975.

Lewis, M., and Solnit, A. J. "Residential Treatment." In Freedman, A. M. et al., Eds., *Comprehensive Textbook of Psychiatry II,* Ch. 40.4. Baltimore, Md.: Williams and Wilkins, 1975.

Lipowski, Z. J. "Review of Consultation Psychiatry and Psychosomatic Medicine. II. Clinical Aspects." *Psychosomatic Medicine, 29,* 201, 1967.

Maguire, G. P., and Granville-Grossman, K. L. "Physical Illness in Psychiatric Patients." *British Journal of Psychiatry, 114,* 1365, 1968.

Malan, D. H. "The Outcome Problem in Psychotherapy Research." *Archives of General Psychiatry, 29,* 719, 1973.

Marmor, J. *Psychiatrists and Their Patients.* Washington, D.C.: American Psychiatric Association, 1975.

May, P. *Treatment of Schizophrenia: A Comparative Study of Five Treatment Methods.* New York: Science House, 1968.

McGarry, A. L., and Kaplan, H. A. "Overview: Current Trends in Mental Health Law." *American Journal of Psychiatry, 130,* 621, 1973.

Meltzer, M. L. "Insurance Reimbursement A Mixed Blessing." *American Psychologist, 30,* 1150, 1975.

Menninger, K. A. *The Vital Balance.* New York: Viking, 1963.

Miller, M. H. et al. "Foreign Medical Graduates: A Symposium." *American Journal of Psychiatry, 130,* 435, 1973.

Modlin, H. C. "Psychiatric Social Service Information." In Freedman, A. M. et al., Eds., *Comprehensive Textbook of Psychiatry II,* Ch. 12.6. Baltimore, Md.: Williams and Wilkins, 1975.

Mora, G. "Historical and Theoretical Trends in Psychiatry." In Freedman, A. M. et al., Eds., *Comprehensive Textbook of Psychiatry II,* Ch. 1.1. Baltimore, Md.: Williams and Wilkins, 1975.

Muller, C., and Schoenberg, M. "Insurance for Mental Health: A Viewpoint on Its Scope." *Archives of General Psychiatry, 31,* 871, 1974.

Murphy, J. "Psychiatric Labelling in Cross Cultural Perspective." *Science, 191,* 1019, 1976.

Musto, D. A. "Whatever Happened to 'Community Mental Health'?" *Public Interest,* No. 39, 53, 1975.

National Center for Health Statistics. *Health Resources Statistics— 1974.* DHEW Publication No. 74–1509. Washington, D.C.: Government Printing Office, 1974.

————. "National Ambulatory Medical Care Survey: May 1973–April 1974." *Monthly Vital Statistics Report,* 24(4), Suppl. 2, HEW Publication HRA 76–1120. Washington, D.C.: Government Printing Office, 1975.

National Institute on Alcohol Abuse and Alcoholism. "First Special Report to the U.S. Congress on Alcohol and Health." DHEW Publication No. (HSM) 73–9031, 1971.

National Institute of Mental Health. Statistical Notes 1–25. Rockville, Md.: National Institute of Mental Health, 1971.

————. Statistical Notes 26–50. Rockville, Md.: National Institute of Mental Health, 1971.

————. "Private Mental Hospitals 1969–1970." *Mental Health Statistics A,* No. 10. HEW Publication HSM 72–9089. Washington, D.C.: Government Printing Office, 1972.

————. "Psychiatric Services in General Hospitals, 1969–70." *Mental*

Health Statistics Series A, No. 11. HEW Publication HSM 72–9139. Washington, D.C.: Government Printing Office, 1972.

———. "Residential Psychiatric Facilities for Children and Adolescents: United States, 1971–72." *Mental Health Statistics Series A,* No. 14. HEW Publication ADM 74–78. Washington, D.C.: Government Printing Office, 1972.

———. Statistical Notes 51–75. Rockville, Md.: National Clearinghouse for Mental Health Information, 1973.

———. "Outpatient Psychiatric Services 1971–1972." *Mental Health Statistics Series A,* No. 13. HEW Publication ADM 74–69. Washington, D.C.: Government Printing Office, 1973.

———. "Staffing of Mental Health Facilities United States 1972." *Mental Health Statistics Series B,* No. 6. HEW Publication ADM 74–28. Washington, D.C.: Government Printing Office, 1973.

———. "Utilization of Mental Health Facilities 1971." *Mental Health Statistics Series B,* No. 5. HEW Publication NIH 74–657. Washington, D.C.: Government Printing Office, 1973.

———. Statistical Notes 76–100. HEW Publication OM 2799. Washington, D.C.: Government Printing Office, 1974.

———. "Characteristics of Federally Funded Rural Community Mental Health Centers in 1971." Statistical Note 101. HEW Publication ADM 74–6. Washington, D.C.: Government Printing Office, 1974.

———. "Patterns in Use of Nursing Homes by the Aged Mentally Ill." Statistical Note 107. HEW Publication ADM 74–69. Washington, D.C.: Government Printing Office, 1974.

———. "Consultation and Education Services in Federally Funded Community Mental Health Centers 1973." Statistical Note 108. HEW Publication ADM 75–158. Washington, D.C.: Government Printing Office, 1974.

———. "Readmissions to Inpatient Services of State and County Mental Hospitals 1972." Statistical Note 110. HEW Publication ADM 75–158. Washington, D.C.: Government Printing Office, 1974.

———. "Provisional Patient Movement and Administrative Data, State and County Mental Hospital Inpatient Services, July 1, 1973–June 30, 1974." Statistical Note 114. HEW Publication ADM 75–158. Washington, D.C.: Government Printing Office, 1975.

———. "The Cost of Mental Illness—1971." *Mental Health Statistics Series B,* No. 7. HEW Publication ADM 76–265, Washington, D.C.: Government Printing Office, 1976.

Ochberg, F. M. "Community Mental Health Center Legislation: Flight of the Phoenix." *American Journal of Psychiatry, 133,* 56, 1976.

O'Toole, A. W. "Psychiatric Nursing." In Freedman, A.M. et al., Eds., *Comprehensive Textbook of Psychiatry II,* Ch. 47. Baltimore, Md.: Williams and Wilkins, 1975.

Ozarin, L. D. "Community Alternatives to Institutional Care." *American Journal of Psychiatry, 133,* 69, 1976.

Plunkett, R. J., and Gordon, J. E. *Epidemiology and Mental Illness.* New York: Basic Books, 1960.

Rabkin, J. "Public Attitudes Toward Mental Illness: A Review of the Literature." *Schizophrenia Bulletin, 10,* 9, 1974.

Reed, L. S. "Utilization of Care for Mental Disorders Under the Blue Cross and Blue Shield Plan for Federal Employees, 1972." *American Journal of Psychiatry, 131,* 964, 1974.

Reed, L. S. *Coverage and Utilization of Care for Mental Conditions Under Health Insurance—Various Studies, 1973–74.* Washington, D.C.: American Psychiatric Association, 1975.

Reed, L. S., et al. *Health Insurance and Psychiatric Care: Utilization and Cost.* Washington, D.C.: American Psychiatric Association, 1972.

Robitscher, J. "Implementing the Rights of the Mentally Disabled: Judicial Legislative and Psychiatric Action." In Ayd, F. J., Jr. et al., Eds., *Medical, Moral and Legal Issues in Mental Health Care,* Ch. 9. Baltimore, Md.: Williams and Wilkins, 1974.

Roemer, R. et al. *Planning Urban Health Services: From Jungle to System.* New York: Springer Publishing Co., 1975.

Rossman, P. L. "Organic Diseases Resembling Functional Disorders." *Hospital Medicine, 5,* 72, 1969.

Rubin, B. "Prediction of Dangerousness in Mentally Ill Criminals." *Archives of General Psychiatry, 27,* 397, 1972.

Shah, S. A. "Dangerousness and Civil Commitment of the Mentally Ill: Some Public Policy Considerations." *American Journal of Psychiatry, 132,* 501, 1975.

Shakow, D. "Clinical Psychology." In Freedman, A. M. et al., Eds., *Comprehensive Textbook of Psychiatry II,* Ch. 46. Baltimore, Md.: Williams and Wilkins, 1975.

Sharfstein, S. S., and Magnas, H. L. "Insuring Intensive Psychotherapy." *American Journal of Psychiatry, 132,* 1252, 1975.

Sharfstein, S. S. et al., "Private Psychiatry and Accountability: A Response to the APA Task Force Report on Private Practice." *American Journal of Psychiatry, 132,* 43, 1975.

Shryock, R. H. "The Beginnings: From Colonial Days to the Foundation of the American Psychiatric Association." In Hall, J. K. et al., Eds., *100 Years of American Psychiatry.* New York: Columbia University Press, 1947.

Spiro, H. R. et al. "Fee-for-Service Insurance versus Cost Financing, Impact on Mental Health Care Systems." *American Journal of Public Health, 65,* 139, 1975.

Spodick, D. H. "The Surgical Mystique and the Double Standard: Controlled Trials of Medical and Surgical Therapy for Cardiac Disease: Analysis, Hypothesis, Proposal." *American Heart Journal, 85,* 579, 1973.

Stanton, A. H., and Schwartz, M. S. *The Mental Hospital.* New York: Basic Books, 1954.

Stone, A. A. *Mental Health and Law: A System in Transition.* National Institute of Mental Health, HEW Publication 75–176, 1975.

Strauss, M. B., Ed. *Familiar Medical Quotations.* Boston, Mass.: Little, Brown, and Co., 1968.

Strecker, E. A. "Military Psychiatry: World War I 1917–1918." In Hall, J. K. et al., Eds., *100 Years of American Psychiatry.* New York: Columbia University Press, 1947.

Sullivan, H. S. *The Interpersonal Theory of Psychiatry.* New York: W. W. Norton, 1953.

Sweet, W. H. "Treatment of Medically Intractable Mental Disease by Limited Frontal Leucotomy—Justifiable?" *The New England Journal of Medicine, 289,* 1117, 1973.

Szasz, T. S. *The Myth of Mental Illness.* New York: Hoeker-Harper, 1961.

Talkington, P. C. *Delivering Mental Health Services: Needs, Priorities and Strategies.* Washington, D.C.: American Psychiatric Association, 1975.

Torrey, E. F. "Psychiatric Training: The SST of American Medicine." *Psychiatric Annals, 2,* 60, 1972.

Torrey, E. F., and Taylor, R. L. "Cheap Labor from Poor Nations." *American Journal of Psychiatry, 130,* 428, 1973.

U. S. Congress. House Committee on Appropriations. Departments of Labor and Health, Education and Welfare Appropriations for 1976. "Part 2 Health Activities Except NIH." Hearings before a Subcommittee, 1975, 966 p. (94:1).

U. S. Congress. House Committee on Interstate and Foreign Commerce. Report by the Subcommittee on Oversight and Investigations. "Cost and Quality of Health Care: Unnecessary Surgery." 1976, 52 p. (94:2).

U. S. Congress. Senate Special Committee on Aging. "Mental Health Care and the Elderly: Shortcomings in Public Policy." 1971, 196 p. (92:1).

Weissman, M. et al. "Treatment Effects on the Social Adjustment of Depressed Patients." *Archives of General Psychiatry, 30,* 771, 1974.

Weston, W. D. "Development of Community Psychiatry Concepts." In Freedman, A. M. et al., Eds., *Comprehensive Textbook of Psychiatry II,* Ch. 43.1. Baltimore, Md.: Williams and Wilkins, 1975.

Wingfield, R. T. "Psychiatric Symptoms that Signal Organic Disease." *Virginia Medical Monthly, 94,* 15, 1967.

Winters v. *Miller* 446 F 2nd 65 (2nd Cir 1971).

Wyatt v. *Stickney* 344 F Supp. 373 (MD Ala 1972).

Zusman, J. "Secondary Prevention." In Freedman, A. et al., Eds., *Comprehensive Textbook of Psychiatry II,* Ch. 43.3. Baltimore, Md.: Williams and Wilkins, 1975.

9

Financing for Health Care

Carol McCarthy

Introduction

Up until now we have been discussing the people and institutions involved in the health care delivery system; we have seen that they interact in complex ways. These relationships are brought about by the medium of money and its exchange for goods and services. In this chapter we turn our attention to the financing of health care delivery: what the money buys, where it comes from, how is it paid out, and how the medical marketplace works. Since constantly rising expenditures have been a feature of the U.S. health care delivery system since such data were first collected in 1929 (except for a few years during the Depression), this topic will also receive attention.

As Table 9.1 shows, it has been estimated that in the fiscal year 1975, $118.5 billion was spent for health purposes in the United States (Mueller and Gibson, 1976), representing 8.3% of that year's Gross National Product (GNP). In 1950, health expenditures had totaled only $12 billion, 4.6% of the GNP; in 1965, $38.9 billion, 5.9% of the GNP. Since 1965, outlays for health have risen, on the average, more than 11% each year. Per capita, in 1975, the United States spent about $550 on health services, in comparison with a 1929 expenditure of about $30. Since that year the population has almost doubled, while expenditures for health care increased thirtyfold. By 1975, the health care industry had become the second largest in the country in terms of expenditures, outranked only by retail trade (Bureau of the Census, Table 610).

What Does the Money Buy?

Each year, statistics on health care financing, gathered by the Office of Research and Statistics of the Social Security Administration (SSA), are published in the *Social Security Bulletin* (in

Table 9.1

Aggregate and Per Capita National Health Expenditures, Selected Fiscal Years, 1929–75

Fiscal Year	Gross National Product (in billions)	Health expenditures								
		TOTAL			PRIVATE			PUBLIC		
		Amount (in millions)	Per Capita	% of GNP	Amount (in millions)	Per Capita	% of Total	Amount (in millions)	Per Capita	% of Total
1929	$ 101.0	$ 3,589	$ 29.16	3.6	$ 3,112	$ 25.28	86.7	$ 477	$ 3.88	13.3
1935	68.7	2,846	22.04	4.1	2,303	17.84	80.9	543	4.21	19.1
1940	95.1	3,863	28.83	4.1	3,081	22.99	79.8	782	5.84	20.2
1950	263.4	12,028	78.35	4.6	8,962	58.38	74.5	3,065	19.97	25.5
1955	379.7	17,330	103.76	4.6	12,909	77.29	74.5	4,421	26.46	25.5
1960	495.6	25,856	141.63	5.2	19,461	106.60	75.3	6,395	35.03	24.7
1965	655.6	38,892	197.75	5.9	29,357	149.27	75.5	9,535	48.48	24.5
1966	718.5	42,109	211.56	5.9	31,279	157.15	74.3	10,830	54.41	25.7
1967	771.4	47,879	237.93	6.2	32,057	159.30	67.0	15,823	78.63	33.0
1968	827.0	53,765	264.37	6.5	33,727	165.84	62.7	20,040	98.54	37.3
1969	899.0	60,617	295.20	6.7	37,682	183.51	62.2	22,937	111.70	37.8
1970	954.8	69,202	333.57	7.2	43,964	211.92	63.5	25,238	121.65	36.5
1971	1,013.6	77,162	368.25	7.6	48,558	231.74	62.9	28,604	136.51	37.1
1972	1,100.6	86,687	409.71	7.9	53,398	252.37	61.6	33,289	157.33	38.4
1973	1,225.2	95,384	447.31	7.8	58,995	276.66	61.8	36,389	170.65	38.2
1974	1,348.9	104,030	484.53	7.7	62,152	294.03	60.7	40,879	190.33	39.3
1975a	1,424.3	118,500	547.03	8.3	68,552	316.46	57.8	49,948	230.57	42.2

Source: M. S. Mueller and R. M. Gibson "National Health Expenditures, Fiscal Year, 1975," *Social Security Bulletin, 39*, February 1976, Table 1. (See Appendix I, A12.)
a Preliminary estimates.

recent years in the February issue). National health care expenditures are considered under two categories: (1) research and
medical facilities construction and (2) payments for personal
health care costs. The latter represent the bulk of outlays, $111.3
billion in 1975 (Mueller and Gibson, 1976, Table 2). Five types
of expenditure accounted for about 80% of the outlays for personal health services (see Table 9.2) : 39% went to hospitals, 19%
to physicians, 9% for drugs and drug sundries, 8% for nursing
home care, and 6% for dentists' services.

The other categories of expenditures are: "other professional"
services, such as podiatry and private speech therapy, 1.8%; eyeglasses and appliances, 1.9%; administrative expenses, 4%; government public health activities, 3%; "other health" services,
2.5%; research, 2.3%; and construction, 3.8%. The costs of medical education are not included in these Social Security Administration figures for total health care expenditures, except insofar
as they are inseparable from hospital expenditures and biomedical research (Mueller and Gibson, 1976, p. 11).

Thus, hospital services are the greatest drain on the health
care dollar. Most appropriately, since the 1976 amendments to
the Social Security Act (P. L. 90-248), interest has focused on
the development of programs for reimbursing hospitals through
federal payment and private insurance mechanisms that incorpo-
rate incentives for economy while maintaining quality of care
(Sigmond; Wolkstein; Bauer; McCarthy). It is also worth noting
the relatively low rate of increase over the years in expenditures
for drugs, given that some of the major advances against morbidity and mortality in this century are attributable to the discovery
and application of such therapeutic agents (Fuchs, 1974, pp.
105–121).

Where the Money Comes From

Ultimately, of course, the people pay all health care costs. Thus,
when we say that health care monies come from different sources,
we really mean that dollars take different routes on their way
from consumers to providers of care. The three major routes are
direct payment from consumer to provider; through government;
and through private insurance companies, profit and nonprofit. In
fiscal 1975, 28% of expenditures were directly out-of-pocket
($33.5 billion) ; the public share was about 42% (about $50 billion), with the federal government bearing about two-thirds of
that, while 26% was paid through insurance companies (about

Table 9.2

Aggregate and Per Capita National Health Expenditures, Selected Fiscal Years, 1929–75

Type of expenditure	1929	1935	1940	1950	1960	1965	1966	1967	1968	1969	1970	1971	1972[a]	1973[a]	1974[a]	1975[b]
Total	$3,589	$2,846	$3,863	$12,027	$25,856	$38,892	$42,109	$47,879	$53,766	$60,617	$69,202	$77,162	$86,687	$95,384	$104,030	$118,500
						Aggregate amount (in millions)										
Health services and supplies	3,382	2,788	3,729	11,181	24,162	35,664	38,661	44,343	49,802	56,327	64,065	71,762	80,548	88,941	97,214	111,250
Hospital care	651	731	969	3,698	8,499	13,152	14,245	16,921	19,384	22,356	25,879	29,133	32,720	36,155	39,963	46,600
Physicians' services	994	744	946	2,689	5,580	8,405	8,865	9,738	10,734	11,842	13,443	15,098	16,527	17,995	19,571	22,100
Dentists' services	476	298	402	940	1,944	2,728	2,866	3,158	3,518	3,920	4,473	4,908	5,364	6,101	6,783	7,500
Other professional services	248	150	173	384	848	989	1,140	1,139	1,217	1,298	1,385	1,509	1,634	1,781	1,927	2,100
Drugs and drug sundries	601	471	621	1,642	3,591	4,647	5,032	5,480	5,865	6,482	7,114	7,626	8,239	8,987	9,612	10,600
Eyeglasses and appliances	131	128	180	475	750	1,151	1,309	1,514	1,665	1,743	1,776	1,810	1,878	1,986	2,160	2,300
Nursing-home care			28	178	480	1,271	1,407	1,751	2,360	3,057	3,818	4,890	5,860	6,650	7,450	9,000
Expenses for prepayment and administration	101	91	161	290	807	1,234	1,446	1,818	1,939	2,066	2,115	2,405	3,645	4,299	4,501	4,593
Government public health activities	89	112	155	351	401	671	731	884	1,001	1,195	1,437	1,698	2,075	2,152	2,625	3,457
Other health services	90	63	92	534	1,262	1,416	1,620	1,940	2,119	2,368	2,625	2,685	2,606	2,835	2,622	3,000
Research and medical-facilities construction	207	58	134	847	1,694	3,228	3,448	3,536	3,964	4,290	5,137	5,400	6,139	6,443	6,816	7,250
Research		58	3	110	592	1,391	1,545	1,606	1,800	1,790	1,846	1,850	2,058	2,298	2,389	2,750
Construction	207	58	131	737	1,102	1,837	1,903	1,930	2,164	2,500	3,291	3,550	4,081	4,145	4,427	4,500

Per capita amount[c]

Total	$29.16	$22.04	$28.83	$78.35	$141.63	$197.75	$211.56	$237.93	$264.37	$295.20	$333.57	$368.25	$409.71	$447.31	$484.35	$547.03
Health services and supplies	27.48	21.59	27.83	72.83	132.35	181.34	194.24	220.36	244.88	274.30	308.81	342.48	380.69	417.10	452.61	513.56
Hospital care	5.29	5.66	7.23	24.09	46.56	66.87	71.57	84.09	95.31	108.87	124.74	139.03	154.64	169.55	186.06	215.12
Physicians' services	8.08	5.76	7.06	17.52	30.57	42.74	44.54	48.39	52.78	57.67	64.80	72.05	78.11	84.39	91.12	102.02
Dentists' services	3.87	2.31	3.00	6.12	10.65	13.87	14.40	15.69	17.30	19.09	21.56	23.42	25.35	28.61	31.58	34.62
Other professional services	2.01	1.16	1.29	2.50	4.65	5.03	5.73	5.66	5.98	6.32	6.68	7.20	7.72	8.35	8.97	9.69
Drugs and drug sundries	4.88	3.65	4.66	10.70	19.67	23.63	25.28	27.23	28.84	31.57	34.29	36.39	38.94	42.15	44.75	48.93
Eyeglasses and appliances	1.06	.99	1.34	3.09	4.11	5.85	6.58	7.52	8.19	8.49	8.56	8.64	8.88	9.31	10.06	10.62
Nursing-home care			.21	1.16	2.63	6.46	7.07	8.70	11.60	14.89	18.40	23.34	27.70	31.19	34.69	41.55
Expenses for prepayment and administration	.82	.70	1.20	1.89	4.42	6.27	7.26	9.03	9.53	10.06	10.19	11.48	17.23	20.16	20.96	21.20
Government public health activities	.72	.87	1.16	2.29	2.19	3.41	3.67	4.39	4.92	5.82	6.93	8.10	9.81	10.09	12.22	15.96
Other health services	.73	.49	.69	3.48	6.91	7.20	8.14	9.64	10.42	11.53	12.65	12.81	12.32	13.30	12.21	13.85
Research and medical-facilities construction	1.68	.45	1.00	5.52	9.28	16.41	17.32	17.57	19.49	20.89	24.76	25.77	29.01	30.22	31.73	33.47
Research		.45	.02	.72	3.21	7.07	7.76	7.98	8.85	8.72	8.90	8.83	9.73	10.78	11.12	12.69
Construction	1.68		.98	4.80	6.04	9.34	9.56	9.59	10.64	12.18	15.86	16.94	19.29	19.44	20.61	20.77

Source: M. S. Mueller and R. M. Gibson "National Health Expenditures, Fiscal Year, 1975," Social Security Bulletin, 39, February 1976, Table 4. (See Appendix I, A12.)

[a] Revised estimates.
[b] Preliminary estimates.
[c] Based on January 1 data from the Bureau of the Census for total U.S. population (including Armed Forces and federal civilian employees overseas and the civilian population of outlying areas).

$30 billion). The balance, 4% ($4.8 billion), was provided by philanthropy and by industry for inplant health services (Mueller and Gibson, 1976, derived from Tables 2 and 5).

Public Outlays

The amount transferred by the public sector in fiscal 1975 ($50 billion, 42% of the total) compares with 24.5% in 1965, 25.5% in 1950, 19.1% in 1935, and 13.3% in 1929 (Table 9-1). The increase is largely due to greater federal expenditures. Proportionately, state and local government outlays have remained rather constant over time, in the 12-13% range. They accounted for 13.6% of the total in fiscal 1975. In contrast, the federal share of outlays rose from 12.8% in 1966 to 25% in 1971, to almost 29% in 1975 (Cooper et al.; Mueller and Gibson, 1976, Table 2). Government spending rose by 22.4% in 1975, close to double the increase in the preceding year, with 72% of this increase accounted for by Medicare and Medicaid.* These programs, Titles XVIII and XIX respectively of the Social Security Act dating from 1965, account for the bulk of federal health expenditures.

Medicare. Medicare was inaugurated on July 1, 1966. It provided a limited range of medical care benefits for persons 65 and over who were covered by the Social Security System. In July 1973 benefits were extended to the disabled, and those suffering from chronic kidney disease (Russel et al, p. 49). Part A of the program, financed by payroll taxes collected under the Social Security System, provides coverage for care rendered in a hospital, an extended care facility or the patient's home. Part B, a voluntary supplemental program that pays certain costs of doctors'

* It happens that proportionately the fastest growing single category of government health care expenditures in fiscal 1975 was for public health activities other than maternal and child health. Between 1974 and 1975, such costs rose 32% to $3.5 billion (Mueller and Gibson, 1976, Table 2). In general, outlays in this category cover government efforts to protect the general public from disease and injury and include a broad range of undertakings, from immunization programs and environmental control to surveillance aimed at occupational safety and consumer protection. Also included are federal and state dollar support for health planning, and federal expenditures in support of the Community Health Centers and migrant health programs. The latter activities, however, were formerly debited to the Office of Economic Opportunity, and this paper change, which took place in 1973–74, accounts for much of the increase (Russel et al., pp. 53–54).

services and other medical expenses, is supported in part by general tax revenues and in part by contributions paid by the elderly (Somers and Somers, p.15).*

Neither Part A nor Part B of Medicare, however, offers comprehensive coverage. Built into the program are deductibles (set amounts the patient must pay for each type of service each year before Medicare begins to pay) and copayments (a percentage of charges paid by the patient). Limitations on the amount of coverage exist as well. Hospital benefits cease after 90 days if the patient has exhausted his lifetime reserve pool of 60 additional days; extended care facility benefits end after 100 days. Home health care visits are limited to 100 (Russel et al., p. 51).

In brief, Medicare provides the elderly with some protection in time of illness but does not pay the whole bill. As Table 9.3 shows, while spending under Medicare rose from $3.4 billion in 1967 to $10.2 billion in 1974, only 38.1% of the $26.7 billion dollars that went for personal health care for the aged in fiscal 1974 was paid for by Medicare. Nor was coverage uniform: 62% of hospital care costs was covered; 51.9% of physicians' charges; 23.7% of "other professional services" and only 3.3% of nursing home expenses.† Even after other government programs and supplementary private health insurance were taken into account, the 1974 per capita out-of-pocket expense for the elderly was over $415, 34.1% of costs (Mueller and Gibson, 1975). The dimensions of the problem emerge when data from the 1970 census are presented: 58% of elderly individuals are in families with less than $5,000 in income; only 18% have family incomes over $10,000.

Medicaid. Unlike Medicare, Medicaid is a program run jointly by federal and state governments: the name is more or less a blan-

---

* The 1972 amendments to the Social Security Act also extend benefits to persons 65 and over who do not meet the criteria for the regular Social Security Program but who are willing to pay a premium for both Part A and Part B coverage. The Amendments provide as well for the establishment of Professional Standards Review Organizations (PSROs) to monitor the quality and quantity of institutional services delivered to Medicare and Medicaid recipients.

† Medicare was intended to stimulate the use of less costly mechanisms for acute care services. Reimbursement was therefore made available on a limited basis to home health care programs and extended care facilities (ECFs). Payments to nursing homes occur in instances where those homes qualify as ECFs (Coe et al.).

Table 9.3

Estimated Amount and Percentage Distribution of Personal Health Care Expenditures for the Aged, Fiscal Years 1972–74

Type of Expenditure	Amount (in millions)					Percentage Distribution				
			PUBLIC					PUBLIC		
	TOTAL	PRIVATE	Total	Medicare	Other	TOTAL	PRIVATE	Total	Medicare	Other
1972 total	$21,649	$8,905	$12,742	$8,364	$4,378	100.0	41.1	58.9	38.6	20.2
Hospital care	9,816	1,632	8,184	6,215	1,969	100.0	16.6	83.4	63.3	20.1
Physicians' services	3,615	1,562	2,053	1,905	148	100.0	43.2	56.8	52.7	4.1
Dentists' services	375	345	30	—	30	100.0	92.0	8.0	—	8.0
Other professional services	360	263	97	77	20	100.0	73.1	26.9	21.4	5.6
Drugs and drug sundries	1,920	1,689	231	—	231	100.0	88.0	12.0	—	12.0
Eyeglasses and appliances	402	396	6	—	6	100.0	98.5	1.5	—	1.5
Nursing-home care	4,981	2,998	1,983	168	1,815	100.0	60.2	39.8	3.4	36.4
Other health services	180	20	160	—	160	100.0	11.1	88.9	—	88.9
1973 total	$23,877	$9,633	$14,244	$9,040	$5,204	100.0	40.3	59.7	37.9	21.8
Hospital care	10,852	1,984	8,868	6,787	2,081	100.0	18.3	81.7	62.5	19.2
Physicians' services	3,854	1,676	2,178	2,016	162	100.0	43.5	56.5	52.3	4.2
Dentists' services	402	371	31	—	31	100.0	92.3	7.7	—	7.7
Other professional services	397	278	119	83	36	100.0	70.0	30.0	20.9	9.1
Drugs and drug sundries	2,064	1,812	252	—	252	100.0	87.8	12.2	—	12.2
Eyeglasses and appliances	425	419	6	—	6	100.0	98.6	1.4	—	1.4
Nursing-home care	5,653	3,073	2,580	154	2,426	100.0	54.4	45.6	2.7	42.9
Other health services	230	20	210	—	210	100.0	8.7	91.3	—	91.3

1974 total[a]	$26,678	$16,082	$10,158	$5,926	100.0	39.7	60.3	38.1	22.2
Hospital care	12,556	10,024	7,778	2,246	100.0	20.2	79.8	62.0	17.9
Physicians' services	3,990	2,250	2,069	181	100.0	43.6	56.4	51.9	4.5
Dentists' services	429	31	—	31	100.0	92.8	7.2	—	7.2
Other professional services	418	141	99	42	100.0	66.3	33.7	23.7	10.1
Drugs and drug sundries	2,260	305	—	305	100.0	86.6	13.5	—	13.5
Eyeglasses and appliances	461	7	—	7	100.0	98.5	1.5	—	1.5
Nursing-home care	6,333	3,113	210	2,903	100.0	50.8	49.2	3.3	45.8
Other health services	231	211	—	211	100.0	8.7	91.3	—	91.3

Source: M. S. Mueller and R. M. Gibson, "Age Difference in Health Care Spending, Fiscal Year 1974," *Research and Statistics Note No. 6, 1975,* (Office of Research and Statistics, Social Security Administration, U.S. Dept. of Health, Education and Welfare, May 13, 1975), Table 2.
[a] Preliminary estimates.

ket label for 50 different programs. Designed specifically to serve the poor, Medicaid provided, as of January 1967, federal funds to states on a cost-sharing basis (according to each state's per capita income) so that welfare recipients could be guaranteed medical services. Payment in full was to be afforded to the aged poor, the blind, the disabled, and families with dependent children for four types of care: (1) inpatient and outpatient hospital care; (2) other laboratory and X-ray services; (3) physician services; and (4) skilled nursing care for persons over 21. By July 1970, home health services and early and periodic detection and treatment of disease for persons under 21 were to be covered.

The 1972 Social Security Act amendments added family planning to the list of "musts." Prescriptions, dental services, eyeglasses, and care in an "intermediate facility" (institutions that do not qualify as skilled nursing homes or those serving the mentally retarded) are allowable "optionals," as is coverage of the medically indigent (those who are self-supporting except for medical care costs). Under the 1972 amendments, coverage of the medically indigent is, by law, tied to their payment of monthly premiums, the amount being graduated by income. Deductibles and copayments are also allowed on all services for the medically indigent and on optional services for welfare recipients (Russel et al., p. 53).

Those who pass a means test (prove that their income is below state-established poverty levels) must be supplied with the five basic services without charge in any state participating in the Medicaid program. Limits on covered benefits are, however, left to the individual state, which, along with the variety of options allowed, has resulted in a wide diversity of operative programs. New York and California, for instance, established such broad programs that in 1971 they received 40% of federal Medicaid outlays despite the fact that both had the lowest federal/state fund-matching rate (Russel et al. pp. 53–54).*

There has been a continuing increase in spending for Medicaid. In 1968, federal outlays for the program totaled $1,805,833,000. By 1975, total federal, state, and local expenditures under Medicaid had reached almost $13 billion, about 54% of it federal (Mueller and Gibson, 1976, Table 3). These monies provided services for approximately 27 million American eligible poor.

* For a further discussion of the principles of Medicare and Medicaid, see Chapter 15.

Excluded from benefits were most working poor, childless couples, the medically indigent in 27 states, and, in 26 states, low-income families with an unemployed father present (Russel et al., pp. 54–56, 64). Estimates made in 1974 by the Office of Research and Statistics of the Social Security Administration indicate that 9 million persons officially designated as "poor" were still excluded from Medicaid coverage (Mueller). Further Medicaid cutbacks will naturally increase that number.

In 1975, Medicaid and Medicare accounted for over 60% of public outlays for health purposes. The next largest expenditure category, general hospital and medical care, totaled $5.5 billion in fiscal 1975—up 8.5% from the previous year. This includes federal dollars expended in support of United States Public Health Service hospitals and the PHS-operated Indian Health Services, and states and local funds used to operate psychiatric hospitals and other long-term care facilities, as well as county and municipal hospitals (Mueller and Gibson, 1976).

Other Public Expenditures. There are five remaining significant health care categories for which government monies are spent: (1) federal outlays for hospital and medical services for veterans ($3.2 billion in 1975, 7% of total public expenditures); (2) provision of care by the Department of Defense for the armed forces and military dependents (in 1975, $3 billion, 7%); (3) general hospital and medical care mentioned above ($5.5 billion, 12%); (4) workmen's compensation medical benefits ($1.8 billion, 4%); and (5) federal, state, and local outlays for public health activities ($4 billion, 9% in fiscal 1975), including those directed at the organization and delivery of health services, Comprehensive Health Planning, Regional Medical Programs, and the National Center for Health Services Research (Russel et al., p. 110), and those used to provide maternal and child health and "other" public health services (Mueller and Gibson, 1976, Table 3).*

The programs of the Veterans' Administration and the Department of Defense are described in Chapter 10. Expenditures for general hospital and medical care include those for the United States Public Health Service and Indian Health Service, state mental and tuberculosis hospitals, and local government hospitals, primarily for the poor. These programs are described in Chapters 7, 8, and 10.

* Beginning in 1974, school health expenditures were included in the education rather than the health category.

Workmen's compensation is an insurance system operated by the states, each with its own law and program, which provides covered workers with some protection against the costs of medical care and loss of income resulting from work-related injury and in some cases, sickness (U.S. National Commission). The first workmen's compensation law was enacted in New York in 1910; by 1948 all states had enacted such laws. The theory underlying workmen's compensation is that all accidents irrespective of fault must be regarded as risks of industry, and that the employer and the employee shall share the burden of the loss: the employer by paying in money and the employee by losing a portion of his/her wages. By 1973, total benefits under the state workmen's compensation programs were an estimated $3.8 billion, of which $2.4 billion was for compensation payments and $1.4 billion for health care. The aggregate cost to employers was $1.19 per $100 of payroll.

On July 31, 1972, the National Commission on State Workmen's Compensation Laws reported on the status of such laws. The Commission recognized the important role the states had played, but found the protection given by such laws to be inadequate and inequitable. The Commission made 13 important recommendations, including compulsory, universal coverage, full coverage for occupational diseases, no limitations on medical care and rehabilitative services, standards for the amount of benefits for death and for permanent and temporary total disability, and principles relating to extraterritorial coverage. The Commission also recommended including all its recommendations as mandates in federal legislation applicable to all employers. In 1976, Congress was considering several bills that would carry out these recommendations (Congressional Research Service).

The relatively low level of government funding for the fifth category, public health activities (part of which, as indicated earlier, is even attributable to a paper change) deserves special attention in view of the growing recognition of the relationship between the environment and health, the importance of preventive care, and the need for planning for a rational system of health delivery. Unfortunately, as experience in all fields shows, voiced interest without dollar support seldom moves beyond the interest stage.

For research and facilities construction, public spending in the mid-1970s was also on the rise. Dollars devoted to construction totaled approximately $1.3 billion in fiscal 1975. Public outlays for research reached $2.75 billion in 1975, with the federal government the source for all but $97 million (Mueller and Gibson, 1976, Table 2). Another $235 million for research came from private sources. Although expenditures for biomedical research represent a small percentage of total health outlays (2.3%), their effects are far-reaching. Federal research dollars not only increase the probability of advancements in disease prevention and control but also provide substantial support for medical schools across the country (Russel et al., p. 24). In 1970, for example, such funds contributed part of the salaries of half the faculty members in medical schools (Strickland, 1972a, p. 249).

Private Health Care Expenditures

The bulk of private health care expenditures comes from two sources: the individual receiving treatment and the private insurer making payment on his behalf. In fiscal 1975, their combined contributions totaled $63.8 billion, 54% of all national health care expenditures (Mueller and Gibson, 1976, Table 2). In 1965, prior to the advent of Medicare and Medicaid, the total private share was 75.5%; in 1935, 80.9%; in 1929, 86.7%. This decline in the private share of total expenditures is due primarily to the sharp drop in out-of-pocket payments which is associated with increased federal spending. In 1950, for example, 68.3% of personal health care expenditures was paid directly by the patient; in 1975, only 28%. Unfortunately, however, because of inflation and other factors, the per capita dollar amount paid directly in 1975 was more than triple what it was in 1950 (Mueller and Gibson, 1976, Table 6).

Private insurers have paid a more or less stable 25% of total health care costs since 1965. Their share was 30.2 billion in fiscal 1975 (26 percent of the total), including profit (or loss) and the costs of doing business (Mueller and Gibson, 1976, derived from Tables 2 and 5). But it is not the dollar figure alone that focuses attention on the private insurance industry. Medicare, and Medicaid to a limited extent, utilize the industry in a middle-man capacity, as a "fiscal intermediary." Several of the major national health insurance plans proposed are based on the private insurance mechanism, as discussed in Chapter 15. Americans questioned on health care problems more often than not cite the expense, confusion, or inadequacies of their insurance policies (Strickland, 1972b). Scholars like Sylvia Law (1974) charge the not-for-profit Blue Cross operation with lack of public responsiveness and accountability. Private insurance is both an important and controversial part of the American system of payment for health care.

Before considering private health insurance in any depth, the manner in which the term "insurance" is used in the health care industry should be clarified. "Insurance" originally meant, and still usually refers to, the contribution by individuals to a fund for the purpose of providing each contributor with protection against financial losses following the occurrence of a relatively unlikely but damaging event. Thus, there is insurance against fire, theft, death at an early age. All of these events occur within a group of people at a predictable rate but are rare occurrences for any one individual in the group.

Medical insurance, when it began, was in this tradition. From 1847, when the first commercial insurance plan designed to defray the costs of medical care was organized, to the 1930s, health insurance consisted essentially of cash payments by commercial carriers to offset income losses resulting from disability attributable to accidents. Sickness benefits (cash payments during sickness) began as an extra, a "frill" on accident insurance policies. As with the latter, emphasis was on the replacement of income lost, in this instance as a result of contracting certain specified and catastrophic communicable diseases—typhoid, scarlet fever, smallpox, and the like (*Source Book of Health Insurance Data*, p. 9). With the origin of Blue Cross and Blue Shield a new policy developed: reimbursing health care costs in general.

Health care utilization is not a rare occurrence. On the average, each person in the United States visits a physician five times a year. One out of every seven Americans is admitted to a hospital at least once a year. Other than coverage for catastrophic illness, a fairly rare event, health insurance has become a mechanism for offsetting expected rather than unexpected costs. The experience of the many is pooled in an effort to reduce expected outlays to manageable prepayment size. Perhaps the term "assurance" more appropriately describes this health care payment system that has evolved. In Britian, "assurance" is used to denote coverage for contingencies that must eventually happen (life assurance) ; "insurance" is reserved for coverage of those contingencies like fire and theft, which may not occur (*Encyclopedia Britannica*, 1970, Vol. 12, p. 337).

Blue Cross and Blue Shield. The establishment of payment

mechanisms to defray in general the costs of illness can be traced to the Great Depression. Previously hospitals had sought to assure reimbursement for their services through public education campaigns directed at encouraging their users, middle-income Americans, to put money aside for unpredictable medical expenses (Law, p. 6). When hard times proved the inadequacy of the savings approach, attention turned to the development of a stable income mechanism. A model was at hand in the independent prepayment plan pioneered in 1929 at Baylor University Hospital in Texas to assure certain area schoolteachers of some hospital coverage. Under the plan, 1,250 teachers prepaid half a dollar a month to provide themselves with up to 21 days of semi-private hospitalization annually.

Like Baylor's, most early plans were for single hospitals. Then, in the early 1930s, in several cities nonprofit prepayment programs offering care at a number of hospitals were organized. The American Hospital Association vigorously supported the growth and development of these plans, soon to be named Blue Cross, and the special insurance legislation which was required for their establishment in each state (Law, pp. 7–8). The AHA set standards for plans and then offered its seal of approval to plans meeting the standards. A provider-insurer partnership was firmly established. Indeed, not until 1972 did national Blue Cross formally separate from the American Hospital Association.

Like Blue Cross, Blue Shield was a child of provider interests born of the Depression. In this instance, the provider was the physician; the professional organization, the state medical society. In 1917, county medical societies in Washington and Oregon had established "medical bureaus" to compete with private doctors and clinics for medical service contracts covering employees of railroads and lumber companies. In 1939, generally recognized as the year Blue Shield began, state medical societies sponsored plans in California and Michigan. Eight additional states followed suit in the period from 1940 to 1942, and in 1943, the American Medical Association established a Council on Medical Service and Public Relations in order to formulate standards and approve state and local Blue Shield plans (Somers and Somers, p. 319). The growth of Blue Shield was less dramatic than Blue Cross following the Depression because physicians in general were in less dire financial circumstances than hospitals were (Anderson, p. 119). Instead, the period of greatest growth for Blue Shield was between 1945 and 1949 when the medical profession sought to stave off movements for federal and state health insurance (Somers and Somers, p. 321).

In other respects, however, Blue Shield mirrors Blue Cross. For example, both are local or statewide undertakings organized for the most part under special state enabling acts. They are incorporated as not-for-profit charitable organizations and therefore relieved of the obligations facing stock and mutual insurance companies—namely, the maintenance of substantial cash reserves and the payment of state and federal taxes (Anderson, p. 123). In most states, the department or commissioner of insurance supervises the Blues, issuing or approving their certificates of incorporation, reviewing their annual income and expenditure reports, monitoring the rates subscribers pay into the program and the rates the programs pay to the providers (Law, pp. 13-18).

In line with their not-for-profit status, both programs, at least initially, were committed to "community rating." Under such a policy, a set of benefits are offered at a single rate to all individuals and groups within a community, regardless of age, sex, or occupation of community members. In essence, the rate represents an averaging out of high- and low-cost individuals and groups so that the community as a whole can be serviced with adequate benefits at reasonable cost (Somers and Somers, p. 309). When commercial for-profit insurance companies entered the field, however, they did so with a policy of "experience rating," charging different individuals and population subgroups different premiums based on their use of services. Low-risk groups could secure benefits at a lower premium. As a result, the Blues also decided to offer a multiplicity of policies with differing rate and benefit structures, and often had to go to experience rating. Had they not, their health insurance portfolios would have comprised adverse risks alone (Krizay and Wilson, p. 40).

Finally, it is the Blues that, by and large, serve as the fiscal intermediaries between the federal and state governments in the Medicare and Medicaid programs (Somers and Somers, pp. 34-35). The role of intermediary is a key one. Under Medicare, for example, the intermediary: (1) determines how much the provider is to be paid; (2) makes the payment; (3) audits the provider's books; and (4) assists in the development and maintenance of utilization review systems designed to check unnecessary costs. In 1971, under Medicare Part A, where the provider chooses the intermediary, Blue Cross handled 93% of the hospitals and 53% of the extended care facilities. Under Part B, where the federal government makes the selection, 60% of provider payments were handled by Blue Shield. Under Medicaid, where state governments select the intermediary, the Blues again had the bulk of the business (Bodenheimer et al., p. 63).

Commercial Insurance. The profit-making commercial insurance companies (Aetna, Metropolitan Life, etc.) entered the general health insurance market cautiously. They had realized losses on income-replacement policies during the Depression; they were leery of the Blues' initial emphasis on comprehensive benefits. However, a Supreme Court decision recognizing fringe benefits as a legitimate part of the collective bargaining process (following as it did upon the freezing of industrial wages during World War II), proved too much of a temptation. Business was shopping for insurance carriers, and the commercials responded (Somers and Somers, pp. 262–263; *Source Book of Health Insurance*, p. 10). By the 1970s, almost 1,000 for-profit companies were offering insurance of one sort or another against the cost of illness (Bodenheimer et al., p. 59).

In the main, Blue Cross offers hospitalization insurance; Blue Shield, coverage of in-hospital physician services and a limited amount of office-based care. The commercials offer both. As in the case of the Blues, commercial hospital and hospital physician coverage is primarily provided to groups through employee fringe-benefit packages negotiated through collective bargaining. Individual coverage can be purchased, but it is usually quite expensive or has limited coverage. The commercials also sell major-medical and cash-payment policies. The former, directed primarily at catastrophic illness, pay all or part of the treatment costs beyond those covered by basic plans. They are sold on both a group and an individual basis. (Blue Cross also sells some group major medical policies.) Cash payment policies pay the insured a flat sum of money per day of hospitalization, and are usually sold directly to individuals, often through mass advertising campaigns. Although the daily cash payment sum is usually small, it can help defray costs left uncovered by other insurance.

Like the Blues, the commercials are subject to supervision by state insurance commissioners, although such supervision does not include rate regulation. The one requirement is that commercials establish premium rates high enough to cover claims made under the insurance they provide. Solvency of the insurer is the principal aim of insurance commission surveillance (Krizay and Wilson, p. 44).

The independent plans. In addition to Blue Cross/Blue Shield and the commercials, a number of so-called independent insurance plans have been established: Kaiser-Permanente, located primarily on the West Coast; the Health Insurance Plan of Greater New York; and the Group Health Cooperative in Washington State are among them. These have been discussed to a certain extent in Chapter 6. Most combine a prepayment mechanism with a captive medical group practice, although comprehensive Foundations for Medical Care (see Chapter 6) and Group Health Insurance in New York use individual practices. Some plans cover inpatient and ambulatory services; some, ambulatory services alone. Sponsors may be industry, employees/unions, community groups, or providers.*

In sum, most independent plans combine to some extent the functions of insurance carrier and provider (Somers and Somers, p. 340-343) : in exchange for premium payments, plan enrollees are entitled to medical services provided by physicians contracting with or employed by the plan. At times, care is provided at sites owned or leased by the plan or in institutions with whom the plan has contracted for services for its enrollees.

Some Health Maintenance Organization (HMOs), if they provide their own prepayment mechanisms rather than using Blue Cross or a commercial carrier, are also classified by the SSA in the independent plan group. However, while sponsors include medical schools, hospitals, unions, consumer groups, government, and other organizations, health insurers are in the vanguard of activity (Salmon). In mid-1974, 55 insurance companies were involved in 71 HMO operations in 25 states. Primarily, insurers are engaged in financial backing, consultation, administrative management, marketing, coverage for hospitalization and/or out-of-area emergency care, re-insurance and acceptance of risk

---

* In arriving at insurance statistics, the Social Security Administration has included in the category of "independent plans" HMOs sponsored by consumer groups, physician groups, hospitals, medical schools, labor unions, and private corporations, when such sponsors are at major financial risk for prepaid care. When the HMO is sponsored by the Blues or a commercial carrier that has accepted financial responsibility for failure, that HMO is included in statistics on the Blues or commercial carriers.

in the event of failure (*Source Book of Health Insurance*, p. 16). Their involvement is an effort to advance the establishment of alternative, less costly delivery systems, utilizing in diverse ways the present insurance framework. Some observers believe that the commercial insurance companies see the development of Health Maintenance Organizations as a positive strategy ultimately leading to the corporate takeover of the health care delivery system (Salmon). (See also Chapter 15.)

Extent of insurance coverage in the United States. Private health insurance coverage for Americans is extensive but uneven. In 1974, approximately three out of every four Americans had at least some coverage for hospital services, surgical physician care, and outpatient X-ray and laboratory examinations, according to the Social Security Administration (whose figures are slightly lower than those of the Health Insurance Association of America) (Mueller and Piro, Table 1). Moreover, 67% of Americans were covered for some out-of-hospital prescription drugs, 60% for some home and office physician visits; 16% for some dental services; 33% for some nursing-home care; and over 60% for some other nursing services.

The proportions of persons with some private health insurance have been increasing over time. By 1962, the proportions of the population having some coverage for hospitalization and physicians' services already stood at a fairly high level: 70% and 65% respectively (Mueller and Piro, Table 7). However, the proportions of the population covered for other services has increased greatly over the years. In 1962, for example, some nursing home coverage was held by only 3% of the population, while for dental care the figure was 0.5%. From 1960 to 1974, the number of Americans with some major medical coverage increased from 29 to 132 million (Mueller and Piro, Table 8). In private insurance, deductibles and copayment abound, as do benefit limits and exclusions.

However, an examination of the proportions of total expenditures covered by private insurance for various types of care tells a different story. As we noted above, in 1975 expenditures made through private health insurance amounted to about 26% of the total. Those private health insurance expenditures that paid for health services (rather than profit or administrative expenses) covered about 27% of all personal health care expenditures in 1975 ($27.3 billion of a total of $103.2 billion) (Mueller and Gibson, 1976, Table 5). There is wide variation in the propor-

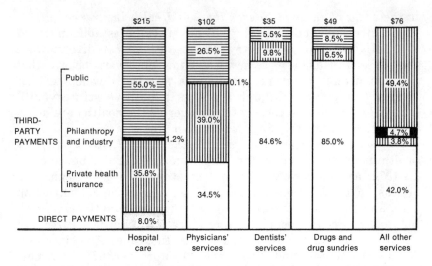

Figure 9.1. Percentage distribution of per capita personal health care expenditures, by type of expenditure and source of funds, fiscal year 1975. (*Source:* M. S. Mueller, and R. M. Gibson, "National Health Expenditures, Fiscal Year 1975," *Social Security Bulletin, 39*, February, 1976, Chart 3.) (See Appendix I, A-12.)

tions of expenditures for the several categories of health care covered by insurance (Figure 9-1). Private insurance covers about 39% of physician expense (primarily for in-hospital care), but only 10% of expenditures for dentists' services, 6.5% of drugs, and less than 4% for "all other services." It is obvious that although many people have some coverage for drugs, doctors' office visits, and "other" services, the coverage doesn't go very far. It is interesting to note that in a 76-page publication of the Health Insurance Institute, which contains data on health insurance in the United States obtained primarily from the Health Insurance Association of America, not one table is devoted to the proportion of total expenditures covered by private health insurance, whereas there are numerous tables citing data on the proportions of persons covered (1975). Table 9.4 compares proportions of persons covered by private insurance for major categories of service with the proportion of total expenditures covered by private health insurance for fiscal 1974.

Retention of premiums in private insurance. The cost to the consumer for insurance coverage—premiums or subscription charges—reached $28.4 billion in fiscal 1974 (Mueller and Piro).

Table 9.4

Private Insurance Coverage, Major Categories of Service, Fiscal 1974

Category of Service	% of Persons with Some Coverage	% of Expenses Covered
Hospital care	78	35
Physicians' services	76	37
Dental care	16	9
Drugs	67	6

Sources: N. Worthington, "National Health Expenditures, 1929–74," Social Security Bulletin, February 1975, Chart 2; M. S. Muller and P. A. Piro, Private Health Insurance in 1974: A Review of Coverage, Enrollment, and Financial Experience," Social Security Bulletin, March 1976, Table 1. (See Appendix I, A-12.)

That same year benefit expenditures by all private insurers totaled $24.8 billion, 87% of premium income. The total operating expenses for the industry were almost $4 billion. Therefore the industry suffered what is called an underwriting loss—the sum of benefit claims and operating expenses exceeded premium income by about $360 million (Mueller and Piro, Table 10). However, different methods of allocation of administrative costs to health insurance are used by different kinds of insurance companies. For example, to sell and process 12% more insurance than the Blues, the commercials reported administrative costs more than three times as high (Mueller and Piro, Table 10). It is thought that some commercial insurance companies allocate to health insurance their sales costs for other kinds of insurance sold to the same beneficiaries. This could considerably alter the "underwriting loss" picture, as could return on investment of premiums, discussed below.

The share of the premium dollar returned in benefits varies widely among the different types of carriers and different types of insurance. In 1974, for example, the Blues returned 94% of monies taken in (96% for Blue Cross, 89% for Blue Shield); commercial carriers, 80% (91% on group and 46% on individual policies, which accounted for about 25% of their business); and the independents, 93% (private group clinics doing the worst at 79% compared with 95% for employer-employee-union plans) (Mueller and Piro, Tables 10, 15).

All insurance companies have the opportunity to make money by investing premium income while they have it. Assuming a going concern, with fairly steady rates of premium income and

Carol McCarthy

benefit payments, $1 billion in premium income annually means about $1 billion in the pot at any one time. That money can be invested. By doing so, in 1974 Blue Cross turned an underwriting loss into a net profit amounting to 1.6% of total income (Mueller and Piro, Table 13). Blue Shield, on the other hand, even with investment income, suffered an overall loss of 1.2% of income in 1974. Unfortunately, net annual income data are not available for the commercial carriers. Thus, one can only guess as to what their true profit picture might be (Jonas, 1974). For 1974, if they made 10% on their investment, their profit, taking into account underwriting losses as they calculate them, was about $1.2 billion. Even if they just took the premium income and put it in a savings bank at 5.5% (day of deposit to day of withdrawal account rate in New York State), they would have cleared over $600 million profit (Mueller and Piro, derived from Table 10).

It is also interesting to compare the difference in operating costs among the different insurers. Blue Cross spent 5.2% of premium income in fiscal 1974, while Blue Shield spent 11.8%, the commercial insurers for group policies 13%, for individual policies 47%, and the independent plans, 7.6% (Mueller and Piro, Table 10). Most notable is the difference in the cost of handling individual as opposed to group policies. The reasons become evident when the functions included under operating costs are outlined: (1) claims handling; (2) statistical services; (3) marketing, including costs of selling and advertising; (4) billing and collection; (5) investment management; and (6) special taxes, licenses, and fees (Krizay and Wilson, p. 45). When the insurance carrier is issuing a single policy to a large group as opposed to diverse individual policies, the costs associated with the first four functions are obviously quite a bit less. However, the question must be raised: are individual policies, which return such a low proportion of premiums to the policy holders as a group, really justified?

For the independent plans, administrative costs are often reduced by employing physicians on a salaried or contract basis to provide a full range of services in return for a set annual payment by enrollees. In such instances, there is no need for billing and collection after each episode of care. Statistical data are more easily collected.

Blue Cross and Blue Shield operate at lower cost than the commercials do because they are exempt from state premium taxes in certain instances and because they pay lower salaries on the average (Krizay and Wilson, p. 46). Finally, Blue Cross, it can be hypothesized, has the administrative-cost edge over all other carriers because it deals *directly* with the *institutional* provider, thereby eliminating the high claims volume characteristic of indirect (via cash payments to the insured) and individual provider (Blue Shield) plans. Once reimbursable services and charges have been determined and incorporated, after negotiation, in the hospital's reimbursement formula, Blue Cross simply pays the hospital the costs of allowable services used by Blue Cross subscribers.

The several insurers hold different shares of the private health care insurance market. In 1974, in all categories of insurance except nursing home care (a small category indeed), commercial carriers served as insurers for over half the Americans covered (Mueller and Piro, Table 3). Although Blue Cross–Blue Shield is most often the target of criticism for failure to utilize the insurance mechanism to promote health care cost-control (Law), that operation captured 40% or less of persons insured for hospital, physician, dental, drug, and nursing services. The commercials are first in premium income too, taking 49%, compared 43% for the Blues and 8% for the independents (Mueller and Piro, Table 10). The order of market dominance—commercials, Blues, then independents—has held since 1950. For those over 65, however, it is Blue Cross–Blue Shield, rather than the commercial carriers, which play the largest role, issuing policies, for the most part, which cover the gaps in Medicare. For the rest, "cash policies" are made available, providing the elderly with specified weekly or monthly payments during periods of hospitalization (Mueller).

The private health insurance industry is extremely influential in the U.S. health care delivery system. In addition to its independent role as a financial agent, which we have analyzed in some detail, its role as the Medicare—and in certain states, Medicaid—fiscal intermediary cannot be forgotten. Its potential as a deliverer of service under national health insurance in the United States is discussed in Chapter 15. Nevertheless, it must be remembered that although more than 75% of Americans have *some* private hospitalization insurance, private insurance covers only 35% of expenditures for hospitalization and slightly more than 25% of *all* expenditures. Is it possible that the industry is being accorded authority to determine future directions for U.S. health care out of proportion to its true importance in the system?

How the Money Is Paid Out
Paying Providers

Health care is a labor-intensive industry, as has been discussed in Chapter 4. About 70% of all expenditures are for personnel (Kramer and Roemer, p. 57). The vast majority of health workers are paid by wages or salary. However, about 400,000 dentists, physicians, osteopaths, optometrists and opticians, chiropractors, psychologists, social workers, speech pathologists, and physicial and occupational therapists, among others, are paid on a fee-for-service basis by their patients or third parties—private insurers or government.

Fee for service. The fee-for-service system has provoked a great deal of controversy. It has been vigorously attacked (Lium; Roemer, 1962; Roemer, 1971) and just as vigorously defended (Sade). Proponents of the fee-for-service system usually argue, especially in relation to fee-for-service reimbursement for physicians, that direct payment cements the necessary bond between provider and patient, a bond on which effective treatment often hinges; that it gives the provider an incentive to work that is not present under any other system; that it is justified by the special life-and-death responsibility that physicians, in particular, must accept.

Opponents claim there is no "natural" justification for the fee-for-service system: it is simply a product of the guild status of physicians, since the majority of health care providers are paid by salary. They point out that the fee-for-service approach creates the two-class system of medical care in the United States about which there is so much complaint. If fees, which some people cannot afford, were not charged at the time of service, then there would be no need to have one set of health care facilities for those who can afford to pay the doctor and a second for those who cannot.

Further, opponents for fee-for-service see the cash exchange as a barrier to utilization and as an interference rather than a help in the provider-patient relationship. As for the argument based on the life-and-death relationship, opponents say that the provider is not usually in a life-and-death relationship with his patient. But even if he were, the airplane pilot does not collect a fee for service, and he certainly has a life-and-death relationship to his passengers. The fireman does not request personal payment before he turns on the water or even after he has put out the fire.

Indeed, when a fireman undertakes a life-and-death responsibility for a person in a burning building, he does not ask for a fee, even though he risks his own life, which doctors rarely, if ever, do.

Finally, opponents argue that with fee-for-service reimbursement, costs go up more rapidly than with other payment mechanisms. They point to the national health insurance experience of other countries such as Canada (Korcok), Australia ("Amendments to Australia's Act"); and Japan (Jonas, 1975). Thinking along the same lines, William Glaser (Ch. 7) cites the unnecessary work so frequently attendant on the fee-for-service system—encouraging the paying patient to return when he wishes, ordering inpatient rather than ambulatory services, and the like. In addition, he indicates that, given the choice of two or more, the practicitioner more often chooses the higher-paid procedure when payment is on a fee basis.

Capitation and salary. The alternative forms of provider reimbursement are capitation and salary. The latter approach is self-explanatory. As indicated earlier, its use as a payment mechanism for health professionals is widespread. Certainly, from the employer's point of view, a salary system has the merit of administrative simplicity. When the employer is the government, there is the added benefit of flexibility: the movement of providers into areas of medical scarcity and unpopular jobs is more easily accomplished under a salary system than under other payment mechanisms. From the provider's point of view, he or she has an income protected from sudden fluctuations in supply and demand, is free of bill collection problems and, usually, benefits from extensive fringe benefits (Roemer, 1962). In a survey conducted by Goldberg, 40% of the physicians interviewed mentioned shorter work weeks, time off to study, rests or vacations without income loss, liberal pension plans, and paid life, health, and malpractice insurance as significant compensations in a salaried system. Finally, salaried providers tend to utilize less costly diagnostic and treatment procedures and to avoid unnecessary utilization of services (Densen et al.; Williams; Roemer, 1962).

However, payment by salary is not without drawbacks. The provider, for example, is faced with a limit on his lifetime income. The comparatively high salaries marking his early years of practice are balanced by the fact that his earnings peak more quickly than the fee-for-service practitioner's (*Harvard Law Review*; Goldberg). In addition, he is subject to administrative constraints on such matters as schedules and vacations and to peer review regarding his performance. Often, he must abandon individual goals in order to conform with his employer's objectives (Shinefield and Smillie; Hayt). To the extent that fee-for-service stimulates quality work, the employer, in turn, must increasingly rely upon the individual physician's dedication, his desire to give fully of his attention and skill to all his patients (Ricketts). From the patient's vantage point the salary system provides few incentives against undertreatment. The physician receives the negotiated salary regardless of the amount of services provided.

Under the capitation arrangement—which is used primarily for physicians providing ongoing care—the physician receives a flat annual fee for each person who agrees to be under his care, again regardless of the frequency with which his services are utilized. Like salary, capitation promotes administrative simplicity—unless, of course, financial incentives are added to base payments to encourage care of the chronic or time-consuming patient. Capitation too removes barriers to care raised by fee requirements for each treatment episode and offers the physician no incentive to undertake more costly rather than less costly medical procedures. In addition, the capitation system advances continuity of care and thus an improved provider-patient relationship (Glaser, Ch. 10).

But there are drawbacks in this system too. With barriers to care reduced, the provider may have to cope with unnecessary calls for treatment. There is also an incentive to increase the number of patients served even if such an increase should result in too little time to offer comprehensive care and needed emotional support (Roemer, 1962).

Paying Hospitals

As stated earlier, payments to hospitals constitute the largest single category of national health expenditures. There are four major modes of hospital reimbursement. The first, oldest, and most rapidly disappearing, is that based on *charges*. This method is used by private, profit, and nonprofit hospitals. A price (which may or may not bear some relationship to the cost of that service) is put on each item of service—a day in bed, use of the operating room, a lab test—and the patient, and/or his insurer under cash-indemnity plans, is billed for that price, usually called a charge.

A more sophisticated reimbursement mode is based on cost.

The determination of cost never involves individual patients. It is a matter for negotiation between hospitals and the major insurance companies in their areas. In certain states, the Insurance Department and/or Department of Health may be a party to the negotiations in either an advisory or approval capacity. Cost reimbursement is used when insured patients receive their benefits as *services* rather than as dollar indemnities. (Almost all group health insurance policies in the United States now provide service benefits rather than dollar indemnities.) In the usual approach, one of several accounting techniques determines the cost of various services per unit of service; the hospital is reimbursed for those costs as it provides the services. Thus, if the agreed bed-day cost figure is $150 for each day of care provided to a patient with Blue Cross insurance, the hospital will receive $150 from Blue Cross. This method is sometimes called "retrospective cost reimbursement."

A still more sophisticated approach, "prospective reimbursement" (Dowling; McCarthy), is used in certain parts of the country. The hospitals and major area insurer get together and attempt to predict, on the basis of previous experience and current rates of cost-increase, what costs will be for the coming year. The hospital then receives that rate per service (or in some instances, per hospital stay or even per time-period without relation to number of units of service actually provided), regardless of its actual cost. There is an obvious stimulus for hospitals to attempt to control costs because under prospective reimbursement they receive a given amount of money for providing a given service without regard to the service at the time it is rendered. This method, particularly when applied to the total hospital budget, obviously approaches annual budgeting for hospitals as related to total program, rather than to individual units of service. However, in most cases reimbursement to the hospitals is still based on the number of items of service delivered.

Finally, government hospitals at all levels operate on total annual budgets, and have always done so. The costs of various inputs, salaries, and expenses, are determined, and a budget is prepared, which is not related to units of service in any way. Although some third-party payments, primarily Medicaid/Medicare, are available to them with reimbursement rates calculated on a cost basis, for most government hospitals the proportion is small. The bulk of government hospital monies comes from tax revenues (Falk et al.). Thus, government hospital budgets are subject to other considerations besides costs and programs. As health care expenditures, particularly for hospitals, continue to rise at a high rate, and as we move toward national health insurance, it is likely that prospective reimbursement or annual budgeting will be applied to increasing numbers of hospitals outside of the public sector in an attempt to control costs, if nothing else.

The Medical Marketplace

Ours is predominantly a market-directed economy: the basic economic questions of what to produce, how, and for whom, are most often answered through the exchange decisions on factors (land, labor, and capital) and products made by individual producers and consumers acting in response to price. According to Samuelson (pp. 44–45) and a host of other noted economists, the distribution of goods and services that results in such instances is difficult to improve upon. Given the way income is apportioned, someone cannot be made better off without making someone else worse off. A condition of optimality is said to exist.

Understood, of course, is a market that, in economic terms, is "perfect" and "competitive"—a situation that rarely, if ever, exists in the health care industry. The industry is, on the contrary, replete with instances of market failure.

Today's medical care cost picture makes it all the more imperative to take a closer look at those failures. When the health care expenditures data presented in the preceding pages are placed against the cost implications for the economy as a whole of employee health care fringe-benefit packages and the knowledge that direct income is foregone to gain protection against the possible cost of illness, the dimensions of the prevailing cost problem emerge. The bulk of private insurance, for example, is obtained through one's place of employment, but employer contributions to employee health plans are not simply written off. The costs involved, allocated from what would otherwise be wages, are passed along to the general public in the form of higher prices for goods and services.

What, then, is a "perfect" market? What are the prerequisites for a "competitive" market? In what specific ways does the medical care market fall short of these ideals that lead to economic efficiency? The requirement for a "perfect" market is simply stated: buyers and sellers must have complete knowledge of market conditions. Price, quantity, quality, and any changes in the same are immediately known to the participants and can be acted upon by them. For a market to be "competitive" three conditions must prevail: (1) there must be a multitude of participants with none so large or powerful that he can exert significant influence on the market itself or on other competitors; (2) there must be no restriction on entry into the market; and (3) the commodity exchanged must be homogeneous—that is, there must be no difference between one seller's product and another's. If conditions one and two are met but not three, one can still speak of "imperfect competition," for price will remain the major determinant of supply and demand (Haveman and Knopf, pp. 140–143).

In the health care industry, however, price is a poor regulator of production and consumption (Fuchs, 1972, pp. 5–8; Mushkin; Klarman, 1965, pp. 10–19). First, unlike the consumer in the general marketplace, the patient is dependent upon the seller, the health care provider, for information about the product he is purchasing, and, in many circumstances, his need for it. At any one time, the patient does not have at his disposal data on the quantity and quality of services offered at a particular price, much less information on changes in quantity, quality, and price. Moreover, he is in no position to make an independent judgment about the most important variable, quality.

The technical nature of medicine, the tremendous uncertainty regarding medical practice outcomes, professional sanctions against advertising, the relative infrequency with which any of the diverse services available are purchased— all work to keep the patient uninformed. In any case, it must be remembered that for the most part, it is the physician, not the patient, who determines what services will be purchased and in what amounts (Fuchs and Kramer, p. 2). Even if one discounts the proven positive correlation between the number of practicing physicians and the number of per capita physician visits per year (Wasyluka), it is impossible to disregard the central role played by the physician in prescribing drugs, other professional services, and hospital and nursing home care. In 1976, this point was stressed by the President's Council on Wage and Price Stability (*New York Times*). Just as there is no "perfect" market, there is no "competitive" market. Because of the skills involved, one appendectomy or tonsillectomy is not necessarily the same as another.

Because of physical facilities, equipment, and manpower resources, a stay at Hospital A may vary considerably from a stay at Hospital B for an identical ailment.

Moreover, although on a national basis there is a multiplicity of "sellers" with none large enough to control the market, in smaller geographic regions both institutions and providers of care may be few enough to dominate the health care delivery system. In some commercial health care operations such as the drug industry, even nationwide market control exists. By product category, the four largest drug firms often account for 50% to 60% of output, with the result that prescription drug prices are seldom responsive to changes in supply and demand (Fuchs, 1974, pp. 105–121).

Finally, as discussed further in Chapter 13, monopolies in the area of education, certification, and licensure of health professions restrict the mobility of manpower both into and within the industry. Licensing prerequisites for physicians, for example, are essentially determined by organized medicine. One of the primary prerequisites is graduation from an approved school. Such schools are those accredited by the Liaison Committee on Medical Education, comprised of representatives of the American Medical Association and the Association of American Medical Colleges. The requirements of institutional accreditation, in turn, place limitations on a hospital's entry into the market.

Even if a "perfect" and "competitive" medical care market existed, however, other industry characteristics would prevent conditions of economic optimality. In the first place, it is largely need rather than demand that occasions the purchase of health services. Those in pain seldom choose health care by rationally weighing the relative merits of all available goods and services. Consider the relation between a family's medical care expenditures and income when illness strikes and stays. When the need factor is added to physician control over the ordering of services, it is easy to understand why a weak relationship exists between consumer demand and price in the medical care industry. Moreover, that relationship is weakened even further by the role of the third-party payor, a role that might be traced, at least in part, to the belief that need should indeed occasion service because health care is a right, as was discussed in Chapter 2. The more frequently and extensively a third party pays, the less often the cost of care enters into decisions of whether or not to seek service (Andersen and Anderson, 1967, pp. 136–140).

Second, a large segment of the industry—particularly the voluntary hospitals—is operated on a not-for-profit basis. Under such circumstances, capital does not flow in and out of the industry in response to market signals. Often, investments are made and resources allocated for other than economic reasons—to improve the quality, availability, and accessibility of care, for example, or because a generous donor wants a particular kind of hospital built or service offered.

Third, at certain times, an individual expenditure in the health care market involves a social utility. Immunization against contagious diseases or treatment for syphilis, for example, benefit the community as a whole. As Mushkin indicates, in instances such as these involving "extra buyer benefits," market price underestimates the total value derived.

The Rising Costs of Health Care

The continually rising cost of health care is one of the most serious problems facing the United States health care delivery system. (It should be pointed out that this problem plagues most capitalist countries [Abel-Smith].) The system has long been viewed as expensive. In 1932, the Committee on the Costs of Medical Care was very concerned with a $3 billion annual rate of expenditure (p. 2), around 4% of the GNP. In 1948, the Director of the Montefiore Hospital in the Bronx, N.Y., was worried because a patient day of care cost $12 and hospital capital construction costs were pro-rated at $20,000 per bed (Bluestone). In 1975, the patient day cost at Montefiore was approaching $200; the pro-rated cost of constructing a teaching hospital bed was approaching $200,000, at the University Hospital, State University of New York at Stony Brook.

Between 1965 and 1975, health care costs increased at an annual rate of between 9 and 14% (Table 9.5). The usual increase was in the 11-12% range. The low occurred in fiscal 1974, when a government price control system, the Economic Stabilization Program (ESP), was in full effect. With the end of the ESP health care cost controls, the rate of increase reached its highest level ever in 1975. Another way to evaluate health care spending is as a percentage of the GNP. This rose sharply from 1965 to 1971, but then leveled off, and even dropped a bit under the ESP. However, in 1975 that indicator took off again too, although one-half of its rise from 7.7 to 8.3% was due to the recession and the resulting slowed GNP growth. If the GNP had continued to rise

Table 9.5

**Total Health Care Expenditures, Annual Percentage
Increase, and Annual Percentage of GNP,
by Fiscal Year, 1965–75**

Year	Amount (in millions)	% Increase over Previous Year	% GNP
1965	39,892	—	5.9
1966	42,109	8.3	5.9
1967	47,879	13.7	6.2
1968	53,765	12.3	6.5
1969	60,617	12.7	6.7
1970	69,202	14.2	7.2
1971	77,162	11.5	7.6
1972	86,687	12.3	7.9
1973	95,384	10.0	7.8
1974	104,030	9.1	7.7
1975ª	118,500	13.9	8.3

Source: M. S. Mueller and R. M. Gibson, "National Health
Expenditures, Fiscal Year 1975," *Social Security Bulletin,*
February 1976. Derived from Table 1. (See Appendix I,
A-12.)
ª Preliminary estimates.

at its 1974 rate, expenditures for health care would have
amounted to about 8% of the GNP (Mueller and Gibson, p. 3).

Health care costs can also be considered in relation to the Consumer Price Index (CPI), a Department of Labor indicator (see
Table 9.6). During the decade 1965–75, the price index for all
medical services rose, on the average, about 18% faster than did
the CPI as a whole. The index for physicians' fees rose about 4%
faster. The drug index rose at about *one-twelfth* the rate, and that
is really an artifact of the relatively sharp rise which occurred in
1975; between 1965 and 1974, the drug index hardly rose at all.
However, the index of hospital semiprivate room rates rose at
about double the rate of overall health care costs and 140% faster
than did the CPI during the same 10-year period.* It is obvious

* There are several other indices used by the Bureau of Labor Statistics for hospital service charges. The operating-room charges index
has closely followed the semiprivate room index. An index of charges
for an upper gastrointestinal radiographic series has moved up much
more slowly than either of the other two. However, a new "total" index
(which we do not discuss in detail because it came into use only in
1973), combining the three previously existing indices with charges for
a group of other ancillary services, in 1975 went up a whopping 27%
faster than did the CPI (*Social Security Bulletin,* March 1976, derived
from Table M-41).

that the cost of hospitalization contributes the most to rising health care costs.

There are five major theories used to explain rises in health care costs in general and hospital costs in particular (Davis and Foster, ch. 1; Davis, 1972; Davis, 1973). The "demand-pull" theory attributes increases to rising income and the growth of insurance, which have enlarged the fund of purchasing power and created new or increased demand on a relatively inelastic supply (Feldstein, 1971). The "labor cost-push" theory states that expenditures rise in response to increased hospital wages and/or lagging productivity gains in the hospital industry. According to the "scientific progress" theory, new, costlier methods of care force prices up. The "waste" theory says that prices rise because of capital investment in costly, expensive-to-maintain facilities that already exist in sufficient supply. Finally, the "cost reimbursement" theory states that increases in supply, equipment, and salary expenditures have occurred with the growth in the number of insurance plans reimbursing at cost. Hospital administrators, it is alleged, have little reason to operate efficiently when costs can be passed on to third-party payors.

In fact, the evidence suggests that all five factors contribute to increasing hospital costs. Let us try to determine which are the most important (see also Chapter 7). It is customary in some quarters to blame the increase in hospitals costs primarily on the

Table 9.6

Consumer Price Indices for All Medical Care Services, Hospital Semi-Private Room Charges, Physicians' Fees, and Prescription Drugs, 1965–75

Year	Consumer Price Index	All Medical Care Services	Hospital Semi-Private Room	Physicians' Fees	Prescription Drugs
1965	89.5	87.3	75.9	88.3	102.0
1966	93.4	92.0	83.5	93.4	101.8
1967	100.0	100.0	100.0	100.0	100.0
1968	106.1	107.3	113.6	105.6	98.3
1969	113.4	116.0	128.8	112.9	99.6
1970	120.6	124.2	145.4	121.4	101.2
1971	128.4	133.3	163.1	129.8	101.3
1972	132.5	138.2	173.9	133.8	100.9
1973	137.7	144.3	182.1	138.2	100.5
1974	150.5	159.1	201.5	150.9	102.9
1975	168.6	178.2	236.0	169.6	109.3

Source: Social Security Bulletin, March 1976, Table M-41. (See Appendix I, A12.)
Note: 1967=100; yearly data are annual averages.

increase in wages, particularly of low-paid hospital workers. For example, Reginald W. Rhein, Jr. of the Washington, D.C. Bureau of *Business Week* said, in reviewing Spencer Klaw's *The Great American Medicine Show*:

> . . . Klaw fails in my view to really come to grips with the increased costs of medical care over the last decade that are primarily due to hospital expenses. Certainly hospital charges account for a major share of the total $118.5 billion health bill.
>
> Klaw devotes only one paragraph, however, to the largest single share of these hospital costs—the wages and salaries of hospital personnel—even though noting that they "account for about 60 percent of the total cost of running a hospital." There is no doubt they also account for much of the rise in hospital costs over the past decade. "In New York City," he says, "orderlies, porters, laundry workers, and other unskilled employees who, fifteen years ago, were earning as little as $28 a week now earn a minimum of $181." Having put his finger squarely on the nub of the problem, he removes it to discuss the more interesting subject (because it makes people angry) of the high costs of drugs and physicians.

Rhein's view is contradicted by an American Hospital Association analysis:

> An American Hospital Association study of the components of hospital cost inflation indicated that, in 1969, 51.3 percent of the increase in hospital expenses per adjusted patient day was due to an increase in the quantity of goods and services purchased [National Hospital Panel Survey and Nonlabor Input Price Index constructed by the AHA Division of Information Services]. Increases in the cost of goods and services contributed only 11.7 percent of the general increase, while the increases in personnel and in average wages contributed 14.3 and 22.7 percent, respectively. It appears that, six years ago, expansion and improvement of services were influences in the increase in costs and the resulting decline in operating margin.
>
> By 1975, however, inflation replaced expansion as a major reason for hospital cost increases. In 1975 44.8 percent of the increase in cost per adjusted patient day was due to increases in the price of goods and services purchased. Increases in the quantity of goods purchased contributed only 11 percent of the overall increase, and increases in personnel and average wages contributed 15.7 and 28.5 percent. (p. 29)

Thus, between 1969 and 1975, wage increases accounted for less than 30% of the total hospital cost increase, and the wages of low-paid workers constitute only one part of a hospital payroll.

Furthermore, the proportion of total hospital expense devoted to payroll has been dropping, from 61% in 1969 (Hospital Indicators, 1971) to 53% in 1974 (Hospital Indicators, 1975). In the mid-70s hospital wages on the whole were rising no faster than general wages. An increasingly important factor was the rises in prices for nonlabor inputs, such as fuel and food (Drake and Raske, 1974).

For earlier periods, like 1962–66 (Davis, 1972) and 1966–68 (Davis, 1973) rising wages were even less influential in rising hospital costs. The Davis data show that only about 10% of the total rise during 1962–68 can be attributed to rises in wages. Major factors were the creation of new expensive services (like open-heart surgical theaters and intensive care units), the addition of new employees to staff them, the increase in the cost of money for capital expansion itself, and, especially after the introduction of Medicare/Medicaid, the availability of new purchasing power to two population groups which, on the one hand, had limited health care purchasing power before 1966, and on the other hand, have higher-than-average health care needs: the poor and the aged. During the 1966–68 period, the greatest increases were found in capital expenditures, and, in particular, in the costs of capital (Davis, 1973). In an era of high interest rates, this latter problem was undoubtedly exacerbated.

Nancy Worthington analyzed "the major factors contributing to annual changes in per capita expenditures for the two largest components of national health spending: hospital care and physicians' services"—hospital care for the 1950–73 period and physicians' services for the 1957–73 period (Worthington, Nov. 1975, p. 3). She found that "real inputs"—that is, new services, often reflecting technological changes—added to each unit of care, had the most important effect on rising costs for both kinds of service. The other major elements—factor prices, the costs of goods and services to the provider, and increased utilization—were less important.

Whereas on the average, hospitals had 178 personnel for every 100 census in 1950, in 1973 the figure was more than 300. In terms of equipment, in 1960, 10% of community hospitals had intensive care units, in which bed costs per day are often more than double that in a semiprivate room; in 1973, the figure was 60% (Worthington, Nov. 1975, pp. 5–6). Physicians have become increasingly specialized, a change in real input. Specialists can get higher fees; unit costs go up. Furthermore, physicians too have added personnel and equipment and use more auxiliary services. These all represent increased real inputs per unit of service (Worthington, Nov. 1975, p. 11). This is not to say that increased factor prices, reflecting general inflation, and increased utilization were not important, but increased real inputs were the most important.

In the spring of 1976, the President's Council on Wage and Price Stability issued a report on rising health care costs (*New York Times*). The report said, in part:

> The nature and extent of services provided is usually determined by the physician in a transaction in which the patient is often a passive participant.
>
> The economic rewards for efficiency and cost-reducing innovation that are characteristic of our economic system seem to be lacking here. Heavy levels of government support have altered the economics of this sector even further. Any attempts to mitigate the rapid rise of inflation in health care must take account of these institutional peculiarities. . . . To the extent these changes [in patterns of care] constitute improvements in the quality or delivery of care, price increases would not be "inflationary" in the technical sense. However, whether such a change is a quality improvement is particularly difficult to evaluate. As a result, there is considerable debate whether the overall quality in delivery of the medical care received by the American people has improved in step with the rapid rise in expenditures and prices.

The *Times* summary added:

> Rising costs, the report said, cannot be explained by increased labor costs, or by the rise in prices that followed a three-year wage and price freeze that held cost relatively stable, or by increased costs on nonlabor items. In short, it said, the increased cost of doing business—general inflation rates—do not account for health price rises. What is peculiar to the health sector and is in part related to the ongoing cost of care, it went on, is the "passive" role of the consumer in health services. When the patient goes to see a doctor, it is the physician who determines how and when he comes back, what other medical services or specialists he

requires, what drugs he needs, and whether he needs to go to the hospital and for how long. Once the patient gets to the hospital, the insurance company picks up the tab and the patient does not feel it, except for the increase in his insurance premiums, which his employee benefits often absorb. . . . The report explored the paradox that in American industry, technology has improved efficiency and lowered manufacturing costs, while in the health sector, technology has improved care and shortened hospital stays but the costs have risen.

Putting all of this information together, the "demand-pull" and "scientific progress" theories seem to be the most useful in explaining that proportion of increased hospital costs and, in turn, increased health care costs which cannot be explained by general inflation. To the extent that "scientific progress" is poorly planned, duplicative, or of questionable utility, and to the extent that new purchasing power is created with minimal attention to cost-control and in a manner that tends to favor utilization of one part of the delivery system (hospitals), the "waste" and "cost reimbursement" theories are applicable.

An understanding of market failures in the medical care industry provides additional understanding of skyrocketing costs. There is little leverage to keep those costs down when neither supply nor demand are allowed the interplay as they do in the ideal, perfectly competitive market. In 1976, the Congressional Budget Office (CBO) estimated that by 1981, depending upon the presence or absence of national health insurance and (if present), the type of NHI, annual health care expenditures would be between $229 billion and $263 billion (*Health Security News*). The CBO predicted that almost any NHI plan would result in lower costs than no plan at all, although others disagree (Davis, 1973; Klarman, 1969).

The complexity of the problem suggests that any recommendation for containing cost inflation must be multifaceted. The aftermath of the Economic Stabilization Program proves the evanescence of cost containment achieved through directly imposed wage and price controls (Worthington). Ways must be found to encourage improved and lasting performance by the private market sector. Certainly, attention should be directed to basic changes in the method of health care delivery, changes that promote cost containment. Effecting a shift away from present reliance upon hospital services, away from almost total dependence upon the physician when medical care is indicated, and toward less costly, equally effective modes of care may well be a first and necessary step.

Conclusion

Money fuels the health care delivery system, but the routes dollars take from consumer to providers can be labyrinthine. Some dollars go directly, some via the government, some through insurance companies. Most health care providers are paid by salary, but some, the higher-income ones for the most part, are paid on a piecework basis. Some institutions get paid on the basis of what they charge, some on the basis of calculated costs per item of service, and some get an annual budget to provide a set of services.

In the United States, in the mid-'70s, a health insurance system that emphasized coverage for hospital care, as well as the practice of having most physicians working both in and out of hospitals, with hospital care generally being more lucrative, "tilted" the system in the direction of utilization and overutilization of the most expensive and inflation-prone component of the system. Without the excessive rate of hospital expenditure increase, total medical care expenditures would probably be rising little faster than the CPI. Technological change, a significant factor in rising health care costs, has been poorly planned and evaluated, with decisions often being made on the basis of emotion, ambition, and pecuniary self-interest, not cost-benefit analysis.

However, as expenditures rise, and as an increasing proportion goes through government hands, the government's interest in cost-control rises. Thus we now turn our attention to various aspects of the role of government in the health care delivery system. It is well known that he who pays the piper calls the tune.

References

Abel-Smith, B. "Value for Money in Health Services." *Social Security Bulletin, 37,* 17, July, 1974.

"Amendments to Australia's National Health Act." *Social Security Bulletin, 34,* 28, December, 1971.

American Hospital Association. "Hospital Operating Margins." *Hospitals, J.A.H.A.*, January 16, 1976, p. 27.

Andersen, R., and Anderson, O. *A Decade of Health Services: Social Survey Trends in Use and Expenditure.* Chicago, Ill.: University of Chicago Press, 1967.

Anderson, O. *The Uneasy Equilibrium.* New Haven, Conn.: College and University Press, 1968.

Anderson, O., and Neuhauser, D. "Rising Costs are Inherent in Modern Health Care Systems." *Hospitals, J.A.H.A.*, February 16, 1969, p. 50.

Bauer, K. G. *Containing Costs of Health Services through Incentive Reimbursement.* Cambridge, Mass.: Harvard Center for Community Health and Medical Care, 1973.

Bluestone, E. M. "Home Care: An Extra–Mural Hospital Function." *Survey Midmonthly, 84,* 99, 133, April, 1948. Reprinted in Committee on Medical Care Teaching of the Association of Teachers of Preventive Medicine, Eds, *Readings in Medical Care.* Chapel Hill: University of North Carolina Press, 1958.

Bodenheimer, T. et al. *Billions for Band-Aids.* San Francisco, Calif.: Bay Area Chapter, Medical Committee for Human Rights, 1972.

Bureau of the Census. *Statistical Abstract of the United States, 1974.* Washington, D.C.: U.S. Department of Commerce, 1974.

Campbell, R. R. *Economics of Health and Public Policy.* Washington, D.C.: American Enterprise Institute for Public Policy Research, 1971.

Coe, R. M. et al. "Impact of Medicare on the Organization of Community Health Resources." *Milbank Memorial Fund Quarterly, 52,* 231, 1974.

Committee on the Costs of Medical Care. *Medical Care for the American People.* Chicago, Ill.: University of Chicago Press, 1932. Reprinted, Washington, D.C.: USDHEW, 1970.

Congressional Research Service. *Workmen's Compensation: Role of the Federal Government.* Issue Brief Number IB75054. Washington, D. C.: Library of Congress, 1976.

Cooper, B. S. et al. "National Expenditures, 1929–73." *Social Security Bulletin, 37,* 1, February, 1974.

Davis, K. "Community Hospital Expenses and Revenues: Pre-Medicare Inflation." *Social Security Bulletin, 35,* 3, October, 1972.

Davis, K. "Hospital Costs and the Medicare Porgram." *Social Security Bulletin, 36,* 18, August, 1973.

Davis, K., and Foster, R. *Community Hospitals: Inflation in the Pre-Medicare Period.* Research Report No. 41. Washington, D. C.: Social Security Administration, 1972.

Densen, P. et al. *Prepaid Medical Care and Hospital Utilization.* Monograph No. 3. Chicago, Ill.: American Hospital Association, 1958.

Derbyshire, R. C. *Medical Licensure and Discipline in the United States.* Baltimore, Md.: Johns Hopkins Press, 1969.

Dowling, W. L. "Prospective Reimbursement of Hospitals." *Inquiry, 11,* 163, 1974.

Drake, D. F., and Raske, K. E. "The Changing Hospital Economy." *Hospitals, J.A.H.A.,* November 16, 1974, p. 34.

Encyclopedia Britannica. "Insurance." Chicago, Ill.: Encyclopaedia Britannica, Inc., 1970. Volume 12, p. 337.

Falk, I. S. et al. *The Costs of Medical Care.* New York: Arno Press, 1972.

Feldstein, M. S. *Economic Analysis for Health Service Efficiency.* Amsterdam, Holland: North-Holland Publicity Co., 1967.

Feldstein, M. S. *The Rising Costs of Hospital Care.* Washington, D.C.: Information Resources Press, 1971.

Fuchs, V. R., ed. *Essays in the Economics of Health and Medical Care.* New York: Columbia University Press, 1972.

Fuchs, V. R. *Who Shall Live?* New York: Basic Books, 1974.

Fuchs, V. R., and Kramer, M. J. "Determinants of Expenditures for Physicians' Sevices in the United States 1948–1968." Pub. No. (HSM) 73–3013. Washington, D. C.: USDHEW, 1973.

Glaser, W. A. *Paying the Doctor.* Baltimore, Md.: Johns Hopkins University Press, 1970.

Goldberg, J. H. "Working for a Paycheck: One MD's Paean. . . . Is Another Man's Pain." *Hospital Physician, 7,* 68, 1971.

Harvard Law Review. "The Role of Prepaid Group Practice in Relieving the Medical Care Crisis." *84,* 948, 1971.

Haveman, R. H., and Knopf, K. A. *The Market System.* New York: Wiley, 1970.

Hayt, E. "The Practice of Medicine by Hospitals." *Hospital Management, 100,* 30, 1965.

Health Insurance Institute. *Source Book of Health Insurance Data, 1975–76.* New York, 1975.

Health Resources Statistics, 1974. Pub. (HRA) 75–1509. Rockville, Md.: National Center for Health Statistics, USDHEW, 1974.

Health Security News. "Forecast—Astronomical Health Cost Increases." April 9, 1976.

"Hospital Indicators." *Hospitals,* J.A.H.A., August 16, 1971, p. 31.

"Hospital Indicators." *Hospitals, J.A.H.A.,* June 16, 1975, p. 26.

Jonas, S. "Issues in National Health Insurance in the United States of America." *The Lancet,* July 20, 1974, p. 143.

Jonas, S. "Japan Strains under Complex Health System." *Hospitals, J.A.H.A.,* September 1, 1975, p. 56.

Klarman, H. E. *The Economics of Health.* New York: Columbia University Press, 1965.

Klarman, H. E. "The Difference the Third Party Makes." *Journal of Risk and Insurance, 36,* 553, 1969.

Korcok, M. "Medicine in Canada." Parts 1 and 2. *American Medical News*, March 20, 1972.

Kramer, C., and Roemer, R. *Health Manpower and the Organization of Health Services*. Los Angeles, California: University of California, Manpower Research Center, Institute of Industrial Relations, 1972.

Krizay, J., and Wilson, A. *The Patient as Consumer*. Lexington, Mass.: D.C. Heath and Co., 1974.

Law, S. A. *Blue Cross: What Went Wrong?* New Haven, Conn.: Yale University Press, 1974.

Lium, R. "Choice, Fees, and Quality." *Harvard Medical Alumni Bulletin, 4*, 1971.

McCarthy, C. M. "Incentive Reimbursement as an Impetus to Cost Containment." *Inquiry, 12*, 320, December, 1975.

Medicare and Medicaid. Committee on Finance, U.S. Senate, 1970.

Mueller, M. S. "Private Health Insurance in 1973: A Review of Coverage, Enrollment and Financial Experience." *Social Security Bulletin, 38*, 21, February, 1975.

Mueller, M. S., and Gibson, R. M. "Age Difference in Health Care Spending, Fiscal Year 1974." *Research and Statistics Note #6–1975*, Office of Research and Statistics, Social Security Administration, USDHEW, May 13, 1975.

Mueller, M.S., and Gibson, R. M. "National Health Expenditures, Fiscal Year 1975." *Social Security Bulletin, 39*, 3, February, 1976.

Mueller, M. S., and Piro, P. A. "Private Health Insurance in 1974: A Review of Coverage, Enrollment and Financial Experience." *Social Security Bulletin, 39*, 3, March, 1976.

Mushkin, S. J. "Toward a Definition of Health Economics." *Public Health Reports, 73*, 785, 1958.

New York Times. "Doctors Strong, Patients Weak, Costs Up." April 26, 1976.

Rhein, R. W. "The Unhealthy State of U.S. Medical Care." *Business Week*, February 2, 1976, p. 6.

Rice, D., and McGee, M. F. *Research and Statistics Note #18–1970*, Office of Research and Statistics, Social Security Administration, USDHEW, October 30, 1970.

Ricketts, H. T. "Forty Years of Full-Time Medicine at the University of Chicago." *Journal of the American Medical Association, 208*, 2069, 1969.

Roemer, M. I. "On Paying the Doctor and the Implications of Different Methods." *Journal of Health and Human Behavior, 3*, 4, Spring, 1962.

Roemer, M. I. "An Ideal Health Care System for America." *Transaction, 8*, 31, 1971.

Russel, L. et al. *Federal Health Spending, 1969–74*. Washington, D.C.: National Planning Association, 1974.

Sade, R. M. "Medical Care as a Right: A Refutation." *New England Journal of Medicine, 285,* 1288, 1971.

Salmon, J. W. "The Maintenance Organization Strategy: A Corporate Takeover of Health Services Delivery." *International Journal of Health Services, 5,* 609, 1975.

Samuelson, P. A. *Economics.* 9th ed. New York: McGraw Hill, 1973.

Shinefield, H. R., and Smillie, J. G. "Prepaid Group Practice and Health Care." *Advances in Pediatrics, 20,* 205, 1973.

Sigmond, R. M. "The Notion of Hospital Incentives." *Hospital Progress, 50,* 63, January, 1969.

Social Security Bulletin. March, 1976. Tables M40, M41.

Social Security Bulletin: Annual Statistical Supplement, 1973. Rockville, Md.: Office of Research and Statistics, Social Security Administration, USDHEW, 1974.

Somers, A. R. *Hospital Regulation: The Dilemma of Public Policy.* Princeton, N.J.: Princeton University Press, 1969.

Somers, A. R. "Recharting National Health Priorities: A New Perspective." *New England Journal of Medicine, 291,* 415, 1974.

Somers, H., and Somers, A. R. *Doctors, Patients and Health Insurance.* Washington, D.C.: The Brookings Institution, 1961.

Source Book of Health Insurance Data, 1974–75. New York: Health Insurance Institute, 1974.

Strickland, S. *Politics, Science and Dread Disease.* Cambridge, Mass.: Harvard University Press, 1972. (a)

Strickland, S. *U.S. Health Care: What's Wrong and What's Right?* New York: Universe Books, 1972 (b).

U.S. National Commission on State Workmen's Compensation Laws. *Report.* Washington, D.C.: Government Printing Office, 1973.

Wasyluka, R. G. "New Blood for Tired Hospitals." *Harvard Business Review, 48,* 66, October, 1970.

Williams, G. "Kaiser: What Is It? How Does It Work? Why Does It Work?" *Modern Hospital, 116,* 67, February, 1971.

Wolkstein, I. "Incentive Reimbursement Plans Offer a Variety of Approaches to Cost Control." *Hospitals, J.A.H.A.,* June 16, 1969.

Worthington, N. "National Health Expenditures, 1929–74." *Social Security Bulletin, 38,* 2, February, 1975.

————. "Expenditures for Hospital Care and Physicians' Services: Factors Affecting Annual Charges." *Social Security Bulletin, 38,* 3, November, 1975.

10

Government in the Health Care Delivery System

Steven Jonas, David Banta, and Michael Enright

Introduction

Thus far we have examined four principal elements of the United States health care delivery system: the people whom it serves, the personnel it employs, the organizational structures and facilities through which care is provided, and the finance mechanisms that enable the system to operate. There is a fifth crucial element of any health care delivery system: government. In our earlier discussions, we have seen some ways in which various components of the government and the health care delivery system interrelate; now we will look more directly at government operations in administration, legislation, regulation, adjudication, planning, quality control, research, and the development of national health insurance. We will also discuss some activities of the private sector in those areas.

In the United States, the government operates neither the health care delivery system nor, as of 1976, the financing system in its entirety; in fact, our government is less involved in health care than the governments of most other industrialized countries. Among the many reasons for this difference, perhaps the most important is the strength of the private sector and its opposition to "government control and interference," except in select areas, such as care of the sick poor, care of the mentally ill, and infectious disease control. Restricted as the government's role is, however, on an absolute scale it looms rather large. This role has developed and expanded gradually over a long period of time.

In the 1940s, the Committee on Medicine and the Changing Order of the New York Academy of Medicine sponsored a series of monographs on the health care delivery system. One—*Medical*

Services by Government: Local, State and Federal, by one of the first medical sociologists, Bernhard J. Stern (1946)—had a preface by W. G. Smillie, one of the noted authorities on public health of the day. The book is fascinating both for its history and for its descriptions of the situation in the mid-1940s. Many of the observations are strikingly relevant to our present situation.

In the preface, Smillie said:

> Our forefathers certainly had no concept of responsibility of the Federal Government, nor of the state government, for health protection of the people. This was solely a local governmental responsibility. When Benjamin Franklin wrote "Health is Wealth" in the Farmers' Almanac, he was saying that health was a commodity to be bought, to be sold, to be conserved, or to be wasted. But he considered that health conservation was the responsibility of the individual, not of government. The local community was responsible only for the protection of its citizens against the hazards of community life. Thus government responsibility for health protection consisted of (a) promotion of sanitation and (b) communicable disease control. The Federal Constitution, as well as the Constitutions of most of the states, contains no reference or intimation of a federal or state function in medical care.
>
> The care of the sick poor was a local community responsibility from earliest pioneer days. This activity was assumed first by voluntary philanthropy; later, it was transferred, and became an official governmental obligation.... (Stern, p. xiii)

Professor Stern continued that line of thought in his introduction:

> Government action in the field has traditionally been limited to the care of the indigent and has been dominated in its scope and administration by the restraining influences of the parochial poor laws. Gradually, and especially after the passage of the Social Security Act and during [World War II], government medical care has increasingly been furnished to some non-indigent groups. New patterns of government medical care are being formulated and the role of local, state, and federal governments in the field is changing. . . . government agencies, after protracted delays and faltering beginnings, are making significant strides in the development of effective administrative procedures and in the provision of skilled and experienced personnel. The attitudes of the medical profession and of the public toward government medical programs will determine whether these resources are to be used

progressively to distribute more medical care of higher quality to the American people. (Stern, pp. 4–5)

Government at all jurisdictional levels in the United States is involved in the health care delivery system to a much greater degree now than in 1946. The kind of involvement has changed too, with such initiatives as Medicare and Medicaid, planning acts, new regulatory powers, and support of biomedical research and health professions education. But certain characteristics have remained unchanged, and they are most significant. To quote Smillie again:

> . . . practically all governmental procedures in medical care stem from the original local community responsibility for the care of the sick poor, and many of our great municipal hospitals, clinics, and health services of today still bear the stigma of pauperism. Two separate types of governmental medicine developed through the years: official public health services, a health department function which attempted to prevent disease, and medical care of the sick poor, which was provided by departments of welfare. Though these frequently impinged and overlapped, they seldom were interrelated, and almost never were fused. (Stern, p. xiv)

The pauper stigma is still attached to much government activity in direct care delivery. It is rooted in the Protestant ethic, which held people directly accountable for their state in life. The legal implementation of the Protestant ethic goes back at least as far as the Elizabethan Poor Laws. Today our society may accept sociological explanations as to why some people are well-off and others are destitute; but attitudes toward the proper role of government in health care are still colored by old values and prejudices.

The Constitutional Basis of Government Authority in Health

To understand how the government operates in the health care delivery system, it is essential to understand the structure of the government itself.* A basic principle of the United States Consti-

---

* The *Public Health Law Manual* by Frank P. Grad (Washington, D.C.: American Public Health Association, 1975) is a valuable guide to the legal basis of government activity in health care and to the many legal procedures involved in the enforcement of public health law.

tution is the sharing of sovereign power between the federal and state governments. The Constitution represents an agreement by the states to delegate some of their powers to the federal government; the states reserve certain inherent powers, among which is police power, the basis of the states' role in health (Mustard, pp. 17–21). As Grad points out:

> The state's police power, i.e., the power "to enact and enforce laws to protect and promote the health, safety, morals, order, peace, comfort, and general welfare of the people" is an attribute of a sovereign government—a sovereign government in this context, being a government with power that derives from its very nature as a government, i.e., with plenary and inherent (rather than delegated) power. Thus, the fifty states are separate repositories of police power, while the national government, which, in its origins, is a government of delegated power, does not possess the police power, at least not in its usual broad sense. (p. 5)

Another basis of the states' authority in health is the tenth Amendment of the United States Constitution, which states: "The powers not delegated to the United States by the constitution, nor prohibited by it to the states, are reserved to the states respectively, or to the people."

Among the states' other inherent powers are those of delegation of authority. The states have used it to create the third tier of the governmental system, local government, and most states have delegated some of their powers in health matters to local governments.

The powers of the federal government in health are not specifically mentioned in the Constitution; they derive from the powers to tax and spend in order to provide for the general welfare, and to regulate interstate and foreign commerce. These powers are stipulated in Article I, Section 8 of the Constitution (Grad, p. 8).

The separation of powers, the clear constitutional division of the federal government into the executive, legislative, and judicial branches, is the second basic principle of the Constitution. Under separation of powers, each branch of the federal government is independent and has its own powers limited by the Constitution through the system of "checks and balances." The tripartite form, with checks and balances, is followed fairly closely by state governments. At the local level, the boundaries between branches become rather blurred: in suburban and rural areas, for example, the chief local executive officer may preside over the local legislative body. Nevertheless, in most jurisdictions, separation of powers is found as a major principle of government.

The Functions of Government in the United States
Health Care Delivery System

The bulk of this chapter deals with the operations of the three jurisdictional levels of government (federal, state, and local) in the delivery of personal health services. However, there are other governmental functions in health, some of which are considered in other chapters. We will briefly review them and indicate in which chapters more detailed discussions may be found.

Licensing, particularly of physicians, is a basic government function in health care. Licensing of individuals determines who may and may not deliver what kinds of health services, and, in theory, establishes minimum standards. Licensing of institutions also sets minimum standards and to some extent investigates the characteristics of owners and providers. Licensing is carried out primarily by the states, and all three branches of government are involved: the legislatures enact the statutes, the executive branches administer them, and the courts interpret and enforce them.

The licensing system, which is discussed in detail in Chapter 13, gives physicians tight control over the central product of the system: medical services. By exercising this control, physicians largely determine the structure of the health care delivery system —how it is organized, the types and functions of the institutions, and the powers of personnel.

Legislatures

In addition to enacting the legal framework within which the health care delivery system functions, legislatures may impose certain requirements for planning and development of the system (see Chapter 12) and for quality measurement and control (see Chapter 13). If the government is to participate in health care financing (see Chapters 9 and 15), or directly deliver service (see this chapter and Chapters 6, 7, and 8), or support research efforts (see Chapter 14), those programs must first be established by legislative acts. Chapter 11 describes legislative functioning in health care at the federal level in some detail.

The Judiciary

The judicial branches in the three levels of government have important powers, but since they cannot apprehend transgressors, or prosecute them, or carry out punishment on their own, they must work in concert with the law enforcement arms of the executive branches. Together they form the civil and criminal justice systems.

The civil and criminal justice systems support the work of the other components of the government in adjudicating disputes related to health care, and in protecting the rights of individuals under the due process and equal protection clauses of the Constitution. Most importantly, although a legislature creates a licensing law for physicians, and an executive branch administers it, the criminal justice system enforces it, if necessary by sending to jail a person who "practices medicine without a license."

Legislatures are passing an increasing number of laws attempting to regulate one or another part of the health care delivery system. Executive branches then interpret those laws and write regulations for their administration. Often one or another provider group, objecting that the new legislation inhibits its prerogatives, turns to the civil justice system for relief. Through litigation, providers avail themselves of the functions of one branch of the government to deal with what they feel are unconstitutional, illegal, or unwarranted intrusions into their work by one or more other branches.

Finally, malpractice litigation is one method by which dissatisfied consumers attempt to get some kind of satisfaction from providers who the consumers feel have wronged them in some fashion. The civil justice system is the arena in which malpractice litigation is carried out (see Chapter 13).

The Executive—An Overview

In speaking of "government in health care," we usually mean the executive branch that administers programs, not the legislature that creates them, or the courts that adjudicate disputes arising from them. In the remainder of the chapter, the term "government" will generally refer to the executive branch of government, but we will use the shorter term because it is common parlance, and much less cumbersome.

The federal government generally delivers personal health services to categories of persons: merchant seamen, American Indians, veterans, members of the uniformed services and their families, and so on. State governments generally provide care for categories of disease: mental illness and tuberculosis. Local governments generally provide care to the lower socioeconomic class and the medically indigent. There are some overlaps: the federal government cares for those afflicted with leprosy and narcotics addiction, and operates St. Elizabeth's Hospital, a mental institution in the District of Columbia; governments at all levels provide care for prisoners; but the distinction holds for the most part.

For community health services, government at all levels is the major provider in such areas as pure water supply and sanitary sewage disposal; food and drug inspection and regulation; communicable disease control; vital statistics and public health laboratory work.* However, there are certain activities which are shared with the private sector. In public health education the voluntary agencies—for example, the Cancer Society and the Heart Association—are very important. Private refuse collectors are important in solid waste disposal. Private organizations are very active in environmental protection. Private institutions of course play a vital role in health sciences education and research.

Government is an important factor in the delivery of combined health services, those which have both personal and community aspects—for example, immunization and treatment of venereal disease and tuberculosis.

Government participates in the financing system in three ways. First, there is spending for governmental delivery of services, personal, community, and combined. This can be direct—as in the federal government's care to veterans in hospitals that it owns and operates—or indirect, as in the federal government's "grant-in-aid" program to state governments to provide care in state tuberculosis hospitals. Likewise, state and federal governments spend directly to collect vital statistics, and give money to local governments to assist them in so doing. Governments also give money by grants and contracts to nongovernmental agencies (and in certain cases, other governmental agencies), for specific projects such as a program in biomedical research, support of health facilities construction, and support for the development of Health Maintenance Organizations. Third, governments pay providers on an item-of-service basis for the delivery of care to third parties, e.g. under Medicare and Medicaid.

* A great deal of valuable detail on government activities in community health services is contained in John J. Hanlon's *Principles of Public Health Administration*, published in periodic editions by The C. V. Mosby Company of St. Louis.

The Federal Government and Health Care Delivery
Introduction

Many federal agencies are involved in the delivery of personal and community health services. About one-sixth of the population, aside from beneficiaries of Medicare and Medicaid, is eligible to receive at least some personal health services from or through the federal government. Table 10.1 shows which agencies have health-related activities, by category of activity, and how much was spent in each category in fiscal 1975. As is to be expected, the USDHEW is the most important federal department in health care activity. Its largest expenditures are for Medicare (SSA) and Medicaid (SRS), two programs in which it is primarily a third-party payor and secondarily a regulator (see Chapters 9 and 15). The Health Services Administration and the Alcohol, Drug Abuse and Mental Health Administration provide significant indirect support for a variety of health services through the grant and contract mechanism. DHEW, through the National Institutes of Health and other agencies, is the largest federal supporter of biomedical research. It is also a significant factor in health sciences education and health facilities construction, as well as health care planning.

The two other federal agencies with large expenditures for health care are the Veterans' Administration and the Department of Defense. They pay primarily for care in their own facilities, but are also involved in research, education, construction, and paying for care for beneficiaries in other institutions. Other federal agencies with significant health-related expenditures include the Department of Agriculture (meat and poultry inspection; food stamps); the Energy Research and Development Administration; and the Department of Labor (the Occupational Safety and Health Act).

The Department of Health, Education and Welfare*

In 1975, the Department of Health, Education and Welfare administered at least 200 programs through 13 operating agencies and 10 regional offices (Miles, pp. 64–65; Wilson and Neuhauser, pp. 104–117); more than 100 of the programs were health or health-related. They were administered through three

---

* The most comprehensive description of the Department of Health, Education and Welfare is Rufus E. Miles, Jr.'s *The Department of Health, Education and Welfare* (New York: Praeger Publishers, 1974).

of the major administrative divisions of the Department: the Public Health Service, which has six major agencies; the Social Security Administration; and the Social and Rehabilitation Service. The operating agencies and the number of personnel employed by each at the end of 1975 were as follows:

Public Health Service	
National Institutes of Health	12,570
Food and Drug Administration	7,263
Center for Disease Control	3,831
Health Resources Administration	1,873
Health Services Administration	16,883
Alcohol, Drug Abuse and Mental	
Health Administration	5,941
Social Security Administration	84,463
Social and Rehabilitation Service	1,854
Total	148,062

The Department underwent a major reorganization in 1973, when the staff of the Assistant Secretary of Health was increased to more than 500. His role is one of potential conflict; he has an empire to protect, but is also supposed to give impartial staff advice on health matters, including Medicare and Medicaid, to the Secretary.

Figure 10.1 shows the organization chart of HEW.

Public Health Service. The organization chart of the Public Health Service, which the Assistant Secretary for Health directs, is shown in Figure 10.2. The Public Health Service has a long and proud history, dating back to the 1798 Act creating the Marine Hospital Service (Schmeckebier, ch. 1; Mustard, pp. 23–81; Stern, pp. 145–154; Wilson and Neuhauser, pp. 105–115, 147–170). In 1878, foreign quarantine activities were added by congressional act, leading to the development of a quasi-military personnel system (the "commissioned corps") in 1889, a group which was largely made up of career medical people. The Public Health Service continued to gain responsibilities gradually, and grew rapidly in the area of communicable disease control during World War II. Since World War II, its responsibilities have grown greatly, with the passage of the Hospital Survey and Construction Act of 1946 (Hill-Burton Act), the rapid growth of the National Institutes of Health, the creation of the Communicable Disease Center in Atlanta (later the Center for Disease

Table 10.1

Federal Agencies Delivering Health Services, by Type of Service, and Amount Spent, Fiscal 1975
(in millions of dollars)

Agency	Indirect Federal Hospital and Medical Services	Prevention and Control of Health Problems	Direct Federal Hospital and Medical Services	Health Research	Training and Education	Construction	Health Planning Activities	Total
Dept. of HEW (total)	$23,002	$639	$255	$1,867	$928	$542	$162	$27,396
Health Services Admin.	578	153	208	9	28	48	11	1,035
Health Resources Admin.	6	12	0	58	528	369	126	1,099
Alcohol, Drug Abuse and Mental Health Admin.	515	96	43	114	152	31	0	950
Center for Disease Control	0	111	0	42	2	0	0	154
National Institutes of Health	0	33	0	1,598	177	82	0	1,889
Food and Drug Admin.	0	172	0	27	0	1	0	201
Asst. Secretary for Health	11	2	4	4	0	2	21	45
Social Security Admin.	14,781	0	0	0	0	0	0	14,781
Social and Rehabilitation Service	6,876	0	1	2	0	0	1	6,879
Other HEW	235	59	0	13	42	9	3	361
Dept. of Defense	567	26	2,261	104	231	96	0	3,285
Veterans' Admin.	211	0	3,018	93	198	122	22	3,665
Dept. of HUD	1	0	0	0	0	164	38	203
Dept. of Agriculture	0	259	0	47	0	1	0	307
Environmental Protection Agency	0	0	0	20	0	0	0	20
NASA	0	3	0	59	0	0	0	62
Energy Research and Development Admin.	0	95	0	143	0	6	0	244

Dept. of Labor	0	81	0	1	9	0	0	91
Dept. of State	1	24	0	0	7	0	12	44
National Science Foundation	0	0	0	44	0	3	0	44
Dept. of the Interior	8	2	0	35	0	3	0	48
Dept. of Transportation	0	23	9	15	2	0	10	60
Dept. of Justice	3	3	23	0	0	3	0	32
Other agencies	40	77	0	31	8	13	71	239
Agency contributions to employee health funds	1,050	0	0	0	0	0	0	1,050
Total	24,883	1,232	5,567	2,459	1,384	949	316	36,790

Source: Special Analyses, Budget of the U.S. Government, Fiscal Year 1977 (Washington, D.C.: Government Printing Office, 1976), p. 215.

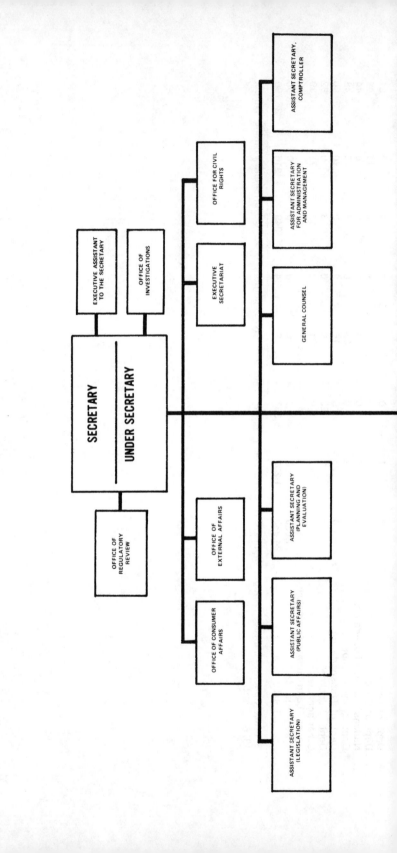

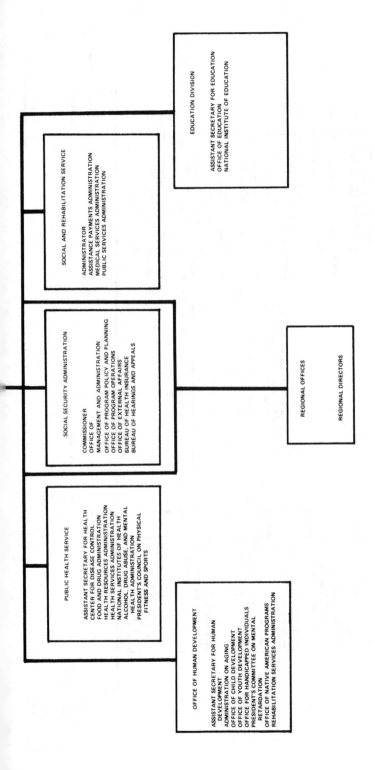

Figure 10.1. Organization chart of the Department of Health, Education, and Welfare

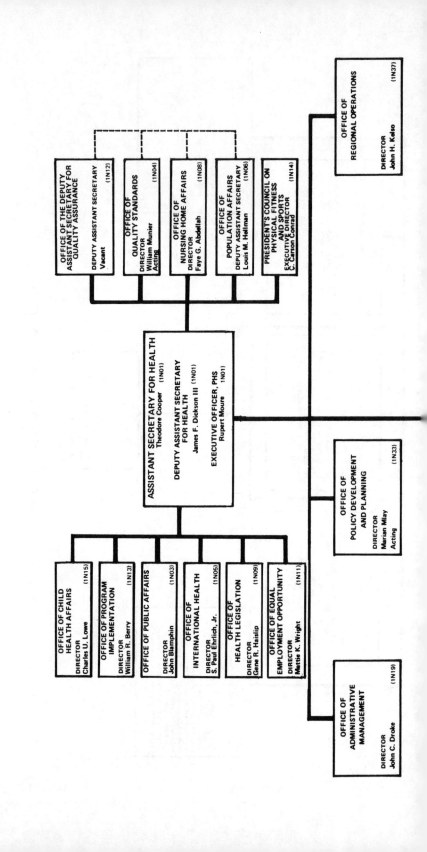

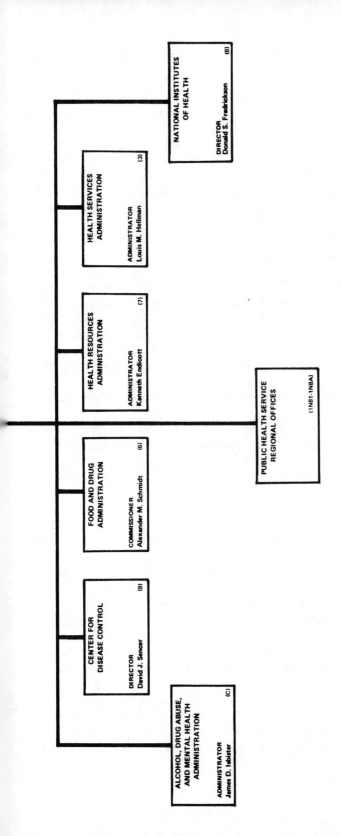

Figure 10.2. Organization chart of the Public Health Service (HEW)

Control), and the development of drug abuse control, mental retardation and mental health centers, and comprehensive health planning. The Public Health Service, however, has suffered a relative decline in recent years for several reasons.

With the passage of Medicare and Medicaid legislation in 1965, the health financing programs began to predominate among federal health activities, and then to compete actively with PHS programs for financial support. Several reorganizations in rapid succession hurt morale. During the 1960s the Budget Bureau (later the Office of Management and Budget) embarked on a crusade to close the PHS Hospitals, which damaged Service morale greatly, and also attempted to abolish the commissioned corps (Miles, pp. 192–200). Further, the unclear role of the Assistant Secretary of Health—and his lack of a top policy analysis staff—have hampered active health leadership from the Public Health Service. In 1968, the functions of the Surgeon General of the PHS were given to the Assistant Secretary for Health (Miles, p. 73), and, after 1973, no Surgeon General was appointed. Most observers feel that the Public Health Service, as a result of the changing nature of government health responsibilities, has largely lost its once great vibrancy and morale.

The Health Services Administration. The Health Services Administration (HSA), with a budget of over $1 billion in fiscal 1975, administers the direct services programs of DHEW, "provides professional leadership in health services delivery programs," especially those with public financing, and administers formula grants which support health service delivery programs. It has two operating arms providing direct health care services: the **Bureau of Medical Services** and the **Indian Health Service** (IHS).

The Bureau of Medical Services' Division of Hospitals and Clinics operates the eight Public Health Service hospitals and 26 independent outpatient clinics. It has a staff of about 5,000 and has 330 physicians on contract in areas in which it has no facilities. Eligible for care under these programs are 200,000 merchant seamen, over 130,000 Coast Guardsmen and their dependents, and active and retired members of all other uniformed services. Because the inpatient load in those facilities is decliniing and quality is suffering, there is some feeling that they are obsolete and should be abolished. The Bureau also operates, under contract, the health services of the Department of Justice's Bureau of Prisons. In addition, it has an alcoholism program for

HSA employees; runs an occupational health service for the entire federal government, and, through the **Division of Emergency Medical Services**, operates a grant program to improve state and local emergency care.

The Indian Health Service was originally in the Bureau of Indian Affairs, part of the War Department until it was transferred to the Department of the Interior in 1849. The IHS was separated out and transferred to the USPHS in 1955. In the 1970 census, of 827,000 persons who identified themselves as Indians, Aleuts, and Eskimos, 527,000 lived on reservations, where the IHS provides service. In the mid-70s, IHS facilities included 51 hospitals with 3,000 beds, 86 health centers, and 300 field stations. The staff included 500 physicians, 200 dentists, 1,200 nurses, and 6,000 allied health personnel. The fiscal 1974 budget was $95 million.

The HSA's **Bureau of Community Health Services** includes many of the indirect service and grant and contract programs, such as maternal and child health, family planning, neighborhood health centers, the National Health Service Corps, the Health Maintenance Organization support program, and Migrant Health. The **Bureau of Quality Assurance** is responsible for setting standards for the Professional Standards Review Organizations and other categorical indirect service programs, such as the one for renal disease.

The Health Resources Administration. The Health Resources Administration (HRA) is also an important agency providing indirect federal health services. In fiscal 1975, its budget was about $1.1 billion. It supports health manpower training through grants and contracts to health professions schools; provides leadership and support for the development of comprehensive health planning; supports activities concerned with health facility development; collects, analyzes, and disseminates data on vital statistics, health resources, and health services utilization; and conducts and supports analyses and research to improve the health services system. The functional divisions of HRA are the **National Center for Health Statistics**; the **National Center for Health Services Research**; the **Bureau of Health Manpower**; and the **Bureau of Health Planning and Resources Development**.

The Center for Disease Control. The Center for Disease Control (CDC), with a $150 million budget (FY 1975) functions primarily to prevent and control communicable disease, to direct foreign and interstate quarantine operations, and to improve the performance of clinical laboratories. It maintains excellent reference laboratories and carries out training programs. It also awards project grants to state and local health agencies to support immunization, particularly for children, and has health education responsibilities.

The Food and Drug Administration. The Food and Drug Administration, with a $200 million budget (FY 1975), functions to protect the public against hazards of various products and to assure potency and effectiveness of such products as drugs. FDA has six divisions, each covering a major type of product: the **Bureau of Foods**, the **Bureau of Drugs**, the **Bureau of Veterinary Medicine**, the **Bureau of Radiological Health**, the **Bureau of Biologics**, and the **Bureau of Medical Devices and Diagnostic Products**. It also includes a **National Center for Toxicological Research**.

The Bureau of Drugs, which has responsibility under the Kefauver-Harris Amendments of 1962 for assuring the efficacy of all drugs, is perhaps the most controversial FDA agency. Some have contended that potentially useful drugs are being kept off the market by a lengthy and expensive approval process. Others feel that such premarket approval is essential to protect the public. Congress, through its consideration of bills to strengthen FDA, and its passage in 1976 of legislation to bring medical devices under similar controls, has shown its belief in the necessity of such assurances of efficacy and safety.

The National Institutes of Health. The National Institutes of Health (NIH), with a budget of about $1.9 billion (FY 1975), is responsible for supporting and carrying out health research through its 11 institutes. NIH has an intramural research program on its campus in Bethesda, Maryland, and supports research through extramural grants and contracts. NIH also fosters research by supporting training, resource development, and construction. In Chapter 14, we consider the NIH in more detail and discuss current major policy issues.

The Alcohol, Drug Abuse and Mental Health Administration. The Alcohol, Drug Abuse and Mental Health Administration (ADAMHA), with a budget approaching $1 billion (FY 1975), is divided into three parts: the **National Institute on Alcohol Abuse and Alcoholism**, the **National Institute on Drug Abuse**, and the **National Institute of Mental Health (NIMH)**.

Each division of ADAMHA supports treatment, rehabilitation, prevention, and research activities in its area of interest. The

National Institute on Drug Abuse has given special emphasis to assuring treatment facilities for heroin addicts; the National Institute on Alcohol Abuse and Alcoholism supports treatment and prevention demonstration programs; the National Institute of Mental Health administers an intramural research program on the grounds of NIH and also controls a large nationwide program of community mental health centers.

ADAMHA is controversial because each of its divisions supports both service and research programs. Many feel that service programs will inevitably erode support for research and doubt that such an agency can support first-class research. A 1976 report from the President's Biomedical Research Panel recommended that ADAMHA's research activities be increased.

The Veterans' Administration

The Veterans' Administration (VA) is an independent agency of the federal government reporting directly to the President. The VA operates the largest centrally directed hospital and clinic system in the United States: in the mid-70s, about 29 million veterans, 13% of the population, were eligible to receive at least a portion of their medical care in a VA medical facility.

The origins of the VA medical services can be traced to a 1776 report of a committee of the Continental Congress established "to consider what provision ought to be made for such as are wounded or disabled in the land or sea service, and report a plan for that purpose" (*Journals of the Continental Congress,* vol. 5, p. 469). The committee had recommended the establishment of a pension system for disabled veterans. (Precedent for such a system can be traced back to an act of the English Parliament in its 1592–93 session which provided relief for veterans of the 1588 war with Spain.) By the time of the American Revolution, every colony had some program to assist disabled veterans (House Committee Print, 1967, p. 29). The federal government took over the responsibilities in 1789.

Following the American Civil War, the federal government established the "National Military and Naval Home" to care for Union Army veterans with service-connected disabilities causing "economic distress." Later, the facilities were made available to all veterans, and "for economic distress" not necessarily related to military service. There were 11 homes throughout the country, primarily for residence, with medical care a secondary consideration.

After World War I, the Public Health Service hospital system was assigned the responsibility of caring for the large influx of disabled veterans. The system was expanded greatly by the addition of certain military hospitals and the construction of new ones—by June 1920, there were 11,639 beds in 52 hospitals. In 1922, the veterans' hospitals were transferred to the Veterans' Bureau, which became the Veterans' Administration in 1930.

In fiscal 1974, the VA was operating 171 hospitals: 138 general hospitals with 70,017 beds (of which about 10% were psychiatric), and 33 psychiatric hospitals with 24,527 beds. There were VA nursing-home units with 6,898 beds in 84 VA hospitals, and 18 domiciliaries with 10,811 beds. The VA employed almost 184,000 persons, 85% of them full-time. The full-time, part-time, and intermittent professional staff included 27,596 physicians, 1,345 dentists, and 24,372 nurses (House Committee Print, 1975, p. ix).

There are four overlapping groups of veterans eligible to receive VA medical care: (1) veterans with service-connected disabilities; (2) recipients of VA pensions; (3) veterans 65 years and older; and (4) "medically indigent" veterans (Levitan and Cleary, p. 73). The latter category includes "any veteran of any war or service after January 31, 1955 for a non-service-connected disability if he is unable to defray the expenses of hospital care" (U.S. Code, Title 38). The means test is self-administered and there are no financial investigations. Over 50% of discharges from VA hospitals in FY 1974 were for patients who had no service-connected disability and drew no VA pension (House Committee Print, 1975, p. 672). A veteran is anyone who has served 90 days or more in an armed service, but he/she must have received an honorable discharge in order to be eligible. Thus, there is a "moral means test."

In fiscal 1974, the VA provided hospital care for 1.14 million patients. In addition, 12.3 million outpatient visits were made to VA staff and fee-basis physicians. Total costs for the medical program were over $2.84 billion (House Committee Print, 1975, pp. 656-659).

Medical staffing in the majority of VA hospitals is provided under a unique arrangement. Following World War II, press reports of abysmal medical care in VA hospitals led to the establishment of affiliation agreements with medical schools under which graduate (and eventually undergraduate) education would be carried out in them, with the VA paying the salaries of the house staff and certain faculty members. These activities are supervised by "Deans' Committees."

The government thus divided its responsibility and authority over its paid VA staff with medical schools and faculty that had neither received government grants or salaries for VA purposes, nor were assigned any accountability for their actions to the government or to the taxpayers; the VA remained ultimately responsible for the quality of services. Neither the schools nor the individual medical personnel were in the employ of the government; nonetheless, the Deans' Committees, since 1946, have controlled the expenditure of many millions of dollars each year for VA residents, interns, full-time and part-time staff, consultants, and attendants, usually from medical school faculties. The committees have, in addition, influenced the annual expenditure of millions of dollars for medical supplies and equipment that, in their judgment, are needed for education, research, and patient care (Lewis, pp. 156–62). Until June 1973, the agreements had been quite informal, and were largely verbal understandings. However, these arrangements generally worked well, and many feel they have been the salvation of the VA system. In 1973, the VA Central Office decided that a little more formality was in order and directed that letters of understanding—quite simple in language and very liberal in policy—be completed. By the mid-70s, 90 VA hospitals had medical school affiliation agreements.

In 1966, federal legislation opened the VA hospitals up for affiliation with other types of health sciences educational institutions. By 1971, VA hospitals had educational agreements with 52 dental schools, 91 graduate departments of psychology, 304 nursing schools, 38 occupational therapy schools, 22 pharmacy schools, 35 physical therapy schools, and 75 social work schools; and in other disciplines the VA had accords with approximately 300 universities, colleges, community and junior colleges, and 100 technical and other types of schools.

Department of Defense

There are 10 million people in the United States (almost 5% of the population) who receive their health care under the auspices of the Department of Defense (DOD). In 1975, some 6.75 million persons were eligible to receive their health care directly in the 131 military hospitals located throughout the continental United States. Another 3.25 million persons, dependents of military personnel, were covered by the Civilian Health and Medical Program of the Uniformed Services (CHAMPUS), an insurance program purchasing care in the private sector.

The basic mission of the military health delivery system is to plan, prepare, and provide medical support for military operations. The entitlement to health care in military hospitals is therefore absolute for the 2.1 million men and women on active duty in the military services. The Congress has also charged the DOD with the provision of health services to dependents and survivors of active duty personnel, to retirees, and to the dependents and survivors of retirees. To these 7.9 million persons, the entitlement to care is a privilege dependent on the availability of space and facilities as well as the capability of the professional staff of a given facility (Cowan, 1974).

The varying missions of the individual services, together with the traditional interservice rivalries, have tended to fragment the health resources of the DOD. The Comprehensive Health Planning Act (P. L. 89–749) included DOD among those responsible for regionalizing medical resources. This requirement, coupled with the growing disparity between the demand for services and the capability to provide them, has proved to be an enormous problem.

Since the end of the draft, DOD has had trouble attracting and retaining qualified medical manpower (McKenzie, p. 3). This problem is being attacked through a variety of programs. First, there is an attempt to reduce the inequities in income differential between military physicians and those in private practice; second, there are educational scholarship support programs that obligate physician graduates to a given term of service; and third, the roles of other medical care providers are being redefined to extend the capabilities of those physicians in service (Cowan, 1975, 1976). All of the services have traditionally relied on medics, particularly in the field, but they are now increasingly turning toward formally trained physicians' assistants and clinical nurse practitioners. Moreover, trained administrators are replacing physician-executives. Finally, under the planned Uniformed Service University of the Health Sciences, the DOD would train its own physicians, as well as other health care providers (*Medical World News*; Boffey).

The Armed Forces Regional Health System is an attempt to reduce the fragmentation of resources by providing health care on an interdepartmental basis. Service personnel and retirees tend to rely on the facilities of their parent service, even if it is not the most appropriate or geographically convenient. The Regional Health System program emphasizes cross-service referrals and encourages personnel to use the most appropriate facility regardless of service connection. There are attempts, particularly in overseas areas, to combine facilities with similar specialties and have the medical specialists assigned to a facility where the specialty is required regardless of the branch of service (Cowan, 1976).

The military medical departments are charged not only with providing a full range of direct health services but also with providing for the environmental health of their communities, an unusual instance of combined preventive and treatment responsibility. A preventive medicine section inspects food and water supplies and is responsible for vector control. (Vectors are carriers of agents of human disease.) Personnel and dependent medical records are scanned to keep immunizations up-to-date. Base commanders are responsible for the upkeep of housing and sanitary conditions, and in many areas are influential in maintaining standards even off-base by declaring establishments that do not maintain a minimum level of sanitation off-limits to military personnel and their dependents. It would be well to extend this model of unitary health services administration to other jurisdictions in which the government provides personal and community health services. The usual model, imposed by custom and/or by the authorizing statute, separates responsibilities for prevention and treatment, a separation we regard as quite artificial.

Other Federal Departments

As noted in Table 10.1, a number of other federal government departments engage in health-related activities not involving the delivery of personal health services. The Department of Agriculture spends most of its health-related money on research and preventive activities. The research focuses on improved production for crops and animals and on environmental health research. Most of the Department's direct health-related expenditures go into meat, egg, and poultry inspection to assure wholesome products. The Department of Housing and Urban Development invests most of its health-related expenditure in construction, especially of rural hospitals and neighborhood clinics; its Federal Housing Authority (FHA) provides mortgage insurance for hospitals, group practice facilities, and long-term care facilities. The Department of Labor invests most of its health-related expenditure in preventive activities in the workplace, through its Occupational Safety and Health Administration (OSHA). OSHA uses criteria developed by the National Institute of Occupational Safety and Health (NIOSH), part of the CDC, to set national standards for occupational safety and health. Enforcement of these standards is intended to eventually be a responsibility of the states. The Environmental Protection Agency conducts research on air pollution control technology and the effects of air pollution on humans, develops criteria and promulgates national standards for pollutants, and enforces compliance with these standards.*

Fragmentation and Reorganization of Health Programs

It has been pointed out that:

> A bewildering array of programs, services, and agencies confronts the individual seeking health care in the United States. Listings of federal assistance programs have revealed hundreds of separate health programs at the federal level of government alone, within the Department of Health, Education and Welfare and other departments. (Roemer et al., p. 2)

This multiplicity of programs leads to fragmented responsibility and provision of services, as well as to overlapping within geographic areas and political jurisdictions. The ultimate result is that "coherent policy, an integrated direction, and coordinated relationships" do not develop (Roemer et al., p. 3).

Robert H. Finch, the first Secretary of the DHEW under President Richard Nixon, put it succinctly: "The tremendous proliferation of federal assistance programs over the years has resulted in a tangled net of programs which now threatens to negate the basic reason for most of the programs: the delivery of services" (Roemer et al., p. 11). Roemer et al. note that these programs have been developed for various reasons:

> The complexity of the health service system in the United States is the result of the accretion of programs and agencies over the

* For further detail on the health programs of other federal government departments, see the Office of Management and Budget's Special Analyses and Louise B. Russel et al., *Federal Health Spending 1969– 1974* (1974).

years as new needs in health services have been recognized, of the specialized and categorical character of these services, of the sheer numbers of individuals and organizations that provide health care, and of the lack of a rational pattern for fitting the many parts into an effective whole. (p. 11)

These programs, then, are generally addressed to real needs, and in many cases the programs' problems stem less from organizational disorder than from lack of money to do the full job. The separation of DOD health programs from categorical HEW programs, for example, is not necessarily a problem. On the other hand, a serious organizational problem does exist in HEW: the separation of the financing programs, Medicare and Medicaid, from the resources development and health planning activities found in the Public Health Service.

There are many possible solutions to these problems, which relate not only to the complexity of the federal government role in health care delivery, but more broadly to the complexity of the structure of government as a whole. "Reorganization" is one commonly proposed solution. As Seidman notes: "Reorganization is deemed synonymous with reform and reform with progress. Periodic reorganizations are prescribed if for no other purpose than to purify the bureaucratic blood and to prevent stagnation" (p. 3). He continues, "Rare indeed is the Commission or Presidential task force with the self-restraint to forego proposing an organizational answer to the problems it cannot solve" (p. 4). During 1976, two instances of this phenomenon occurred: the Diabetes Commission suggested placing diabetes activities under a National Diabetes Advisory Board in the Office of the Assistant Secretary for Health (National Diabetes Commission on Diabetes) and the President's Biomedical Research Panel suggested a special presidential Biomedical and Behavioral Research Panel to advise the President (President's Biomedical Research Panel).

These two proposals illustrate a tendency on the part of special interest groups to favor reorganization that will raise the bureaucratic level of the office supervising the program in which they are interested. This effort to gain more attention for their own area of concern at the expense of other important areas can only add to "the tangled net of programs."

The most important problems addressed by reorganization, however, are overlapping and duplication, and confused or broken lines of authority and responsibility. Rational organization should assure that "(1) Each function is assigned to its appropriate niche within the Government structure; (2) Component parts of the executive branch are properly related and articulated; and (3) Authorities and responsibilities are clearly assigned" (Seidman, p. 5). As described in the federal Reorganization Act of 1949, reorganization should result in more effective management, economy, and efficiency; however, these goals are often incompatible. Because truly effective reorganization is difficult to achieve, form rather than substance is often emphasized. As Seidman notes: "Frequently studies of executive branch structure degenerate into sterile box-shuffling and another version of the numbers game" (Seidman p. 12).

It is difficult to apply organizational theory to the executive branch because such a structure inevitably "reflects the values, conflicts, and competing forces to be found in a pluralistic society" (Seidman, p.13). "Rational organization" can mean excluding some elements of society from effective participation in the system and an equitable share of its benefits. The organization of the executive branch has an organic function that may not be perceived by even the wisest reformers. For example, some overlapping of programs in different parts of the organization may assure plurality of funding that acts against dogmatic program development. Categorical programs or specific programs, while tending to fragment the executive branch, do elicit congressional and public support—thus the change in the name of the National Microbiological Institute to the National Institute of Allergy and Infectious Diseases (Seidman, p. 34). This continual jousting for programs support and power is part of the real world. It is true, however, that such jurisdictional problems have probably been the main force preventing reorganization.

In outlining some of the drawbacks of reorganization, we do not argue against it per se. Reorganization is often valuable and even critical: the old organizational framework may become anachronistic, and, for political reasons, a controversial program may be buried deep in the bureaucracy, or a prestigious one brought into public view.

A variety of reorganization plans were being considered for HEW in 1976. The most sweeping proposal of the early 1970s was President Nixon's plan to consolidate the Departments of Interior, Commerce, Labor, HUD, HEW, and Transportation, plus some other functions, into four new departments: Community Development, Natural Resources, Human Resources (including health activities), and Economic Affairs (Fox). Programs would have been organized around functional goals (e.g., health services delivery) rather than clientele (e.g., Indians), and the secretary would have been given increased managerial authority and staff. This is a typical attempt to make organization more hierarchical, that is, more responsive to the managers and to the President himself. However, this plan was too sweeping to be accepted. Its underlying philosophy was partially followed in the "Mega Proposal" developed by Secretary Richardson of HEW in 1972.

Briefly, the Mega Proposal entailed establishing special revenue-sharing programs to replace the scores of categorical programs, intensifying efforts to build state, local, and private agency capability for providing services while reducing federal money, and replacing Medicare and Medicaid with a maximum liability (or catastrophic) health insurance plan (Miles, p. 285). As will be discussed in the next section, the shift to revenue-sharing has been accomplished to some extent. The remainder of much of the Mega proposal resurfaced in the Ford health message and 1977 budget presented in January 1976.

Congressman Paul Rogers, the Chairman of the Subcommittee on Health and the Environment of the House Committee on Interstate and Foreign Commerce, has been particularly interested in developing a Department of Health, recognizing that health is important enough as a federal activity to have its own department and that the size of the expenditures make it more and more necessary. This proposal has been endorsed by a former Assistant Secretary of Health (Edwards). A proposal by Senator Herman Talmadge to develop an Assistant Secretary of Health Care Financing—who would administer the health programs now in the SSA (Medicare) and the SRS (Medicaid), plus others—represents a possible step in that direction. Before this proposal becomes viable, however, the close relationship between welfare and health benefits provided by the federal government must be considered. A comprehensive compulsory national health insurance program would make this simpler; however, such a plan would tend to abolish scores of categorical programs now providing service to needy people, such as neighborhood health centers (Seggel, p. 93).

It is worth pointing out that NIH, FDA, and CDC have all had considerable stability over a number of years, and will probably continue in much their present form whatever form government health programs take. It is the service and manpower programs which have changed the most. After the disruptive impoundments, vetoes, and attempts at program abolition of the Nixon years, it seems best to continue those programs until a consensus on policies has emerged.

State and Local Governments
Introduction

Like the federal government, state and local governments have multiple functions in health care delivery. The state and local governments are involved, to varying degrees, in administration of laws, including regulating providers and financing agencies; in direct delivery of both personal and community health services; and in financing—through direct spending for their own programs, grants, and contracts to other agencies for support of various programs and as third-party payors to providers on an item-of-service basis for care given to individual patients.

Other branches of government—the legislatures, and the criminal and civil justice systems—also function at the state and local levels in relation to health care. State governments have licensing power, which may be the single most important element in determining the character of the United States health care delivery system (see Chapter 13).

Unfortunately, our knowledge concerning the activities of local and state governments in health is incomplete, as Miller pointed out:

> . . . there is no available directory of local health departments or of their directors; there is no central repository of information concerning them, and they have not been the subject of any recent intensive published study. In 1968, Myers published a report on medical care as offered by local health departments. [*] That report was drawn from a survey sample taken from a registry then maintained by the Department of Health, Education, and Welfare. That registry was discontinued in 1971.
> The Association of State and Territorial Health Officers

---

* Myers, B. A. et al. "The Medical Care Activities of Local Health Units." *Public Health Reports, 83*, 757, 1968. See Chapter 6 for further discussion.

recently completed a study of programs within the jurisdiction of state health departments. [*] A group at the University of North Carolina has established a registry of local health departments, and surveys are in progress on their funding, staffing, administrative authorities, legislative mandates, and relationship to other local and state interests. Surveys are also in progress at The University of Texas School of Public Health. (Miller, p. 1330)

To shed light on the states' and localities' roles in health care, let us first examine some aspects of their relationships with the federal government.

Federal-State-Local Relationships for Health Services

Money transfers from the federal government to state and local governments began very early in the history of the United States, but did not become significant until after World War II. As late as 1950, such transfers for all purposes totaled only $2 billion (Office of Management and Budget p. 236). After 1960, the amount rose rapidly, with an expected 1976 expenditure of $56 billion. That was about 22% of total state and local government expenditures (Office of Management and Budget, p. 235).

About $20 billion of the total (36%) came from the DHEW. Health expenditures showed the most dramatic growth, rising from 4% of federal aid in 1961 to 16% in 1976. The estimated federal expenditures for health services' aid to the state and local governments approached $9 billion (Table 10.2). The increase has been largely due to the Medicaid program (see Chapters 9 and 15). Most recently, increases in the health area have been due to general revenue-sharing and environmental protection. Income security, a separate but important health-related function, accounted for more than $12 billion in federal aid to state and local governments in 1975.

Federal aid developed as "categorical" grants to support specific activities. (Categorical programs are those developed to aid certain groups, such as the maternal and child health (MCH) program or the tuberculosis control program.) The first such program was created by the Sheppard-Towner Act of 1921. Enacted over the bitter opposition of the AMA, it provided for grants-in-

* Association of State and Territorial Health Officials. *Initial Report on Programs and Expenditures of State and Territorial Health Agencies: Fiscal Year 1974.* Washington, D.C.: Health Program Reporting System, May, 1975.

Table 10.2

Federal Aid to State and Local Governments for Health Functions, by Federal Agency

Agency	Amount (in millions)
Dept. HEW	
Health Service Admin.	$527
Center for Disease Control	52
Alcohol, Drug Abuse and Mental	
Health Admin.	457
Health Resources Admin.	580
Medicaid	7,156
Dept. of the Interior: Mine Safety	1
Dept. of Labor: OSHA	43
Special Action Office for Drug	
Abuse Prevention	1
Total	8,818

Source: *Special Analyses, Budget of the United States Government, Fiscal Year 1976* (Washington, D.C.: Government Printing Office, 1975), p. 248.

aid to the states, setting the pattern for future categorical federal programs (Stern, pp. 123-124; Mustard, pp. 73-77; Burrow, pp. 157-165).

By the late 1960s, however, there was increasing concern about uncoordinated programs, excessive federal requirements on the funds, and rigid funding arrangements that prevented local innovation and decision-making. James Haughton wrote rather vehemently:

> The worst way to finance health care is by categorical grants. Categorical grants tend to attract programs to where the money is rather than where the need is . . . rather than developing services on a broad basis so that people get the services they need, categorical grants tend to stimulate programs that match the money that is available. (Haughton, p. 773)

Reforms instituted by the Nixon Administration in the early 70s included: (1) decentralization of decision-making to federal field offices in 10 regions; (2) simplification of federal grant administrative requirements; (3) maximum possible sharing of planning and management functions with state and local governments; and (4) consolidation of overlapping federal grant programs (Office of Management and Budget, p. 239). This led to the development in 1973 of what was called "general revenue-sharing," designed principally to get away from the categorical approach, to give money to states based on a formula reflecting population and relative economic status, and then, within very broad program guidelines, to let the states—and through them the local governments—decide how to spend the money, based on their knowledge of specific community needs. However, in the Nixon approach, general revenue-sharing had other goals, in particular to slow the growth of federal aid to states (Whitman). The 1976 estimate of outlays for general revenue-sharing was $6.3 billion (Office of Management and Budget, p. 249); the amount would have been considerably higher if earlier trends had continued. Concomitant reductions in numerous grant programs are likely to lead to reduced levels of social services, especially to the poor, and to less innovative government activity in urban areas (Whitman). Thus, revenue-sharing was partially in conflict with the state goals of the earlier reforms.

These changes attempt to redefine the appropriate role of government and the relationship between state and federal government. An overall reduction in spending implies that the public wishes to have fewer programs. A shift to state and local initiative indicates a growing awareness that not all governmental programs can be administered from Washington. It makes good sense to decentralize as many functions as possible, if the states are capable of handling them; but many experts are skeptical on this point (Seggel, pp. 110-112). Federal program administration has also been largely decentralized to Regional Offices, despite congressional opposition. Indications are that these offices lack the expertise required to furnish technical assistance, a critical federal role (Martin; Seggel, pp. 112–113).

Another consideration is equity. The history of welfare programs in the United States is not reassuring in this regard. Welfare has been run through grants-in-aid to the states, but as Burns points out (p. 49), states have been required to carry some of the costs, on the assumption that this will help to assure responsible administration. Purely local program development can lead to great inequities because of unequal resources, because of the traditional pauper stigma, and because of racial prejudice. The innumerable different state benefits, exclusions, and unreasonable eligibility requirements have led to proposals to federalize welfare. Proponents point to the Supplemental Security Income (SSI) program for Social Security Beneficiaries, a partial federalization of welfare. It has relieved the states of responsibility for about $1 billion annually in expenditures for public assistance to the aged, blind, and disabled, and simultaneously abolished the inequities (Seggel, p. 71).

The Medicaid program is also plagued with inequities. Although President Ford proposed early in 1976 that more of the administrative and financial responsibility for this program should be turned back to the states, the above considerations make that unlikely. In fact, the federalization of Medicaid has been proposed in several national health insurance bills, and seems inevitable. Several NHI proposals, however, have included state administration.

Thus the debate continues. A concept of policy direction from Washington—along with considerable financial assistance, in the federal government's role as income-transfer agent—has evolved, but the specifics of this philosophy applied to each program will have to be worked out over time. It is clear that this will remain one of the critical policy issues of American government.

Health Services by State and Local Governments

Available information regarding the activities of state and local governments in the delivery of both community and personal health services is quite limited, as was pointed out above.* By 1976, there had been only one national survey of state government health activities, carried out by the Health Program Reporting System of the Association of State and Territorial Health Officials (ASTHO, 1975). This survey was limited to the single department in each state and territory designated by the state government as the State Health Agency (SHA). However, at the state and local levels, just as at the federal level, there are many different agencies involved in health services (Wilson and Neuhauser, p. 180). For example, in most state governments, two of the most important state health functions, providing mental hospital services and operating the Medicaid program, are run by departments other than the SHA (ASTHO, pp. 2,7), perpetuat-

---

* Roemer et al. provide particularly useful detailed discussions of four prototypical public health functions in which state and local health departments play an important part: maternal and child health, mental health, emergency medical care, and health facilities planning and regulation (1975, chs. 4–7). The standard text in the field is John J. Hanlon's *Principles of Public Health Administration*, published in periodic editions by the C. V. Mosby Company of St. Louis.

ing Finch's "tangled net of programs." Licensing of health manpower often resides in the education department, vocational rehabilitation in a special agency, occupational health in the labor
department, school health in the local boards of education, and in
some states environmental protection programs are found in a
special agency too. Most states also have a Board of Health, usually appointed by the Governor, which has varying administrative, policy, and advisory functions.

The National Commission on Community Health Services recommended consolidation of official health services in a single
state health agency. One state that has attempted such consolidation is Massachusetts, which until recently had classical public
health programs plus certification of need and licensing of private health facilities in a Department of Public Health, but had
the following programs in other agencies as well:

1. Rate-setting—the Office of Administration and Finance
2. Regulation of health insurance—the Commissioner of Insurance
3. Licensing and standard-setting for health personnel—Office of Consumer Affairs
4. Administration and standard-setting for the Medicaid
   program—Department of Public Welfare
5. Health planning activities—Office of Human Services

These functions were reorganized into a Health Systems Regulation Administration in 1974 (Executive Office of Human Services).

In Chapter 6, in our consideration of the role of local health
departments in ambulatory care, we discussed the political struggles with the private practitioners in the 1920s that led to the
departments being generally limited in functions to Haven
Emerson's "Basic Six": vital statistics, public health laboratories, communicable-disease control, environmental sanitation,
maternal and child health, and public health education (Wilson
and Neuhauser, p. 180). Local governments (usually not local
health departments, however) were also given responsibility for
providing general medical services for the poor. State governments were generally confined to the Basic Six as well (excluding
general medical care for the poor), but also ran the public mental
hospitals. In recent years, additional responsibilities have been
given to state governments (and on occasion to large local gov-

ernments) in regulation and quality control, rate-setting, institutional licensing, planning, and acting as a third-party payor under Medicaid. The ASTHO has reported on those activities carried out by State Health Agencies (1975).

Activities of state health agencies. The ASTHO study covered the designated State Health Agencies (SHAs) in the 50 states, the District of Columbia, Guam, Puerto Rico, and the Trust Territory of the Pacific Islands, referred to generically as "states."

The SHAs were asked to report their activities and expenditures under four major program headings: (1) personal health services, (2) environmental health services, (3) health resources, and (4) other programs, services, and administration. Capital expenditures were excluded. For fiscal 1974, they reported expenditures of $4.9 billion, about 47% of which was for Medicaid and 6% for "special social services" (e.g., adoption services in California and juvenile delinquent services in Maryland) (ASTHO, pp. 2-3). In 10 states, including Guam, Puerto Rico, and the Virgin Islands, the SHA was the designated Single State Agency for Medicaid. Thus SHAs spent about $2.3 billion to support their own health services in fiscal 1974.

About 75% of all expenditures were for personal health services (Table 10.3). Major services delivered or supported by a majority of SHAs are: laboratory, public health nursing, maternal and child health, family planning, crippled children, immunization, tuberculosis and chronic respiratory disease control other than in institutions, and venereal disease control. These are traditional public health services.

Large amounts of money were spent on certain other services in a limited number of SHAs. For example, seven SHAs spent funds on the noninstitutional care of mental illness, but over $150 million of the total of $167 was spent in California (ASTHO, Appendix Table 20). Five SHAs operated general hospitals—the District of Columbia, Puerto Rico, the Virgin Islands and the Pacific Trust Territories, and Hawaii. Eight SHAs—including those of Hawaii, Puerto Rico, and the Virgin Islands—operated mental hospitals. Twelve SHAs operated tuberculosis and respiratory disease hospitals. Twenty-one SHAs operated alcoholism and drug abuse programs.

Of all expenditures, $169 million (7%) went for environmental health services (Table 10.4). More than 70% of the money went for general environmental health and sanitation services, general consumer protection, and water control. All but four SHAs

Table 10.3

Personal Health Services Delivered by SHAs, Fiscal Year 1974

Program Area	No. of SHAs Reporting	Expenditures (in millions)	(%)
General, supporting, and other[a]	55	$251	15
Maternal and child health, crippled children, and family planning	54	310	18
Communicable disease control[b]	55	89	5
Dental services	51	19	1
Chronic disease[c]	47	37	2
Mental health[d]	30	318	18
State-operated institutions[e]	24	711	41
Total	55	1735	100

Source: ASTHO, *Programs and Expenditures of State and Territorial Health Agencies* (Washington, D.C.: Government Printing Office, 1975), pp. 3–8.

[a] Includes laboratory, public health nursing, programs of care not primarily in institutions, local health department support, emergency medical services, migrant health, disability, and other.
[b] Includes immunization, tuberculosis and chronic respiratory disease control other than in institutions, venereal disease, general, and other.
[c] Includes cancer, cardiovascular disease, renal disease, general, and other.
[d] Includes alcoholism and drug abuse, mental illness, mental retardation, general, and other. Excludes care in state-operated institutions.
[e] Includes general, chronic disease, tuberculosis and respiratory disease, and mental hospitals, institutions for the mentally retarded, and other.

reported some activity in environmental health (ASTHO, p. 8). An additional $129 million (6%) was spent on "Health Resources Programs" which included: planning and development, facilities and services regulation, manpower regulation, and vital and health statistics (ASTHO, p. 10). With the exception of vital statistics (the responsibility of the SHA in all jurisdictions but Idaho and the District of Columbia), these activities represent the newer and expanding functions of SHAs in planning and regulation.

In 29 states, the Comprehensive Health Planning agency was located in the SHA, while in 48 states the Hill-Burton Agency was there (see Chapter 12). Certification-of-need powers (see Chapters 12 and 13) were lodged in an indeterminate number of SHAs. SHAs were particularly important in the regulation of health facilities by standard-setting, licensing, and/or certification. In addition, 45 SHAs were involved in regulating inpatient facilities, clinical laboratories, blood banks, ambulatory treatment centers, home health agencies, child day-care centers, and

Table 10.4

Environmental Health Services Provided by SHAs

Program Category	No. of SHAs Reporting	Expenditures (in millions)	(%)
General environmental health	33	$40.0	23.8
General sanitation	30	33.5	19.9
General consumer protection	29	27.3	16.2
Water and water quality	29	20.4	12.1
General	4	3.0	1.8
Potable water	22	6.5	3.9
Water quality	15	10.9	6.5
Laboratory services	24	15.3	9.1
Air quality	18	10.7	6.4
Solid wastes management	14	7.1	4.2
Occupational health	25	6.5	3.9
Radiation control	33	5.8	3.5
Other	9	1.3	0.8
Total	51	168.0	100.0

Source: ASTHO, *Programs and Expenditures of State and Territorial Health Agencies* (Washington, D.C.: Government Printing Office, 1975), p. 9.

boarding homes. Four SHAs were involved in cost-control and four had medical audit and/or utilization review programs (ASTHO, p. 10). It remains to be seen what will happen to the development and distribution of these state powers under the National Health Planning and Resources Development Act of 1974, which requires certificates of need in all states, but requires review at the local level (see Chapter 12).

Local government health services. All states but Rhode Island, Vermont, Delaware, and Hawaii have local health departments. (Neither the District of Columbia nor any of the four territories has them.) As of 1966, the most recent year for which figures are available, there were about 1,700 such departments, operated by several types of local government jurisdiction (Myers et al.). The departments run on a combination of federal funds that the states funnel to them, state funds (provided by all but 3 of the 46 states with local health departments), and local budgetary support. There are wide variations in the degree of supervision and technical assistance provided to local health departments by the states.

As noted above, there is no general catalogue of local government health services in the United States. Local health departments tend to be limited to the Basic Six, although some of them in recent years have become involved in the direct delivery of

ambulatory services to the poor (Wilson and Neuhauser, p. 182).
Local health department personal health services were discussed
in Chapter 6.

Following the state and federal model, local health services are
provided by various agencies other than health departments. For
example, cities and counties are likely to place their hospitals for
the poor and their mental health services in separate agencies.
Local government hospitals, which are extremely important for
health care of the poor in many areas of the country, are discussed in Chapter 7. Water supply, sanitary sewage and solid
waste disposal, and pollution control are also likely to be in separate agencies, if they are not handled by the private sector.

Conclusion

It should be quite clear that government is heavily involved in the
health care delivery system in the United States. Our constitutional structure and our economic system determine and limit the
nature of that involvement to a great extent. Government provides the legal underpinning for the system through the licensing
laws, and regulates its workings through covering financing and
quality of care. Government is a direct financier and a direct
provider of service. It is preeminent in community health services and plays an important part in supporting health sciences
education and research. However, the resistance to "government
interference in the practice of medicine" is still very prominent
among private medical practitioners, and in many laws concerning the health care delivery system—for example, the Social Security Amendments establishing the Medicare program—such interference is expressly prohibited. Nonetheless, most providers recognize the reality of the situation—that government is already
heavily involved in the practice of medicine—and they welcome
participation in certain critical areas: licensing; care of the
mentally ill, the tubercular, and the poor; and community health
services.

We now face the problem of determining the precise role of
government in the health system: what proportion of payment
for health services will be public money, who shall plan how
funds are used, who shall assure quality of care in physicians'
offices, and so forth. The "tangled net of programs," with multiple jurisdictions and interests, leading to overlapping coverage
for many people and lack of any coverage for others, presents a
major difficulty. But a more serious problem is defining the rela-

tion between government and the private sector. What we need is not a "government takeover," but a rational division of labor between the public and private sectors; a cooperative effort aimed at benefiting the citizenry rather than aggrandizing either sector. However, it is easier to state the need for this alliance than to identify the programs and procedures that can bring it about.

In the remaining chapters we will examine how government is and will be involved in solving our health care problems in legislative action, planning, quality control, research policy, and in national health insurance.

References

American Hospital Association. *Hospital Statistics*. Chicago, Ill.: American Hospital Association, 1975.

American Public Health Association. "The State Public Health Agency." An Official Statement Approved by the Governing Council, October 17, 1965.

———. "The Role of Official Local Health Agencies." A Position Paper Approved by the Governing Council, October 23, 1974.

Association of State and Territorial Health Officials. *Initial Report on Programs and Expenditures of State and Territorial Health Agencies: Fiscal Year 1974*. Washington, D.C.: Health Program Reporting System, May, 1975.

Ball, R. "Background of Regulation in Health Care." In *Controls on Health Care*, papers of the Conference on Regulation in the Health Industry, January 7–9, 1974. Washington, D.C.: National Academy of Sciences, 1975.

Boffey, P.M. "Military Medical School: It Survives Despite All Efforts to Kill It." *Science, 190*, 860, 1975.

Burns, E. *Health Services for Tomorrow*. New York: Dunellen, 1974.

Burrow, J. G. "AMA: Voice of American Medicine." Baltimore, Md.: Johns Hopkins Press, 1963.

Cowan, J. R. "The Role of Military Medicine." *Urban Health*, October, 1974, pp. 25–26.

Cowan, J. R. "Retention Biggest Problem for DOD." *U.S. Medicine*, January 15, 1975, pp. 17–20.

Cowan, J. R. "Volunteer Force: DOD Successful." *U.S. Medicine*, January 15, 1976, pp. 7–9.

Edwards, C. Testimony before the President's Biomedical Research Panel, July 28, 1975, Washington, D.C.

Elazar, D. "The New Federalism: Can the States Be Trusted?" *Public Interest, 35,* 89, Spring, 1974.

Executive Office of Human Services, Commonwealth of Massachusetts. "Statement of Rationale for the Health Systems Regulation Administration." Proposed in House 6120, July 17, 1973, Boston.

———. "Statement of Rationale for the Health Systems Regulation Administration." July 17, 1974. Mimeograph.

Finch, R. H. Hearings before Subcommittee on Intergovernmental Relations. 91st Cong., 1st Sess., September, 1969.

Fox, D. "President Nixon's Proposals for Executive Reorganization." *Public Administration Review, 34,* 487, 1974.

Grad, F. P. *Public Health Law Manual.* Washington, D.C.: American Public Health Association, 1975.

Haughton, J. G. Heargings before the Subcommittee on Executive Reorganization of the Committee on Intergovernment Operations. U.S. Senate, 90th Cong., 2nd Sess., July, 1968.

Herman, H., and McKay, M. "Community Health Services." Washington, D.C.: The International City Managers' Association, 1968.

House Committee Print No. 4. *Medical Care of Veterans.* 90th Congress, 1st Session. Washington, D.C.: Government Printing Office, April, 1967.

House Committee Print No. 1. *Operations of Veterans Administration Hospital and Medical Program.* 94th Congress, 1st Session. Washington, D.C.: Government Printing Office, 1975.

Journals of the Continental Congress. Volume 5.

Levitan, S. A., and Cleary, K. A. *Old Wars Remain Unfinished: the Veteran Benefit System.* Baltimore, Md.: Johns Hopkins University Press, 1973.

Lewis, B. J. *Veterans Administration Medical Program Relationship with Medical Schools in the United States.* House Committee Print No. 170, 91st Congress, 2nd Session. Washington, D.C.: Government Printing Office, 1970.

Martin, J. Statement of the General Accounting Office (GAO) before the Subcommittee on Health, Committee on Labor and Public Welfare, U.S. Senate, on the Implementation of the Health Maintenance Organization Act of 1973. November 21, 1975, Washington, D.C.

McKenzie, V. Testimony before Subcommittee No. 2, Committee on Armed Services. 93rd Congress, 2nd Session, October 26, 1974. H.A.S.C. No. 93–70, 1974.

Medical World News. "Military Medical Schools Launched." *16,* No. 17, p. 32.

Miles, R. *The Department of Health, Education and Welfare.* New York: Praeger Publishers, 1974.

Miller, A. "Issues of Health Policy: Local Government and the Public's Health." *American Journal of Public Health, 65,* 1330, 1975.

Mueller, M., and Gibson, R. "National Health Expenditures, Fiscal Year 1975." *Social Security Bulletin, 39*, 3, 1976.

Mustard, H. S. *Government in Public Health.* New York: The Commonwealth Fund, 1945.

Mueller, M., and Gibson, R. "National Health Expenditures, Fiscal Year 1975." *Social Security Bulletin, 39*, 3, 1976.

Mustard, H. S. *Government in Public Health.* New York: The Commonwealth Fund, 1945.

Myers, B. A. et al. "The Medical Care Activities of Local Health Units." *Public Health Reports, 83*, 757, 1968.

National Commission on Community Health Services. *Health Is a Community Affair.* Cambridge, Mass.: Harvard University Press, 1966.

National Commission on Diabetes. *Report to the Congress of the United States.* HEW Pub. No. NIH 76-1018. Washington, D.C.: USDHEW, 1975.

Office of Management and Budget. *Special Analyses, Budget of the United States Government, Fiscal Year 1976.* Washington, D.C.: Government Printing Office, 1975.

President's Biomedical Research Panel. *Report Submitted to the President and the Congress of the United States.* HEW Pub. No. OS 76–500. Washington, D.C.: USDHEW, 1976.

Roemer, R. et al. *Planning Urban Health Services: From Jungle to System.* New York: Springer Publishing Co., 1975.

Russel, L. et al. *Federal Health Spending 1969–1974.* Washington, D.C.: National Planning Association, 1974.

Schmeckebier, L. F. *The Public Health Service.* Institute for Government Research. Service Monographs of the U.S. Government No. 10. Baltimore, Md.: Johns Hopkins Press, 1923.

Seggel, R. "Social and Human Service Functions." In S. Humes and G. Graham, Eds., *Policy Formulator,* pp. 61–116. Fort Lauderdale, Fla.: Nova University Press, 1975.

Seidman, H. *Politics, Position, and Power.* New York: Oxford University Press, 1970.

Senate Finance Committee. *Medicare and Medicaid: Problems, Issues, and Alternatives.* Report of the Staff. Washington, D.C.: Government Printing Office, 1970.

Stern, B. J. *Medical Services by Government: Local, State, and Federal.* New York: The Commonwealth Fund, 1946.

U.S. Code, Title 38, Chapter 17, Sec. 610.

Whitman, R. D. "The Future of Revenue Sharing." *Challenge,* July–August, 1975, p. 14.

Wilson, F. A., and Neuhauser, D. *Health Services in the United States.* Cambridge, Mass.: Ballinger, 1974.

11

The Federal Legislative Process and Health Care

David Banta

Introduction

Most national public policies are established by legislative enactment, although some policy-making powers do lie with the executive branch and the courts (Lindblom, pp. 72–73). In the previous chapter, we described the major functions of government in the delivery of health care services. To illustrate how legislative branches function, this chapter describes the role of Congress in the health care delivery system and its modus operandi in decision-making and the establishment of policy.

Policy may be defined as "any set of values, opinions, and actions which moves decision-making . . . in certain directions" (Anderson). Those who analyze policy generally think in terms of rational objectives, such as eliminating poverty or curing cancer (Rivlin). But thinking of the policy process as rational "fails to evoke or suggest the distinctively political aspects of policy-making, its apparent disorder and the consequent strikingly different ways in which policies emerge" (Lindblom, 1968, p. 4). In particular, rational planning is difficult to achieve in a democracy. Planning seeks to maximize the public good, but different groups within the society have a different concept of "public good" (Lindblom, p. 17). Moreover, rational policy-making is stymied because Congress, like the country it represents, is complex. It is chaotic, decentralized in its functioning, and difficult to understand, even superficially. Committee jurisdiction, which divides the health effort into many parts, acts against the goal of sound, comprehensible policy formation.

The constitutional separation of powers also complicates the policy-making process, as pointed out in Chapter 10. The executive is more likely to be integrative, comprehensive, and national in its policy development than is the Congress; its goals often conflict with the provincial interests of congressmen. These conflicts are exacerbated when different political parties control the White House and the Congress. As chief administrative officer of the executive branch, the President obviously has important policy functions. Even in the legislative arena, the President may (and usually does) propose legislation; he presents the budget; and he must approve, and may veto legislation.

Of course, governmental health policies are not determined only at the federal level, as was discussed in Chapter 10. States and localities retain considerable power in the health field and may have philosophies and plans that may conflict with federal policies. Policy is molded by a variety of societal forces beyond those of the policy-making system, such as the wealth of the nation and its social structure. The fact that major elements of the health system remain largely in private and disparate hands not only limits federal influence on the health system but makes the development of health policies based on rational planning difficult.

Nonetheless, the broad outlines of a national health policy for the United States are beginning to emerge (Anderson; Geiger; Kisch; McNerney; Somers; Weinerman; White). There is agreement on certain critical needs concerning the organization of medical and health care: the need to assure access to primary health care services; to plan and organize health services in a region; to foster group practice and team medicine; to train health manpower to carry out the tasks of the future; and to establish a national health insurance system. In dealing with all of these questions, the role of government must be carefully defined. In particular, the society must grapple with the appropriate method of assuring an effective public-private mix in health services. If Edwards is correct in saying that the private health sector has failed to accept leadership responsibility, functioning instead merely as an array of special interests, a deeper penetration of government in medicine is likely (1975).

Although the public generally favors limiting the federal budget, polls carried out in the mid-70s indicated that the public is willing to pay higher taxes for expanded health services with government involvement. Indeed, in one poll in 1975, 22% of persons interviewed supported a totally nationalized health system; another 35% supported national health insurance to guarantee each person as much care as needed; only 13% endorsed keeping things as they are (Walters). Such opinion is certain to have increasing impact on Congress, accelerating the trend toward planning and development of comprehensive health systems that began in 1967 (Kissick).

The Congress and Its Organization

The Congress has been evocatively described: "It is organized quite differently from the conventional bureaucracy, which Casual Observer professes to despise, but which he and his friends comprehend. Instead of having a single head, Congress looks like the hydra (or perhaps the Medusa) of Greek mythology. Instead of neatly delegating work downward and responsibility upward, Congress is a complex, redundant, not always predictable, and purposely unwieldy network of crisscrossing and overlapping lines of authority and information" (Polsby, 1971, p. 3).

Basically, Congress has the following functions: (1) legislating, (2) overseeing government programs, (3) expressing public opinions, and (4) servicing constituents (Mayhew, 1974, p. 8). These functions, however, do not coincide with the main interests of an individual congressman. Indeed, a congressman's three primary goals have been said to be (1) getting re-elected, (2) achieving influence in Congress, and (3) making good public policy, perhaps in that order (Fenno, 1973). Studies have indicated that a substantial part, perhaps as much as half, of the factors determining the outcome of a congressional election are local: for this reason, a congressman must be attuned to his constituents. On the other hand, the average voter has a limited awareness of the voting records and general effectiveness of his representative, so the congressman takes special note of the opinions of those active in politics, particularly if they are prominent. (It is also worth noting that different groups vote at different rates, with the poor, least educated, and least involved in the community voting the least [Schattschneider, p. 105]). The congressman values campaign contributions as much to prevent an opponent from receiving them as because he or she needs them. Valuing organizations that can produce volunteers for the campaign, he or she tends to move toward the positions of organized groups. Thus, the electoral process connects a congressman primarily to important persons and groups of people with strong feelings on particular issues (Mayhew, pp. 40–42).

Certain ingrained structural characteristics tend to weaken Congress, while others strengthen it. Congressmen are *formally* equal to each other, which distinguishes them from members of hierarchically ordered organizations. This formal equality tends to fragment the Congress, as does the committee structure. Forces acting to preserve and strengthen the institution include the political parties and certain committees, especially in the House of Representatives. The complex rules of the House control the fragmentation and moderate the power of interest groups (Mayhew, pp. 146–155).

The much-maligned seniority system is an important mechanism for maintaining institutional integrity. More than half of Congress has been elected since 1970. Seniority assures that those in positions of leadership have knowledge of the government, as well as knowledge of specific policy issues in such areas as health. Key leaders in the health subcommittees have been active in Congress for more than 10 years. Because of the seniority system, most leadership positions are held by members from "safe" districts. They tend to be less concerned about re-election, and are able to use their judgment more (Fenno, 1973).

The two houses of Congress operate in quite different ways. The House of Representatives, with 435 members, is a large, unwieldy body, controlled by complex rules and divided into groups of specialists. Each member is assigned to only one or sometimes two committees, where he or she may spend years. This specialization is believed to reduce conflict (Fenno, 1973). Floor debate in the House is generally limited to committee members, who are expected to concentrate their attention on the area of jurisdiction of their committee.

The Senate is less structured. Senators are fewer, more prominent socially, may be quite wealthy, serve longer terms, and, except for states with small populations, represent larger areas. The Senate, much more than the House, is the place of the individual, and much of the business is done by unanimous consent (Huitt, p. 91). "The essence of the Senate is that it is a great forum, an echo chamber, a publicity machine" (Polsby, p. 3, 1971). Each senator serves on many committees and subcommittees; few specialize. The Senate tends to develop policies, and in recent years has been likely to pass legislation dealing with a new issue much more quickly than does the House.

Congressional Committees: Structure and Function

The congressional committees are important loci of power; indeed, in the House, they have been referred to as the "backbone of the decision-making structure" (Fenno, 1973, pp. 64–65).

There are 22 standing committees in the House and 18 in the Senate. At the beginning of the 93rd Congress (1973), there were 143 subcommittees in the Senate and 132 in the House (Mayhew, p. 94).* The principal committees and subcommittees with health functions and the names of the chairmen and ranking minority members are shown in Table 11.1.

Changes resulting from the Legislative Reform Acts of 1946 and 1970, as well as from alterations in the Democratic Party caucus, have given such prerogatives as budgets and staff to subcommittee chairmen. Subcommittees have also become more important because of the complexity of the issues. In the mid-70s, the House Democrats had a rule that no member could have more than one subcommittee chairmanship, which makes a significant number of members chairmen. The Senate had no such rule, and with only 100 Senators, in the mid-70s, most Democrats were committee or subcommittee chairmen (Mayhew, pp. 96–97).

Role of Staff

Congressmen's claims to expertise derive from their own knowledge *plus* that of their staffs, the staff having much more policy input than is generally recognized. Congressional staff is divided into office staff—which works directly for a congressmen or senator, primarily on constituent problems and requests—and committee staff—which identifies problems, provides facts and questions, and carries out the day-to-day work of the committee, such as writing reports. In practice, the line between these two types of staff can be very fuzzy. Both types have expanded rapidly with the increasing complexity of the federal government, becoming quite large (Taaffe; Seidman, 1970). For example, by 1975 there were 26 professionals, including four physicians, on the staffs of the four Senate and House authorizing committees and two appropriations subcommittees that write the great majority of federal health legislation (Inglehart).

The role of staff differs considerably in the two houses. Since representatives are much better versed on the technical issues, their staff has a limited role. In the Senate, where members tend to spread themselves thin, committee staff especially have considerably more autonomy. Few senators are interested enough in

---

* Congressional committees and subcommittees are listed periodically in the *Official Congressional Directory*, published by the Government Printing Office.

Table 11.1

Some Key Congressional Committees and Subcommittees with Health Functions, 1976

Committee/ Subcommittee	Area of Health Activity	Chairman (Dem.)	Ranking Minority Member (Rep.)
Senate:			
Committee on Labor and Public Welfare		Harrison Williams (N.J.)	Jacob Javits (N.Y.)
Subcommittee on Health	Most health legislation, jurisdiction over the Public Health Service Act (Most programs in DHEW)	Edward M. Kennedy (Mass.)	Richard Schweiker (Pa.)
Committee on Finance	Taxes, Social Security	Russell B. Long (La.)	Carl T. Curtis (Neb.)
Subcommittee on Health	Medicare, Medicaid	Herman Talmadge (Ga.)	Robert Dole (Kans.)
Committee on Appropriations		John McClellan (Ark.)	Milton Young (N. Dak.)
Subcommittee on Labor, Health, Education, and Welfare	Allocation of tax funds in the Budget —DHEW health programs except Medicare and Medicaid	Warren Magnuson (Wash.)	Edward Brooke (Mass.)
House of Representatives:			
Committee on Interstate and Foreign Commerce		Harley Staggers (W. Va.)	Samuel Devine (Ohio)
Subcommittee on Health and Environment	Most health programs in DHEW, including Medicaid and Part B of Medicare	Paul Rogers (Fla.)	Tim Lee Carter (Ken.)
Committee on Ways and Means	Taxes, Social Security	Al Ullman (Ore.)	Herman Schneebeli (Pa.)
Subcommittee on Health	Medicare, Part A	Dan Rostenkowski (Ill.)	John Duncan (Tenn.)
Committee on Appropriations		George Mahon (Tex.)	Elford Cederburg (Mich.)
Subcommittee on Labor, Health, Education, and Welfare	Allocation of tax funds in the Budget —DHEW health programs except Medicare and Medicaid	Daniel Flood (Pa.)	Robert Michel (Ill.)

health to spend a great deal of their time on it, so the task of creating and constructing legislation is delegated almost entirely to staff. Of course, staff works within limits defined by each senator.

In addition to the two types of staff described, Congress has technical resources available, although these are miniscule in comparison to those of the executive branch. The Congressional Research Service of the Library of Congress has several health experts, as do the new Offices of Technology Assessment and of Congressional Budget. The General Accounting Office, part of the legislative branch, employs about 200 people to carry out yearly program evaluations in the health field, and is the primary tool for carrying out congressional "oversight" of executive branch programs. And the Office of the Legislative Counsel has expert legal help for drafting bills; there are also experts in health law.

The Legislative Process

During each two-year congressional term, approximately 25,000 legislative proposals are introduced by members of the House and Senate, with as many as 2,000 in health or health-related fields. Any member of either house can submit a bill for consideration by his house on any subject. These bills can be written by the member, his or her staff, lobbyists, members of the executive branch, constituents, or anyone else designated by the member.

During the mid-1960s, perhaps 90% of health legislation originated with the executive branch, and was actively pushed by testimony in favor of that proposal and against other related proposals, by reports and letters, and by personal contact and lobbying by members of the Administration (Lawton). Until the late 1960s, Congress responded to the proposals of the executive branch, and demonstrated little inclination to initiate substantive policy-oriented legislation. Legislation establishing Regional Medical Programs, Medicare, Medicaid, and Comprehensive Health Planning was essentially fashioned by the executive. However, the Nixon/Ford Presidency (1969–77) saw considerable conflict between the White House and the Congress, and Congress began to attempt to establish independent positions. With more activist chairmen of the several health subcommittees, plus increased staff, some proposals are originating in the Congress. For example, the Senate Labor and Public Welfare Committee bill on health manpower in the 93rd Congress (1973–1974) largely originated in the Health Subcommittee.

Most legislative work is spent renewing expiring authorities, except on the appropriations committees. Authorization measures establish programs and provide for spending goals, while appropriations, which require separate votes, specify exactly how much money is to be made available for a particular authorized program. Almost all authorizing legislation is written with a time limit, usually two or three years. The renewal process gives Congress a chance to review programs, collect testimony, and consider changes. For example, health manpower legislation has been substantively altered each time it has been considered, beginning in 1960. The 1968 act involved little more than an attempt to insure financial viability of health professions schools. The 1971 act, in addition to providing per capita support for students, included requirements for the schools—for example, that they expand enrollment and institute special programs in such areas as primary care. The legislation passed in 1976 required further changes in medical school policies in return for the "capitation" payments. The renewal process also affords Congress an opportunity to carry out "oversight" on federally funded programs. The legislative process on these renewals is essentially identical to that for new legislation. That process requires consideration of the bill by subcommittee and committee, passage by both houses, a conference to reconcile the differences between the two bills, and presidential signature.

After introduction, each bill, whether for a new program or a renewal, is assigned to the standing committee that has jurisdiction over the subject area of the bill. Most bills dealing with health programs are assigned in the House to the Committee on Interstate and Foreign Commerce and in the Senate to the Committee on Labor and Public Welfare, both of which have health subcommittees (see Table 11.1). However, the bulk of federal health spending is in the Medicare and Medicaid programs (see Chapter 9), which fall under the jurisdiction of the Committee on Finance in the Senate. In the House, Medicaid falls under the jurisdiction of Interstate and Foreign Commerce, as does Part B of Medicare. This strange split in jurisdiction resulted from the so-called "Hansen reforms" of 1975, when a compromise proposal for House reorganization left all payroll-tax funded programs—such as Part A of Medicare—with the Ways and Means Committee, while shifting all other health programs to Interstate and Foreign Commerce.

Jurisdictional disputes are common. An important one in 1975 centered on the question of which of the two main authorizing committees in the House would control national health insurance legislation—the Committee on Ways and Means, or the Interstate and Foreign Commerce Committee. Such disputes often block potentially valuable legislation, as occurred with a Senate proposal to use the leverage of Medicare and Medicaid funds to force changes in medical residency training programs. The interest in changing medical residency training rests with Labor and Public Welfare, along with jurisdiction over health manpower legislation, while, as noted, Senate Finance has jurisdiction over health care financing.

Lack of space prevents our describing in detail each of the committees involved in health policy. The committees have their own personalities, which tend to be stable over time (Fenno, 1973). For example, Labor and Public Welfare has been a very liberal committee for more than 10 years, and has been referred to as the "conservative's graveyard."

In addition to the four authorizing committees (Labor and Public Welfare and Finance in the Senate; Commerce and Ways and Means in the House), a number of others have jurisdiction over some health or health-related program. Particularly important ones controlling the authorization of health care expenditures are the Armed Services and Veterans' Affairs Committees. As noted in Chapter 10, the Department of Defense expended approximately $3.3 billion on health activities in 1975; those funds were authorized by the Armed Services Committees. The Veterans' Administration expended almost $4 billion in 1975, falling under the jurisdiction of the Veterans' Affairs Committees.

After a bill is referred to the appropriate committee or subcommittee, if the leaders consider it important, public hearings will be held. Interested organizations and individuals, including executive branch officials, will be invited to express their opinions. Approximately 10% of bills presented in Congress receive hearings (Fenno, 1965). After hearings, a subcommittee "markup" session will be held, during which the bill is rewritten by the members, taking into account testimony heard in hearings. This mark-up may take months in the House, where Congressmen are very involved in the details of the legislation, but in the Senate the process generally takes less time. The bill will also be considered by the full committee, which may also hold hearings. Then, if it is favorably endorsed by the committee, it is reported to the floor of the respective house.

In the health area, floor votes are generally predictable. Members are likely to defer to the judgment of the committee unless there is great controversy, ideological conflict, or a split committee (Fenno, 1965). With a few recent exceptions, notably national health insurance and health manpower legislation, health has not been a controversial area; Congressmen know that their constituents favor an expansion of the government role. Nonetheless, important committee decisions can be overturned on the floor: in 1974, the Kennedy-Javits health manpower bill was rejected, and an amendment offered by Senator Beall, in effect substituting a different bill, was accepted. The Kennedy-Javits bill included a controversial provision requiring national service for all medical school graduates.

Often, problem areas will be the subject of similar, but not identical, bills passed by each house. In that case, what is called a "conference committee" will be necessary to reconcile the areas of difference. If agreement is reached, the Conference Committee Report, essentially a revision of the bill passed in each house into a mutually acceptable version, must be resubmitted to both houses for approval. If no agreement can be reached, the bill "dies in conference," as did health manpower legislation in December 1974.

Once the final common bill has passed both houses, it is sent to the President for signature. He may sign it, allow it to become law without his signature, or veto it within 10 days. If Congress adjourns during the 10-day period, he may allow it to die by neither signing it nor vetoing it; this is known as a "pocket veto."

The Budgetary Process

As previously mentioned, authorization and appropriation functions are separated in Congress. Authorization does not assure a program a place in the budget. The authorization committees are by far the most publicly visible, but the appropriation committees are obviously crucial, as a "policy" is meaningless without monetary support. Each January, the appropriation process begins when the President presents his budget, which is as close to a national policy statement as the country has. This budget is the end result of activities which consume many months in all departments of the executive branch. The process begins in the summer before the fiscal year for which it is being prepared*

* Since 1976, the federal fiscal year has begun on October 1; before then, it began on July 1.

when the Office of Management and Budget (OMB), an executive agency which oversees the budget under the President's direction, sends predetermined budget ceilings to all departments and agencies. Each department and agency then produces its own budget proposals, beginning at the program level. These are aggregated and modified, with the involvement of the staff to the secretary, in the case of HEW, until they come back to OMB as departmental budgets in August. Final development of the President's budget is done by OMB an agency which has become more and more powerful as the budget has become more and more complicated.

Appropriations bills are first considered by the House Appropriations Committee and its 13 subcommittees. The budget is reviewed line by line and is often changed considerably. The budgets proceed through hearings and mark-ups to passage by the full House. The bill is then considered by the Senate, where the process is similar. As with authorization measures, differences between the House and Senate versions must be reconciled by conference committee. The budget is not passed *in toto* but in parts: the budget for the Department of Health, Education, and Welfare is a separate piece of legislation, as are the budgets for the other major government departments. Thus, although the President proposes his budget as a single document, the final budget appears as a series of separate legislative appropriation acts.

During the late 1960s, because of the complexity of budgetary decisions and the conflict between the President and the Congress, Congress commonly did not finish the budget by the beginning of the fiscal year. Since all federal expenditures are budgeted for only one fiscal year at a time, this situation left the agencies in considerable uncertainty about what they could and could not spend for much of the year. Departmental operations were maintained by "continuing resolutions" and "extensions of legislative authorization," which left them ticking over at the previous year's level of activity. Congress, aroused by presidential "impoundments,"* passed the Budget Control Act of 1974. New budget committees were established to determine the total amount of the federal budget, including the size of the deficit, a task of balancing expenditures, resources, and priorities that had

---

* President Richard Nixon claimed the right to refuse to expend funds appropriated by Congress for authorized programs, a process called "impoundment."

formerly rested largely with the executive branch. The budget process is described in full detail elsewhere (Wildavsky, Blechman, et al.).

The "Cozy Triumvirates"

The legislative process does not operate in a vacuum. Influencing the process are the "cozy triumvirates," a term used to denote a coalition between an outside pressure or interest group, professionals working on a particular program in the Administration, and a like-minded group in Congress. The clearest example in the health area is biomedical research, where researchers and concerned lay people make alliances with staff at the National Institutes of Health and staff and members of Congress to assure growth of certain research areas. The "War on Cancer" of the early 1970s is a particularly prominent example (Strickland). Coalitions have also formed on lung diseases, environmental health problems, Sickle Cell Disease, and diabetes. These coalitions do not consider broader questions, such as overall health programs or budget limitations: they lobby specifically for expansion of one particular program.

To initiate such an alliance, agency bureaucrats take their proposals directly to the Congress, usually secretly. In the early 1970s, the Administration tried very hard to stamp out this practice, with some success. Interest groups are an inevitable part of the democratic process, as concerned constituents and physicians cannot be prevented from contacting a congressman. On the other hand, the President does need some control over the executive bureaucracy if he is to lead. Any rational planner would be opposed to this inefficient pulling and tugging; however, Lindblom has argued that what he calls "muddling through" is quite natural in a democracy, especially in dealing with social programs (1968). Maddox points out that the process of muddling through yields some important advantages: (1) making politically feasible decisions, (2) avoiding or minimizing major mistakes, and (3) allowing for maximum participation (1971). Several case studies have described how this process works for specific issues (Bowler; Strickland; Redman; Marmor).

Role of Lobbyists

Many interest groups set up their own offices to "lobby" the Congress and the executive branch; sometimes they hire a professional lobbying firm. In the health area, the best known lobbying groups are the American Medical Association (AMA), the Association of American Medical Colleges, the American Hospital Association, and the American Federation of Labor/Congress of Industrial Organizations. The American Academy of Family Physicians, the American College of Radiology, the American Cancer Society, and many others also have lobbying offices.

A legitimate difference exists between "special interest" groups and "public interest" groups. A special interest is shared by a few members of society, whereas a public interest is shared by a substantial number of citizens of the community or nation (Schattschneider, pp. 23–25). In practice, this distinction is often difficult to make, for special interest groups universally use the language of public interest. For example the AMA's public concern for the quality of medical care is little different from the argument of organized business that profits are the best guarantee of the public good. A characteristic shared by both types of interest groups is their elitist bias; they are led by and responsive to the educated and the affluent, making for a *de facto* exclusion of the poor and powerless from participation in the system.

It would be an oversimplification to state that policy results from the contentions of special interest groups. Special interests certainly influence legislation, perhaps excessively, but their power is limited once an issue becomes a matter of public controversy (Schattschneider, p. 40). They work best "behind the scenes," and thus they try to keep issues out of the public arena.

Interest groups are aware that the important work of Congress takes place in committee, and focus their attention accordingly. Besides seeking directly to influence votes, they supply valuable information; they may draft bills and contribute to research and other technical committee work; appear at public hearings; and they serve as a bridge from committees to Administration experts, who may not be easily identified without such help. The lobbyist informs the groups he represents about Washington events. Some health lobbies have been very powerful in affecting policy, notably the AMA. However, by the mid-1970s, its influence was being strongly rivaled by that of the Association of American Medical Colleges (*The New Physician*).

The Legislative Role of the Executive Branch

The President has important legislative powers: he presents the budget; he may present legislation; and he approves, and may veto, legislation. The Department of Health, Education, and Welfare has about 50,000 people working in the health area, any one of whom may have an idea for legislation. These suggestions are sent up through channels, and sometimes become part of legislative proposals. At the top layers of the Department are the political appointees, who have the basic responsibility for policy development. Important appointees in the HEW include the Assistant Secretary for Health and the Assistant Secretary for Legislation. Legislative proposals are discussed within the Department, and eventually proposed, after clearance by OMB and perhaps the White House. Thus, new proposals may originate anywhere in the Department, but are most likely to come from the political appointees who are most in tune with the policies of the Administration.

Implementation

After legislation is passed, it must be implemented, and the first step is generally the development of what are called "regulations," which describe how the law is to be administered. During the early stages of regulation writing, personnel in the designated agency generally consult with the groups involved, including congressional members and staff, officials of state and local governments, and lobbyists. In effect, this is a legislative process with all the forces contending, but it is a hidden process compared to the rather open congressional operations. Draft regulations are published in a daily official publication called the *Federal Register*, with invitations to all interested parties to comment. Final regulations are then published, usually 90 days after the appearance of the draft regulations. They have the force of law.

Outlook and Discussion

Since Congress will doubtless become increasingly involved in the health care delivery system, it is critical that health professionals have some understanding of the legislative process. After the long ascendancy of the "powerful presidency," which commenced with Franklin Roosevelt, Congress began reasserting its authority during the Nixon years, attempting to establish an independent power base. It also began to develop technical resources to give it the capability of dealing with the complex issues in the health area. It is difficult to predict how this struggle for independence from the executive will be resolved.

Congress does have serious problems in meeting modern challenges. We have said it lacks the national perspective characteristic of the executive branch. The decentralization, fragmentation, and specialization in Congress all militate against this integrated perspective. There have been moves to provide a more centralized mechanism, as with the development of the congressional budget committees. But the dilemma facing Congress is that any such move reduces its democratic basis and accessibility to the people.

The organizational problem is also severe. In the health area, supervision of activity, even that within HEW, is fragmented between several committees. If this country is to adopt a positive national health policy, such as Canada's, Congress must reorganize its health activity to be effective.

Finally, the health of the democratic system depends on citizen involvement and respect for governmental processes. Without a more informed citizenry, this cannot be expected, and the continued evolution of Congress will be slowed or prevented.

References

American Hospital Association. "A Summary of Federal Legislative Process and the Process of Federal Program and Regulation Development." *Washington Developments, 3,* 1974 (Supplement).

Anderson, O. "Influence of Social and Economic Research on Public Policy in the Health Field, a Review." *Milbank Memorial Fund Quarterly, 44,* 11, 1966 (Part 2).

Blechman, B. et al. *Setting National Priorities, The 1975 Budget.* Washington, D.C.: The Brookings Institution, 1974.

Bowler, K. *The Nixon Guaranteed Income Proposal.* Cambridge, Mass.: Ballinger Publishing Company, 1974.

Congressional Quarterly. The Washington Lobby. Washington, D.C., 1974.

Edwards, C. C. "The Federal Involvement in Health: A Personal View of Current Problems and Future Needs." *New England Journal of Medicine, 292,* 559, 1975.

Fenno, R. "The Internal Distribution of Influence: The House." In Truman, D., Ed., *The Congress and America's Future.* Englewood Cliffs, N.J.: Prentice-Hall, 1965.

Fenno, R. *Congressmen in Committees.* Boston: Little, Brown, 1973.

Geiger, H. "Health Services in the Concentration Camp." In Blumstein, J., and Martin, E., Eds., *The Urban Scene in the Seventies.* Nashville, Tenn.: Vanderbilt University Press, 1974.

House of Representatives. *How Our Laws Are Made.* Washington, D.C.: Government Printing Office, 1971.

Huitt, R. "The Internal Distribution of Influence: The Senate." In Truman, D., Ed., *The Congress and America's Future.* Englewood Cliffs, N.J.: Prentice-Hall, 1965.

Huntington, S. "Congressional Responses to the Twentieth Century." In Truman, D., Ed., *The Congress and America's Future.* Englewood Cliffs, N.J: Prentice-Hall, 1965.

Inglehart, J. "Health Report/Congress Expands Capacity to Contest Executive Policy." *National Journal Reports, 7,* 730, 1975.

Isaacs, S. "Senators Found Using Committee Personnel for Own Work." *Washington Post,* February 16, 1975, p. 1 (and following articles on February 17, 18, 19, 20, 21, 23, and 24).

Jewell, M., and Patterson, S. *The Legislative Process in the United States.* New York: Random House, 1966.

Kisch, A. "The Health Care System and Health: Some Thoughts on a Famous Misalliance." *Inquiry, 11,* 269, 1974.

Kissick, W. "Health-Policy Directions for the 1970s." *New England Journal of Medicine, 282,* 1343, 1970.

Lawton, S. Address to the Federal Bar Association, June 27, 1975, Washington, D.C.

Lindblom, C. *The Policy-Making Process.* Englewood Cliffs, N.J.: Prentice-Hall, 1968.

Maddox, G. "Mudding Through: Planning for Health Care in England." *Medical Care, 9,* 439, 1971.

Marmor, T. *The Politics of Medicare.* Chicago, Ill.: Aldine, 1970.

Mayhew, D. *Congress: The Electoral Connection.* New Haven, Conn.: Yale University Press, 1974.

McNerney, W. "Health Care Financing and Delivery in the Decade Ahead." *Journal of the American Medical Association, 222,* 1150, 1972.

New Physician, The. Special Issue. "The AAMC: Medicine's New Superpower." October, 1974.

Polsby, N. *Congress and the Presidency.* Englewood Cliffs, N.J.: Prentice-Hall, 1964.

Polsby, N. "Strengthening Congress in National Policymaking." In Polsby, N., Ed., *Congressional Behavior,* p. 3–13. New York: Random House, 1971.

Redman, E. *The Dance of Legislation.* New York: Simon and Schuster, 1973.

Rivlin, A. M. *Social Policy: Alternate Strategies for the Federal Government.* Washington, D.C.: The Brookings Institution, 1974.

Schattschneider, E. *The Semi-Sovereign People.* Hinsdale, Ill.: The Dryden Press, 1960.

Seidman, H. *Politics, Position and Power: The Dynamics of Federal Organization.* New York: Oxford University Press, 1970.

Somers, A. "Some Basic Determinants of Medical Care and Health Policy." *Milbank Memorial Fund Quarterly, 46,* 13, 1968.

Stevens, R. *American Medicine and the Public Interest.* New Haven, Conn.: Yale University Press, 1971.

Strickland, S. *Politics, Science, and Dread Disease.* Cambridge, Mass.: Harvard University Press, 1972.

Taaffe, W. "The Costs of Keeping Congress Exceed Other Inflation." *Washington Star,* November 12, 1975, p. 1.

Walters, R. "Patrick Caddell: Whiz Kid Pollster—What America Thinks." *Parade (Washington Post),* November 30, 1975, pp. 4–5.

Weinerman, E. "Anchor Points Underlying the Planning for Tomorrow's Health Care." *Bulletin of the New York Academy of Medicine, 41,* 1213, 1965.

White, K. "Organization and Delivery of Personal Health Services: Public Policy Issues." *Milbank Memorial Fund Quarterly, 46,* 225, 1968.

Wildavsky, A. *The Politics of the Budgetary Process.* Boston: Little, Brown, 1974.

Woodcock, L. "Testimony re National Health Insurance." Testimony before the Subcommittee on Health, House Committee on Interstate and Foreign Commerce, December 8, 1975.

12

Planning for Health Care

Carol McCarthy

In this chapter, we turn to a consideration of health care planning, an activity for which government has historically borne a major responsibility. After discussing the basic principles and problems of health care planning, we examine the major planning efforts that the federal and state governments have undertaken over the past 50 years.

Principles and Problems of Planning

Planning involves a series of steps. First, needs and demands are delineated so that long-term and short-term objectives can be determined. Then alternative plans for meeting these objectives are developed and a course of action is chosen. After an action plan has been implemented, it is evaluated in terms of effectiveness and efficiency.

Health care planning, however, must keep in mind certain assumptions which have been summarized as follows: (1) resources are scarce; thus ways must be found to secure optimum value from allocations devoted to health; (2) health care serves social purposes and should, therefore, be valued above activity undertaken in pursuit of economic or other social ends; (3) an effective health care system is rooted in responsiveness to consumer needs and requires public accountability (Gottlieb).

Moreover, organized efforts to make rational health care plans do not operate in a vacuum. Planners may attempt to follow a certain model, but each planning step—goal formulation, program development, implementation, and evaluation—is affected by certain facilitating and hampering factors. These include situational realities, political imperatives, and the technical state of the planning art.

346

Situational Realities and Political Imperatives

Situational realities and political imperatives can be considered separately, but they are intrinsically related in the arena of health care delivery. As this book has shown, our delivery system is fragmented. Although private entrepreneurship dominates the provider scene, government at every level plays a role, as do religious and other voluntary associations, industry, labor, insurers, consumer groups, and the schools. The drug and medical supply industries and the insurance industry also play important parts. Moreover, health care delivery is intimately linked with its environment—cultural and religious beliefs, systems of education, transportation, land use, and the like.

Planners must thus take into account a plethora of needs and interests when setting goals, the primary step in health planning. Different goals are bound to exist within this fragmented system; for successful planning, common goals must be negotiated and interdependent programming must take place (Sigmond). Political considerations are central to goal formation and cannot be ignored; in attempting to achieve goal consensus, it has been suggested that planners develop skills in assessing and mobilizing public opinion (Taylor).

Political considerations and situational realities have a major effect on program development and implementation. The planner must cast aside the myth that there is one ideal plan (Tell) and direct his attention to specifying the organizational framework, personnel, and facilities required to launch different plans, as well as to calculating their respective costs and benefits. He must present this information to those responsible for plan implementation, his role being to propose, not dispose (Thomas). If the planner has taken care to discover, reveal, and utilize goals "generated by the community," one of several plans will usually be accepted, once the implications of each has been made clear. The outlook for acceptance probably also improves when policy makers, program inplementers, and the concerned general public are allowed to contribute to developing the alternative plans.

Once implemented, programs must be evaluated. Taylor (1972) indicates the need for a two-pronged approach: evaluation for administrative purposes (Are targets being met within specified time frames and in accordance with standards set?) and evaluation for plan revision (Are original goals appropriate?

Are the necessary resources being developed as anticipated?).
Five levels of evaluation have been outlined:

1. Activity. Is the program operative?
2. Criteria. Is the program operating according to standards
   (of quality, access, etc.)?
3. Cost. Are program costs in line with those agreed upon?
   Can unit cost be improved?
4. Effectiveness. How well is the program achieving the desired output?
5. Outcome validity. To what extent has the program realized
   the ultimate goal for which it was designed? (Blum, 1974)

Avoiding biased measures of outcome is a primary concern.
Indeed, the literature on laboratory and field experiments is
replete with cautions against evaluator contamination. Program
designers are advised against evaluating their own programs,
evaluation designers against implementing their own designs.
But evaluator contamination is also traceable to the promotion of
"outside" interests. Tabb, for example, doubts computerized
retrieval systems will find meaningful use in state government
decision-making (1971). The computer, he warns, provides data
on accomplishments without regard to the distribution of political power. Morehouse's discussion is even more pointed. Evaluations fail in two ways, he says: for methodological reasons and
for failure to produce "acceptable" findings—that is, those consistent with the policy maker's commitment to program success.
A planning imperative thus becomes clear. The shifting power
structure in health must be given attention (Elling) and a coalition of support for thorough and factual program evaluation,
regardless of political repercussions, must be formed.

The Technical State of the Art

The fragmented health care delivery system in the United States
affects the nature of the technical planning process. In brief, the
science rather than the art of planning consists of collecting and
using data. The data needed depend on the existing level of health
knowledge and planning knowledge, on the particular health care
delivery system at issue, and on characteristics of the larger
social framework. Since the planning process is a continuous,
cyclical whole (Sigmond) all categories of data are relevant

throughout the planning process, although one may be more heavily relied upon at a particular stage than another.

Planning for personal health services requires knowledge of (1) the population to be served, (2) its health status, and (3) existing health care resources and their utilization. Without such information, one cannot determine whether the consumer demand for medical services is greater than, equal to, or less than the quantity of services health professionals estimate are required. The difference between consumer demand and professional estimates must be taken into account in national planning (Jeffers et al.). If planning is based on professional estimates only, and demand falls short of these estimates, excess capacity will result. If services are designed on the basis of demand only, capacity may prove either inadequate or excessive.

Measures of health. Demographic data on populations to be served (Susser and Watson; Zola; Chapman and Coulson; Reinke and Baker) are discussed in Chapter 3. A population's health status is assessed through measures of mortality and morbidity or combinations of the two. Traditionally, mortality has been the primary indicator—infant, perinatal, maternal, and other age-adjusted death rates. Such measurements are used in international health comparisions and, of course, in identifying major causes of death in the population and in particular subgroups. Mortality indices, however, are less than optimal measures of health. Their interpretation is confounded by multiple causes of death, poor reporting systems (Guralnick), and the shift from acute to chronic diseases as the major killers of our time. Without a major research breakthrough, additional significant declines in mortality are unlikely. Moreover, infant mortality is no longer a sensitive indicator of sanitary conditions and standard of living (Moriyama).

Measures of morbidity (the presence of a disease condition or active pathology) and disability (restricted performance of normal roles) also present problems. There are a limited number of reportable diseases, and selective reporting leads to inaccurate data (Blum, 1974; Sullivan). In addition, the definition and classification of morbidity states entail difficulties. The same clinically defined disease presents with different complaints in different ethnic populations (Zola). A cross-culturally valid index for each disease is needed, one that will encompass physical, emotional, and social causal factors, incidence (the number of new cases in a specified time period), prevalence (the number of extant cases in specified time period), duration, and severity.

In the National Health Survey (outlined in Chapter 3), disability is measured in terms of the number of days of restricted activity in the six months preceding the study interview. Data are gathered from a random sample of civilian, noninstitutional households. In the survey conducted by the Social Security Administration, respondents are classifed along a continuum based on the extent of their work limitations. Although the resultant "functional limitations index" provides a greater degree of specificity about disability (Haber), highly sensitive measures of acute and chronic disability are still unavailable.

A variety of other health status indicators have been used to attempt to define the health of a population adequately. Activity counts (USDHEW, 1969), the Q value developed by the Indian Health Service (J. E. Miller), an index of physical, mental, and social health devised by the Human Population Laboratory in Berkeley, California (Meltzer and Hochstim), and diverse mathematical models (National Center for Health Statistics) are among them.*

Health care resources. The profile of the health care consumer constructed from sociodemographic data and health status indicators must be matched against an inventory of existing health care resources and their utilization rates. Resources are of three kinds: human, physical, and financial. The number, age, sex, education, specialization, type of practice, productivity, and geographic location of available manpower must be determined, along with the output of operating and approved training programs. Sites of care must be inventoried as to number, type, distribution, and characteristics such as size, services offered, physical condition, approvals, policies, financial solvency, and referral patterns. For each facility, patient characteristics must be noted and utilization measures compiled—the number of patient visits, average daily census, percent occupancy, length of stay. (The two vantage points from which utilization can be measured are discussed in Chapter 3.) Financial data concerning the number and types of insurance mechanisms, government-supported

---

* Fanshel and Bush have done some promising work in developing health status indicators, as have Balinsky and Berger. Goldsmith provided a good review.

programs, median family income, and sources of philanthropy must be obtained.

Available resources constitute the supply side of the planning equation; sociodemographic factors, health status measures, and professional assessments of undetected problems, the demand side. By using the mathematical tools and subjective estimates at his or her command, the planner weighs one against the other and both against established standards to identify problems requiring attention. Her or she then works for the formation of realistic goals and alternative approaches to goal realization.

Realistic goals are rooted in sound priority-setting; sound priorities depend on the vulnerability of a health or health care problem to attack. To the extent feasible, the health planner quantifies vulnerability so that priorities are defensible (Ahumada). In program planning, he or she is careful not to neglect time-series graphs and curve-fitting techniques (Prest and Turvey) as well as cost-benefit analysis (Bright). All three planning tools take into account the time span between planning and implementation and the "objective" merits of viable program alternatives.

Finally, without planning data, there is no baseline against which the impact of implemented programs can be measured. Information is needed on the extent to which anticipated changes in health status occur, at what cost, and with what positive or negative spillover. Indeed, baseline data provide the foundation for systems of continuous feedback, systems that must be in place if inappropriate goals or inadequate work activities are to be identified and corrected.

Early History of Regional and Comprehensive Health Planning in the United States

The use of the health planning techniques outlined above, as well as efforts at regional health planning (planning across several political jurisdictions) and comprehensive health planning (planning for more than one disease category, population, or facet of the health care delivery system), are relatively recent. Diverse forces have affected our health delivery system over the past 50 years. Planning has been stimulated by advances in health care technology and the lag between the development and general availability of such advances; by more widespread education and a concomitant rise in consumer health care expectations; by the

arrival of organized third-party payors and unionized health care
workers; by urbanization and increased health hazards; by suburban sprawl and resultant accessibility problems; by a shortage
of medical manpower; and by skyrocketing health care costs.

Recognition of the need for regional and comprehensive health
care planning can be traced back to the establishment in 1927 of
the Committee on the Costs of Medical Care, to which we have
referred elsewhere. To review, the 42-man committee had been
formed in response to the desire of leading physicians, public
health personnel, and economists for sound studies on the economic and social aspects of health services. Supported by 1 million dollars from six foundations, the Committee and its staff
studied the incidence of disease and disability in the United
States, health care facilities open to the general public and those
organized to serve particular population groups, family expenditures for health care, and income earned by providers of care
(Anderson). Citing the rising costs of diagnosis and treatment
and the inequitable distribution of health services across the
nation, the final report of the majority of the Committee, published in 1932, recommended support for group medical practice
and group prepayment for health care services, or health insurance. The strong reactions that report elicited stimulated a series
of changes in health care financing and delivery. Equally important from the vantage point of regional and comprehensive
health planning was the Committee's call for the coordination of
primary and specialty services within defined geographic areas
(Committee on Cost).

At first the call was picked up locally. Efforts were few in
number, however, and generally limited to exploring the feasibility of a "regionalized" or three-tiered system of institutionalized
care. Regionalization in this context denoted integrated net-
works, with primary care delivered through rural or outlying
hospitals and clinics, secondary (more specialized, consultant
care) at district or "intermediate" hospitals, and tertiary (highly
specialized, technologically based care) at medical centers
(Mountin et al.). In rural New England, for example, the
Bingham Associates Fund worked to coordinate medical services
for area residents. To that end, program linkages were established between the Pratt Clinic, New England Center Hospital,
and Tufts Medical School (Gartland). In Michigan the Hospital
Survey Commission explored that state's bed needs in the context
of regionalization (Commission on Hospital Care).

Only in 1944, when the American Hospital Association's (AHA) Committee on Postwar Planning took up the standard, was regionalized planning for health services promoted on an nationwide basis. A Commission on Hospital Care was established by the AHA and local, district, and state councils formed to work in conjunction with "the official state planning agency." The outcome was a recommendation to coordinate the regionalization of hospital services, equipment, and personnel. The Commission was explicit in its report:

> The haphazard development of hospital services of the past should not be extended to the future. The public must be made aware of, must assume its responsibility for the development and support of adequate hospital care on a communitywide basis. The expansion and development of individual institutions must be in accord with an overall planned program for the community. Direct benefits will accrue to both hospitals and public through organized effort in the intelligent planning of hospital care. (p. xi)

Legislation for Areawide Planning
The Hill-Burton Act

The first attempt by the federal government to translate a generalized health planning concept into action came in 1946 with the passage of the Hospital Survey and Construction Act, better known as the Hill-Burton program, after its sponsors, Senator Hill of Alabama and Congressman Burton of Michigan. The stated intent of the act was to improve the hospital bed-to-population ratio in rural areas and to upgrade facilities and standards. Federal grant assistance was authorized to the states for surveying their needs and developing state plans for hospital facilities based on those surveys. With plans in existence and minimum standards for hospitals incorporated in state licensing laws, federal funds were to be made available on a matching basis (up to one-third federal) to construct and equip public and voluntary nonprofit general, mental, tuberculosis, and chronic disease hospitals and public health centers (Public Law 79–725).

The American Medical Association (AMA) also viewed the legislation as a capital subsidy approach to the problem of physician maldistribution. The Association believed that building hospitals in rural areas would attract needed doctors (Bugbee). Whether the AMA's vision of Hill-Burton potentialities was a broadly held position, however, or merely the attempt of a conservative professional society to divert federal activity away from the domain of private medical practice remains a moot question.

Clearly, however, the Hill-Burton mandate for a state health facilities plan and the requirement that a single state agency assume responsibility for plan development and program implementation were important. (The word "survey" in "Hospital Survey and Construction Act" was added only after the work of the Commission on Hospital Care and the "regional plan" or three-tiered concept of the Public Health Service were discussed in hearings on the bill.) For the first time, a determination of need was to form the basis of priorities for action, and such priorities were to be explicitly stated. Centering the responsibility for such action in a single authority was also new. However, the law's emphasis on construction alone, rather than construction and coordination of facilities, supports the interpretation that the single agency requirement was adopted primarily for orderly management of funds.

Between 1949 and 1970, the Hill-Burton program was amended to provide additional grants, loans, and loan guarantees to improve geographic bed distribution. Moreover, from 1956, the United States Public Health Service received appropriations under the law for research and demonstrations relating to the development, utilization, and coordination of hospital services, facilities, and resources.

From the planning standpoint, however, the most significant additions to the Hill-Burton program came in 1964 with the Hospital and Medical Facilities Amendments. Along with 1.34 billion dollars for the construction, modernization, and replacement of health care facilities, project grants were made available to develop comprehensive plans for health and health-related facilities on a regional, metropolitan, or other basis. Furthermore, the arbitrary bed-to-population ratio utilized in determining priorities for grant and loan requests was abandoned. A new formula, incorporating known hospital utilization data, projected population estimates, and a desirable (80%) standard of occupancy was instituted as a more sensitive measure of area hospital needs.

The legislation that continued the Hill-Burton program into the seventies maintained the grant program and provided both guaranteed and direct loans for construction, modernization, or replacement purposes. In addition to hospitals, neighborhood health centers and emergency room facilities were made eligible for funding, a major departure from the original law. With regard to areawide planning, the continuing legislation stipulated that, in order to be approved, projects must comply with plans established by state or areawide planning agencies, creations of the Comprehensive Health Planning Act of 1966, described below.

Thus, the Hill-Burton legislation was a landmark program in two ways. It provided the stimulus and the means for a much-needed building and reconstruction program. In 1944, the American Hospital Association's Committee on Governmental Aid for Postwar Reconstruction had estimated a deficiency of 180,000 beds in the United States delivery system (Bugbee). By June of 1970, projects approved under the Hill-Burton program included construction of 334,438 hospital beds, 93,749 long-term care beds, 1032 outpatient facilities, 520 rehabilitation facilities, 1258 public health centers, and 41 state health laboratories (USDHEW, 1970). Moreover, efforts were concentrated in those areas where shortages were most acute. The program also introduced new approaches to facilities planning and development. Each of the 53 states and possessions, for example, had established plans and methods for establishing priorities. Documentation of need, however general, was no longer a totally untried concept.

From the standpoint of the planning principles outlined earlier, however, the Hill-Burton program was not an unqualified success. It was a regional rather than comprehensive approach to remedying health delivery system inadequacies. Its overwhelming emphasis on bed scarcity indicates the absence of a goal-setting process rooted in identified community needs. In fact, Hill-Burton program planning involved minimal interaction between provider and consumer and between Hill-Burton and other planning activities (Gottlieb).

Nor did Hill-Burton planning procedures encompass the total hospital field. Because of the law's emphasis on underserved rural areas and "conforming beds" (those adhering to specified standards of designs, equipment, and structure), and its exclusion of proprietary institutions, only 25% of the nation's hospital beds were involved in the program (Hilleboe et al.). Promoters of hospital projects denied Hill-Burton support could raise funds elsewhere. In brief, Congress and supporters of the bill—the AMA and AHA, in particular—were amenable to federal dollar support but not to federal control over the essentially voluntary hospital system. Finally, the Hill-Burton program did not achieve the same results in physician redistribution that it did in bed redistribution (Clark and Koontz).

Certification of Need

The states initiated laws controlling the need for hospital beds and services. Certificate-of-need laws began with New York's 1964 Metcalf-McCloskey Act and 1965 Folsom Act (Curran). Essentially, certificate-of-need programs establish criteria of public need for health care institutions and programs against which requests for changes in plant and, in certain states, program offerings of individual health care institutions, are reviewed, approved, or disapproved (Dorsey; Havighurst, 1974). In 1968, with the support of the American Hospital Association, a nationwide drive to institute certificate-of-need laws began. By mid-1975, 23 states had certificate-of-need legislation covering at least some health facilities (Bicknell and Walsh).

Like all regulatory mechanisms, certification-of-need has its limitations (Havighurst, 1973). Furthermore, whether it actually controls unwarranted health care and institutional growth and development is unclear. A study in New York, the state that provided the model for certification-of-need programs, seriously questioned their value (Rothenberg). Moreover, certification-of-need is a negative rather than positive health planning tool. It allows a health planning agency to prevent projected changes proposed by institutional health care providers that do not accord with established health plans. It does not increase the agency's ability to implement desired changes that require public and political support.

Regional Medical Programs

Just as the Hill-Burton Act provided for planning on the structural level (bricks and mortar), Public Law 89-239—which established Regional Medical Programs (RMPs)—facilitated functional planning (i.e., planning new or improved working arrangements for health care delivery). The law, passed in 1965, was an outgrowth of three of the major recommendations of a presidential commission headed by Dr. Michael DeBakey (Russell). President Johnson had appointed the Commission to develop a "realistic battle plan leading to the ultimate conquest of three diseases—heart disease, cancer, and stroke" (President's Commission p. ii).

After identifying two major problems—inadequate federal support for basic and clinical research and limited application of the knowledge then available—the Commission proposed 35 courses of remedial action.

The original draft version of Public Law 89-239 strongly echoed the intention of Commission members. A nationwide series of "regional medical complexes" were to be established, one each for heart disease, cancer, and stroke. Each complex was to include a research center, a medical center, and diagnostic and treatment "stations" within a defined geographic area. The medical members of the DeBakey Commission came almost exclusively from the research and academic establishments and their proposed solutions to the problems reflected their professional affiliations (Jonas, 1967).

However, as a result of organized opposition during the legislative process by the American Association of General Practice and the American Medical Association, the "regional complexes" concept was replaced by "regional medical programs" which were to make the latest scientific advances in the "killer diseases" available at the grassroots level without interfering with "the patterns or methods of financing of patient care or professional practice" (Public Law 89–239). This approach specifically proscribed the creation of chains of new, academically dominated, research/treatment centers (Jonas, 1967).

Thus, largely through the efforts of organized medicine, mandates for new institutional arrangements on a regional basis were replaced by incentives for voluntary efforts at joint problem-solving. On the basis of applications received, the country was divided into 56 regional medical program areas. At times, existing political boundaries were honored, and an RMP served distinct counties within a state or the state itself. At other times, such boundaries were ignored in favor of established patterns of patient flow (Komaroff).

Within each region, a public or nonprofit institution, agency, or corporation was designated grantee or fiscal agent. Originally, universities served as the grantees for 34 of the Regional Medical Programs, other nonprofit corporations for 18, and medical societies for 4 (Office of Planning and Evaluation). Overall program guidance was the responsibility of the RMP's Regional Advisory

Group (RAG), a voluntary body comprising local providers, representatives of public organizations, and consumers (Creditor and Nelson).

Core staffs, consisting of physicians, nurses, health planners, allied health personnel, health service administrators, statisticians, demographers, and others were paid through grant funds (Komaroff). They were to work with the individual Regional Advisory Groups to set regional priorities and objectives, develop programmatic approaches, review local applications for grant monies, submit selected projects to a 20-member National Advisory Council of nonfederal reviewers in Washington, and guide and evaluate operational projects. In brief, RAG and core staff were to provide the technical assistance required to forge planned linkages among the various elements of the health delivery system.

In many instances RMP efforts resulted in institutions and agencies working together to increase available resources and improve utilization. For example, the University of California San Francisco Medical Center under an RMP grant assisted hospitals in 11 counties in designing coronary care units, training necessary personnel, and coordinating delivery of services (Office of Planning and Evaluation of RMP, 1971). Indeed, the Public Accountability Reporting Group, spokesman for the 53 RMPs in existence in 1973, cites the following accomplishments for that year: approximately 27,000 providers took part in RMP medical-audit programs designed to promote quality assurance; 9 million Americans received health care services directly from RMP-funded activities; an estimated 12 million derived benefits from the 150,000 health professional using new skills acquired through RMP-supported training programs (Public Accountability Reporting Group).

Some of these accomplishments are traceable to the expansion of RMP's original categorical mandate (Miller, 1972). Public Law 91-515, passed in 1970, called for RMP efforts for all major diseases and conditions, and for prevention and rehabilitation as well as diagnosis and treatment. Attention to the delivery of primary care and to improving manpower utilization were promoted. Closer ties to comprehensive planning were assured by requiring that areawide planning agencies review and comment on RMP grant requests.

In sum, despite numerous phase-out orders and presidential impoundment of appropriated funds in 1972 (Ward), individual

RMPs made possible the regionalization of certain services and the introduction of innovative approaches that hold promise for reforms in the organization and delivery of care. On the other hand, RMPs have been criticized for the "anticomprehensiveness" of RMP regionalization (Bodenheimer) and for concentrating on developing cooperative relations among interested providers instead of on reorganizing the delivery system (Bodenheimer; Creditor). The merits of the criticism can be debated, but the accomplishment of RMP—facilitating cooperative health care planning—should not be slighted.

Although few Regional Medical Programs across the country employed operations researchers or systems analysts (Shuman), the program cannot be charged with minimal use of technical planning techniques. The publications of the Minnesota Northlands Regional Medical Program, from 1968 to 1972 alone, belie the charge (W. R. Miller). During that period, 44 planning and feasibility studies were completed—resource inventories, studies of migration, attitudinal surveys, medical practice profiles, current need estimates, and projections of need over time, to name but a few.

Comprehensive Health Planning Agencies

In addition to the Regional Medical Program, the 89th Congress signed into law another outgrowth of DeBakey Commission recommendations, Public Health Service Act Amendments of 1966, Public Law 89-749 on comprehensive health planning. Along with Public Law 90-174, passed the next year, these amendments to the Public Health Service Act created what was called the "Partnership for Health Program." It was designed to stimulate planning for health service through involvement of and cooperation among diverse community interests. Section 314(a) of P.L. 89-749 outlines the objectives of the program:

> The Congress declares that fulfillment of our national purpose depends on *promoting and assuring the highest level of health attainable for every person, in an environment which contributes positively to healthful individual and family living*; that attainment of this goal depends on an effective partnership, involving close intergovernmental collaboration, official and voluntary efforts, and participation of individuals and organizations; that Federal financial assistance must be directed to support the marshalling of all health resources—national, state and local—to assure comprehensive health services of high quality for every

person, but *without interference with existing patterns of private professional practice of medicine, dentistry, and related healing arts*. [*Author's emphasis*]

The program was to be a distinct departure from categorical approaches to health planning, which are directed at specific diseases, population groups, or types of health services. However, the single largest segment of the U.S. health care delivery system, private practice, was left untouched, just as it had been under RMP.

Public Law 89–749 established five avenues to reach set goals. Section A of the law provided formula grants to a single state agency for comprehensive health planning at the state level. (Formula grants are monies divided among qualified applicants according to some set formula, in this case, on the basis of population and per capita income.) Section B provided project grants for developing comprehensive health plans at the regional level and for coordinating existing and planned health facilities, manpower, and services. (Project grant awards are made on the strength of the application submitted in support of a particular project.) Section C allocated grant monies for projects designed to train health planners. Section D provided formula grants to states for public health services. Section E created project grants for the development of health services (Jacobs and Froh; Stebbins and Williams). From the standpoint of comprehensive health planning, the first three avenues are of particular interest.

Under section A, a state had to submit to the Public Health Service office in its region a "plan for comprehensive health planning" that indicated the state agency selected to administer the planning operation. (The single state agency requirement had had its genesis in the Hill-Burton program.) The state agency was to be assisted by the State Advisory Council representing a variety of health interests—voluntary groups, public agencies, general planning agencies, universities, and practitioners, with consumers of health services a majority.

The state, or A agency (so-called because of the section of P.L. 89–749 under which it was authorized) with its advisory council was to: establish state and areawide health goals; define the health needs of communities in relation to those goals; inventory relationships among local, state, and national governmental and voluntary programs and assist these programs in marshalling resources for a greater impact on health care problems; provide data, analyses, and recommendations that would assist the governor, communities, and other health programs in allocating health care resources more effectively (Office of CHP, 1967; Hilleboe and Schaefer). In brief, A agencies were not charged with developing detailed plans. Rather they were to review and integrate into a state plan the efforts of local, regional, and other state health planning groups dealing with health services, manpower, and facilities.

Unlike RMP operations, which were totally federally funded, section B project grants to public or nonprofit agencies engaging in areawide planning required 25 to 50% local matching funds. These B agencies were charged with both comprehensive planning and project development, although the state A agency retained final responsibility for approving areawide plans and proposed developmental projects. Like the state agency, areawide agencies operated with the assistance of advisory councils made up of health interests, the majority of whom were consumers.

Project grants to Comprehensive Health Planning C agencies were designed to provide the manpower needed for health planning. Grant recipients could be public or nonprofit agencies. In 1973, 23 university-based programs were training health professionals and others interested in acquiring health planning skills (Stebbins and Williams).

The 1967 amendments to P.L. 89–749, which extended the act into the 1970s and made additional funding available, also contained provisions designed to advance the planning process. First, assistance was made available to health care facilities for the development of capital expenditures programs to replace, modernize, or expand facilities. Second, grant funds were provided to underwrite research or demonstration projects aimed at innovations in health services, facilities, and manpower that could be incorporated into health plans. Third, local government representation in the areawide planning process was required for federal funding, thus assuring at least the promise of plan implementation.

In 1973, under a mandate from the Secretary of Health, Education and Welfare, the Division of Comprehensive Health Planning in Washington, D.C., undertook a nationwide assessment of both A and B agencies (1974). Their interim analysis, compiled in early 1974, summarized 48 B agency assessments and 9 developmental plans. The analysis indicated strengths in the following areas: developing a functioning orga-

nization; identifying existing data resources and inventories of
area health needs; reviewing proposed facility and program
changes; and cooperating with other planning organizations.
Deficiencies were noted, however, in the critical areas of community education, assessment of health delivery system inadequacies, planning, and sensitivity to needed changes in agency
direction. In sum, most of the CHPs reporting were still organizing themselves for planning and securing support for their
agency as the health planning body in the community. Ardell
reports similar conclusions following the review of all assessment reports (1974). He attributes CHP's failure to four factors: insufficient financial resources; less-than-adequate training
of staff and volunteers; an uncertain legislative mandate and
minimal enforcement powers; and blurred lines of responsibility
regarding other federally funded programs.

Others have suggested alternative reasons for the failure of
comprehensive health planning to move beyond infancy under
Public Law 89–749. Roseman, for example, believes CHP
involvement in certificate-of-need programs diverted agency
efforts from the planning task. Although few states had such programs throughout CHP's life span, certainly CHP involvement in
the general review and comment process worked against the fulfillment of the planning mandate. By 1973, A and B agencies
were reviewing projects submitted for funding under at least 13
different federal programs, state mental retardation proposals,
and capital expenditures for health care facilities reimbursed
under Medicare, Medicaid, and the Maternal and Child Health
programs (Block, McGibony, and Assoc.). The time required
for adequate review was substantial; staff resources, in general,
were limited.

The failure of B agencies has also been attributed to poor management of the political aspect of the planning process. In many
cases boundaries of these agencies were drawn regardless of
actual or potential delivery system resources (Creditor). The
game was over before it began because appropriate participants
were not invited to play. Even when boundaries were appropriate, plan development and implementation were tied to achieving
a consensus for action among advisory council members. According to Roseman, providers dominated the councils through their
"superior knowledge," despite the 51% consumer membership
requirement. Providers espoused a policy of avoiding conflict in
formulating goals and succeeded in making talk rather than

action the hallmark of areawide operations. In addition, the requirement for local matching monies resulted in endless hours devoted to fund-raising, and promoted inactivity because of conflict of interest.

The 51% consumer requirement was an attempt by the federal government to induce changes in the health care delivery system by changing the cast of characters involved in planning that system (Evans; Hilleboe et al.). Why did changes not occur? The data suggest that several factors worked against change: the clause in the law allowing ex-officio membership on areawide advisory councils, a membership almost exclusively of providers; the working definition of "consumer" that concentrated on an individual's occupation, thus permitting hospital trustees, health facility auxiliaries, and the like to participate (Evans, 1974); and the failure to organize and train consumers to participate in the planning process (Schwebel et al.).

National Health Planning and Resources Development Act of 1974

Late in 1974, the 93rd Congress, perhaps responding to the minimal progress under the Partnership for Health Program, passed the National Health Planning and Resources Development Act, Public Law 93-641. Under the law, single state and areawide health planning agencies were created to perform the functions of Hill-Burton programs, Regional Medical Programs, and Comprehensive Health Planning organizations. The new agency was faced with the considerable task of merging the operations of a state-dominated program (Hill-Burton), a program with both state and federal reporting requirements (CHP), and one reporting to DHEW in Washington but dominated by medical schools (RMP). P.L. 93-641 was a federal attempt to end fragmentation in health planning.

The provisions of P.L. 93-641 were embodied in new titles XV and XVI of the Public Health Service Act. Part A of Title XV was a first in the annals of federal health care legislation. It required the Secretary of DHEW to issue national health planning goals based on the health priorities made explicit in the law. Previously, health planning had been characterized by mandates for rational planning without reference to any goals (Daniel). To assist the Secretary in setting goals, the act established a National Council on Health Planning and Development, with rather vague, nondirective, advisory powers.

Part B of Title XV created the units that were the core of the whole program: the Health Systems Agencies (HSAs). State governors were required to designate health planning areas within their states according to a rather complex set of guidelines. Designated areas, each with a federally funded HSA, were to: (1) reflect consideration of the different health planning and developmental needs of metropolitan as opposed to nonmetropolitan areas; (2) not divide Standard Metropolitan Statistical Areas (SMSAs), a stipulation honored mostly in the breach; (3) be coordinated with areas for Professional Standards Review Organizations and areas for existing regional and state planning efforts. Each was to contain no fewer than 500,000 and no more than 3 million residents, unless the entire state population was less, or the population of an SMSA more. In each area, there was to be at least one center capable of providing highly specialized health services. The first four of these requirements indicated a sensitivity to the difficulty of collecting data for health planning. They represented an attempt to advance planning efforts under P. L. 93-641 by coordinating them with ongoing data retrieval activities.

HSAs could be public or private nonprofit entities, but not educational entities, thus excluding the medical schools that had dominated RMP operations. Existing RMPs, CHPs, local and county health departments, and other areawide and hospital planning councils all scrambled to be designated as HSAs. In certain areas, the outcome was productive; in others, the old antagonisms among various health care sectors continue to interfere with the planning process.

Under Section 1513 of P. L. 93-641, HSAs were charged with:

1. gathering and analyzing suitable data
2. establishing health systems plans (long-range) and annual implementation plans (short-range), abbreviated as HSPs and AIPs
3. providing either technical and/or financial assistance to those seeking to implement provisions of the plans
4. coordinating activities with PSROs and other appropriate planning and regulating entities
5. reviewing and approving or disapproving applications for federal funds for health programs within the area
6. assisting states in the performance of capital expenditures reviews (certification-of-need)

7. assisting states in reviewing existing institutional health
   services with respect to the appropriateness of such services; and annually recommending to states projects for the
   modernization, construction, and conversion of medical facilities in the area

Except for powers relating to plan development and disbursement of federal funds, the emphasis is on "assist," "recommend,"
"gather," and "coordinate." Nevertheless, the HSA is to carry
out these tasks for critical purposes: (1) improving the health
of residents of [the] health service area, (2) increasing the
accessibility . . . acceptability, continuity, and quality of . . .
health services . . . (3) restrain[ing] increases in . . . cost . . .
and (4) prevent[ing] . . . unnecessary duplication of health resources" (P. L. 93-641, Section 1513 (a)).

An incongruity exists in P. L. 93-641 between broad goals and
limited powers. This gap has been characteristic of almost all
health services planning legislation in the United States. Thus, in
the long run, the most significant aspects of this law may turn
out to be the health services data-gathering requirement (Section
1513 (b) (1)). The requirements for establishing health status
measures, utilization data, health care resources data, and measures of the relations between health and health care on a
national basis could be as significant as the establishment of uniform vital statistics reporting was earlier in the century.

P.L. 93-641 also created two planning bodies at the state
level (P. L. 93-641, Part C). The first, called the State Health
Planning and Development Agency (SHPDA), is an agency of the
state government designated by the governor, with the approval
of the Secretary of DHEW, and supported by federal grant
monies. The SHPDA uses input from the areawide Health Systems Agencies to create a statewide health plan. It also reviews
institutional services in the state and operates a certificate-of-
need program.

The second state-level planning body is the Statewide Health
Coordinating Council (SHCC). The Council, aided by the
SHPDA, reviews and coordinates Health System Agency plans,
reviews their budgets, and reviews state applications for federal
funds under the Public Health Service Act, the Community
Mental Health Centers Act, and the Alcoholism Control Act of
1970. Each HSA is represented on the Council. At least 50% of
the Council's members are consumers, and at least one-third of

its provider members are "direct providers"—that is, individuals delivering health care or administering health care institutions.

DHEW provides technical assistance to HSAs and HPDAs in defining the minimum data needed to determine health status, health resources, and service utilization, and in planning methodologies, policies, and standards. DHEW is also empowered to establish systems for uniform cost-accounting, utilization, determination, and rate-setting in hospitals, nursing homes, and other institutional settings (P. L. 93-641, Section 1533).

Title XV repeated many planning strategies from earlier legislation, but it also broke new ground. As in CHP, the governing boards of area HSAs and State Health Planning and Development Agencies have consumer majorities. The boards of the HSAs and the SHCC also contain elected and appointed public officials and providers of care. Both the presence of public officials and the clear definition of the population to be served were viewed as mechanisms for increasing public accountability (Daniel). As in the case of Regional Medical Programs, broad provider representation was built into the system to encourage cooperation, accommodation, and the implementation of plans.

The most noteworthy departure from prior legislation is the establishment under P. L. 93-641 of close relations between the federal government and areas within states. In grants review, HSAs were empowered to review and *approve* or *disapprove* requests for funds under the Public Health Service Act and other acts. The review and comment procedures associated with CHP operations—that is, local area recommendations but state disposition—are retained only in the areas of certificate-of-need, Medicare and Medicaid capital controls, and decisions on the appropriateness of institutional health services. Conflicts between the state agency and HSAs over area matters are subject to resolution by the Secretary of DHEW. The relationship between the SHCC and the HPDA provides further indication of the power of the HSA in relation to the state agency. The Council is empowered to "prepare and review and revise" at least annually a state health plan (a reconciliation of HSA plans in the state) and approve or disapprove state applications for funds under the Public Health Service Act and other acts. The HSAs of each state collectively hold a majority of the seats on the SHCC.

Title XVI of P. L. 93-641, Parts A through E, effected minor revisions in the old Hill-Burton program, and related construction activities more closely to the comprehensive health planning process. Part F authorized developmental grants for further implementation of approved HSA Annual Implementation plans. The American Association for Comprehensive Health Planning had argued for including developmental activities in the law. Undoubtedly, they had the RMP experience in mind when they argued that with such monies, they could convince providers to take on mandates to alter the delivery system, mandates for which other funds were not available (Daniel).

Conclusion

Assessing how far the United States has traveled along the health planning road is difficult. Certainly, the absence of any requirement in P. L. 93-641 to avoid interfering with established patterns of medical practice is a step forward, as is the stipulation that areawide planning agencies be given federal grant review and approval powers. Continuing support for the developmental function, establishing specific requirements for a data base, and drawing areawide planning boundaries that encourage data system sharing are also positive steps.

Legislative restrictions, one barrier to constructive alteration of the health care system, have been removed. Work has been done that can provide a firmer technical foundation for both regional and comprehensive community health care planning. The structure of the planning process has been reinforced by adding developmental dollars and approval powers to the purely suggestive powers of CHP.

Such surface changes can be easily catalogued; foreseeing the impact of underlying changes is more difficult, however. One may question, for example, whether the health care consumer can be best served by placing the planning, development, and regulation of health services under a single agency's jurisdiction. Experience with federal regulatory commissions has, more often than not, indicated the dangers of eliminating competition and the cross-checking of claims that retard self-aggrandizement (Huntington; Havighurst, 1973). It is not clear whether combining the three functions will reduce the degree to which self-interests are advanced and overcome the coordination problems long inherent in our pluralistic health care system. Perhaps even greater powers or changes outside the health planning realm are required. Congressional figures behind the passage of the 1974 Health Planning and Resources Development Act saw it as a prerequisite to national health insurance. Perhaps the reverse is true: perhaps a comprehensive and flexible national health insurance scheme must be established before health planning directed at making our health care system work rationally can be accomplished. If reimbursement problems no longer plague providers, it may be possible to establish a set of values that encourages mutual adjustment for the common good. Unfortunately, there are many possibilities, but few certainties.

References

Ahumada, J. et al. *Health Planning: Problems of Concept and Method.* Washington, D.C.: Pan American Health Organization, Scientific Publication No. 111. 1965.

Anderson, O.W. "Influence of Social and Economic Research on Public Policy in the Health Field—A Review." *Milbank Memorial Fund Quarterly, 44,* (Suppl.), 11, 1966.

Ardell, D. B. "The Demise of CHP and the Future of Planning." *Inquiry, 11,* 233, 1974.

Arnold, M. F. "Basic Concept and Critical Issues in Health Planning." *American Journal of Public Health, 59,* 1686, 1969.

Balinsky, W., and Berger, R. "A Review of the Research on General Health Status Indexes." *Medical Care, 13,* 283, 1975.

Bicknell, W. J., and Walsh, D. C. "Certification of Need: the Massachusetts Experience." *New England Journal of Medicine, 20,* 1052, 1975.

Block, McGibony and Associates, Inc. "A Discussion of Health Issues." *Special Report,* Jan. 1973.

Blum, H. L. *Notes on Comprehensive Health Planning.* San Francisco: Western Regional Office, American Public Health Association, 1967.

Blum, H. L. *Planning for Health: Development and Application of Social Change Theory.* New York: Human Sciences Press, 1974.

Bodenheimer, T. S. "Regional Medical Programs: No Road to Regionalization." *Medical Care Review, 26,* 1125, 1969.

Branch, M. C. *Planning: Aspects and Applications.* New York: Wiley, 1966.

Bright, J., ed. *Technological Forecasting in Government and Industry.* Englewood Cliffs, N.J: Prentice-Hall, 1968.

Bugbee, G. "The Hill-Burton Construction Bill." *Journal of the American Medical Association, 127,* 657, 1945.

Chapman, J., and Coulson, A. "Community Diagnosis: An Analysis of Indicators of Health and Disease in a Metropolitan Area." *International Journal of Epidemiology, 1,* 75, 1972.

Clark, L. J., and Koontz, T. L. "Analysis of the Impact of the Hill-Burton Program on the Distribution of the Supply of General Hospital Beds and Physicians in the United States 1950–1970." Paper delivered at Annual Meeting of American Public Health Association, 1973, San Francisco.

Cohen, H. S. "Regulating Health Care Facilities: the Certificate-of-Need Process Re-examined." *Inquiry, 10,* 3, 1973.

Colt, Avery M. "Elements of Comprehensive Health Planning." *American Journal of Public Health, 60,* 1194, 1970.

Commission on Hospital Care. *Hospital Resources and Needs, The Report of the Michigan Hospital Survey.* Battle Creek, Mich.: Kellogg Foundation, 1946.

———. *Hospital Care in the United States.* New York: The Commonwealth Fund, 1947.

Committee on the Costs of Medical Care. *Medical Care for the American People.* Chicago, Ill.: University of Chicago Press, 1932. Reprinted: Washington, D.C., USDHEW, 1970.

Conant, R. W. *The Politics of Community Health.* Washington, D.C.: Public Affairs Press, 1968.

93rd Congress, House of Representatives. *Conference Report,* Number 93–1640, December 19, 1974.

Corbett, R. M. "Health Planning: Some Legal and Political Implications of Comprehensive Health". *American Journal of Public Health, 64,* 136, 1974.

Creditor, M. C. "A Modest Proposal: Let CHP and RMP Run the System." *Modern Hospital, 119,* 101, 1972.

Creditor, M.C., and Nelson, D. "Regional Medical Programs and Office Management and Budget—Parallel Philosophies." *New England Journal of Medicine, 289,* 239, 1975.

Curran, W. J. "A National Survey and Analysis of State Certificate of Need Laws for Health Facilities." In Havinghurst, C. C., *Regulating Health Facilities Construction,* Ch. 3. Washington, D.C.: American Institute for Public Policy Research, 1974.

Daniel, S. L. "Issues Raised by Pending Comprehensive Health Planning Legislation." *Health Politics, 4,* 3, 1974.

Division of Comprehensive Health Planning, Health Resources Administration. "Interim Analysis of Results of CHP Agency Assessments," CHP Program Letter 74–14, May 29, 1974 (E. J. Rubel, Director of the Division). Rockville, Md. 20852.

Division of Hospital and Medical Facilities, U. S. Public Health Service, Department of Health, Education and Welfare. *Principles for Planning the Future Hospital System: A Report on Proceedings of Four Regional Conferences.* Washington, D.C.: Government Printing Office, 1959.

Dolfman, M. L. "Health Planning—A Method for Generating Program Objectives." *American Journal of Public Health 63,* 238, 1973.

Dorsey, J. L. "Certification of Need Laws." *Archives of Surgery, 106,* 765, 1973.

Elling, R. H. "The Shifting Power Structure on Health." *Milbank Memorial Fund Quarterly, 46,* Suppl., 119, 1968.

Evans, R. D. "Representational Standards in Comprehensive Health Planning." *American Journal of Public Health. 64,* 549, 1974.

Fanshel, S. and Bush, J. W. "A Health Status Index and Its Applications to Health Service Outcomes." *Operations Research, 18,* 1021, 1970.

Gartland, J. E. *An Experiment in Medicine: A History of the First 20 Years of the Pratt Clinic and the New England Center Hospital of Boston.* Cambridge, Mass.: Riverside Press, 1960.

Goldsmith, S. B. "The Status of Health Status Indicators." *Health Services Reports, 87,* 212, 1972.

Gottlieb, S. "A Brief History of Health Planning in the United States." In Havighurst, C.C., Ed., *Regulating Health Facilities Construction,* Ch. 1. Washington, D.C.: American Institute for Public Policy Research, 1974.

Guralnick, L. "Some Problems in the Use of Multiple Causes of Death." *Journal of Chronic Diseases, 19,* 979, 1966.

Haber, L. "Identifying the Disabled: Concepts and Methods in Measurement of Disability." *Social Security Bulletin 30,* 17, 1967.

Havighurst, C. C. "Regulation in the Health Care System." *Hospitals, 48,* 65, 1974.

———. "Regulation of Health Facilities and Services." *Virginia Law Review, 59,* 1143, 1973.

Hilleboe, H. E., and Schaefer, M. "Administrative Requirements for Comprehensive Health Planning at the State Level." *American Journal of Public Health, 58,* 1039, 1968.

Hilleboe, H. E. et al. *Approaches to National Health Planning,* Public Health Papers #46. Geneva, Switz.: World Health Organization, 1972.

Huntington, S. P. "The Marasmus of the ICC: The Commission, the Railroads and the Public Interest." *Yale Law Journal, 61,* 467, 1952.

Jacobs, A. R., and Froh, R. B. "Significance of Public Law 89–749." *New England Journal of Medicine, 279,* 1314, 1968.

Jeffers, J. et al. "On the Demand vs. Need for Medical Services and the Concept of 'Shortage'." *American Journal of Public Health, 61,* 46, 1971.

Jonas, S. "Heart Disease, Cancer and Stroke—Regional Medical Programs." *Journal of the National Medical Association, 59,* 7, 1967.

Jonas, S. "'74 Planning Act Is Dubbed 'Sleeper'; The Prospective from the Campus." *The Nation's Health, 5,* June, 1975.

Kissick, W. L. "Health Policy Reflections for the 1970's." *New England Journal of Medicine, 282,* 1343, 1970.

Komaroff, Anthony L. "Regional Medical Programs in Search of a Mission." *New England Journal of Medicine, 284,* 750, 1971.

Le Breton, D. P., and Henning, D. A. *Planning Theory.* Englewood Cliffs, N.J.: Prentice-Hall, 1961.

Lindblom, C. E. *The Intelligence of Democracy.* New York: The Free Press, 1965.

May, J. J. *Health Planning: Its Past and Potential.* Health Administration Perspectives #A5. Chicago, Ill.: Center for Health Administration Studies, Graduate School of Business, University of Chicago, 1967.

Meltzer, J. W., and Hochstim, J. R. "Reliability and Validity of Survey Data on Physical Health." *Public Health Reports, 85,* 1075, 1970.

Miller, J. E. "An Indicator to Aid Management in Assigning Program Priorities." *Public Health Reports, 85,* 721, 1970.

Miller, W. R. "A Five Year Perspective of NRMP." *Minnesota Medicine, 55,* 9, 1972.

Morehouse, T. A. "Program Evaluation: Social Research versus Public Policy." *Public Administration Review, 32,* 868, 1972.

Moriyama, I. M. "Problems in the Measurement of Health Status." In Sheldon, E. and Marie W., Eds., *Indicators of Social Change.* New York: Russell Sage Foundation, 1968.

Mountin, T. W. et al. *Health Service Areas: Requirements for General Hospitals and Health Centers.* Public Health Service Pub. No. 292. Washington, D.C.: USDHEW, 1945.

National Center for Health Statistics. *An Index of Health: Mathematical Models.* U.S. Public Health Service Pub. No. 1000. Washington, D.C.: Government Printing Office, 1965.

Office of Comprehensive Health Planning, USDHEW, Public Health Service. *Information and Policies on Grants to States for Comprehensive Health Planning.* Washington, D.C.: Government Printing Office, 1967.

Office of Planning and Evaluation of the Regional Medical Programs Service, Health Services and Mental Health Administration, USDHEW. *Fact Book on Regional Medical Programs: A Special Report to the National Advisory Council of the Regional Medical Programs Service.* Washington, D.C.: Government Printing Office, 1971.

Prest, A. R., and Turvey, R. "Cost-Benefit Analysis: A Survey." *The Economic Journal, 75,* 683, 1965.

President's Commission on Heart Disease, Cancer and Stroke, *A National Program to Conquer Heart Disease, Cancer and Stroke.* Washington, D.C.: Government Printing Office, 1964.

Public Accountability Reporting Group. *Regional Medical Programs Benefiting People and Implementing Local Health Services.* Boise, Idaho: Public Accountability Reporting Group, 1974.

Public Law 79–725. *Hospital Survey and Construction Act.* August 13, 1946.

Public Law 89–239. *Amendment to the Public Health Service Act. Title IX—Education, Research, Training and Demonstration in the Fields of Heart Disease, Cancer, Stroke and Related Diseases.* October 6, 1965.

Public Law 89–749. *Comprehensive Health Planning and Public Service Amendments of 1966.* November 3, 1966.

Public Law 93–641. *National Health Planning and Resources Development Act.* January 4, 1975.

Rienke, W. A. "An Overview of the Planning Process." In Rienke, W. A., Ed., *Health Planning: Qualitative Aspects and Quantitative Techniques,* Ch. 5. Baltimore, Md.: Johns Hopkins University Press, 1972.

Rienke, W. A., and Baker, T. D. "Measuring Effects of Demographic Variables on Health Service Utilization." *Health Service Research, 2,* 61, 1967.

Roseman, C. "Problems and Prospects for Comprehensive Health Planning." *American Journal of Public Health, 62,* 16, 1972.

Rosenfeld, L. S. "Problems in Planning Community Health Services." *Bulletin of the New York Academy of Medicine, 44,* 165, 1968.

Rothenberg, E. "Evaluating the Impact of Certificate of Need on Hospital and Health Facilities Planning Outcomes: the New York State Experience." Ph.D. dissertation, New York University, 1975.

Russell, John M. "New Federal Regional Medical Programs." *New England Journal of Medicine, 275,* 6, 1966.

Schwebel, A. I. et al. "A Community Organization Approach to the Implementation of Comprehensive Health Planning." *American Journal of Public Health, 63,* 675, 1973.

Seder, R. M. "Planning and Politics in the Allocation of Health Resources." *American Journal of Public Health, 63,* 774, 1973.

Shuman, R. "The Role of Operations Research in Regional Health Planning." *Operations Research, 22,* 234, 1974.

Sigmond, R. M. "Health Planning." *Milbank Memorial Fund Quarterly, 46,* Suppl., 91, 1968.

Stebbins, E. L., and Williams, K. N. "History and Background of Health Planning in the United States." In Rienke, W. A., Ed., *Health Planning: Qualitative Aspects and Quantitative Techniques,* Ch. 1. Baltimore, Md.: Johns Hopkins University Press, 1972.

Stewart, W. H. *Report on Regional Medical Program to the President and the Congress.* Washington, D.C.: Government Printing Office, 1967.

Sullivan, D. F. *Conceptual Problems in Developing an Index of Health.* DHEW, National Center for Health Statistics, *Vital and Health Statistics,* Ser. 2, No. 17, Washington, D.C. 1966.

Susser, M. W., and Watson, W. *Sociology in Medicine*. London: Oxford University Press, 1962.

Tabb, W. K. "Data Retrieval Systems, the University and State Decision-Making." *Public Administration Review, 31*, 435, 1971.

Taylor, C. E. "Stages of the Planning Process." In Rienke, W. A., Ed., *Health Planning: Qualitative Aspects and Quantitative Techniques*, Ch. 2. Baltimore, Md.: Johns Hopkins University Press, 1972.

Tell, R. "A Realistic Approach to Health Planning." *Hospital Administration, 14*, 90, 1969.

Thomas, W. "Health Planning and Realism." *Hospital Administration, 14*, 16, 1969.

Treolar, A., and Chill, D. *Patient Care Facilities: Construction Needs and Hill-Burton Accomplishments*. Chicago, Ill.: American Hospital Association, 1961.

U.S. Department of Health, Education and Welfare. *Congressional Hearings Data Book, Fiscal Year 1970*. Rockville, Md.: Health Services and Mental Health Administration, Community Profile Data Center, 1969.

U.S. Department of Health, Education and Welfare, Public Health Service. *Facts About the Hill-Burton Program: 1 July 1947—30 June 1970*. Washington, D.C.: U.S. Government Printing Office, 1970.

Ward, P. W. "The Curious Odyssey of Regional Medical Programs." *Western Journal of Medicine, 120*, 425, 1944.

Weinerman, E. R. "Anchor Points Underlying the Planning for Tomorrow's Health Care." *Bulletin of the New York Academy of Medicine, 41*, 1213, 1965.

Zola, I. K. "Culture and Symptoms: An Analysis of Patients Presenting Complaints." *American Sociological Review, 31*, 615, 1966.

13

Measurement and Control of the Quality of Health Care

Steven Jonas

Why Be Concerned with Quality of Care?

A number of measures show that health care delivered in the United States varies sharply in quality. There is an extensive literature on the subject of the approaches aimed at ensuring good care, but before beginning to review that literature in some detail, we might address ourselves to the question, "Why be concerned about the quality of health care at all?"*

First, perhaps, is the principle *primum non nocere*, "primarily, do no harm." This precept is at least as old as the Hippocratic Oath, of which it is a part. As our consideration of the results of quality determinations below will demonstrate, this is an important consideration in a health care delivery system in which a substantial minority of care delivered is of less than good quality and could be harmful.

Second, as pointed out in Chapter 9, our society devotes a significant and increasing portion of its economic resources to providing health services. Americans have a strong interest in obtaining a good product for the money spent. Further, there are social and humanitarian motivations to see that the large sums of money spent actually help those persons who are receiving the services.

---

* In this chapter we are concerned primarily with the quality of *medical* care, the subject of the bulk of the literature. However, many of the principles, although not all of the practices, apply to *health* care in general.

Portions of this chapter are taken from a paper entitled "PSRO: Issues in Quality Review and Regulation," delivered by the author at the annual meeting of the American Public Health Association, New Orleans, Louisiana, October 22, 1974.

Third, from the providers' point of view, a major motivation for doing good work in health care is professionalism. The concepts of "profession" and "professionalism" are related to quality. A profession is, in part at least, a field of human endeavor in which the practitioners themselves control entry and exit, in which a common body of knowledge exists, and in which the practitioners attempt to expand and develop that body of knowledge to improve the quality of human life and extend the understanding of man's existence. The last aspect of professionalism, aside from personal pecuniary and self-protective interests, adds a strong impetus to the thrust of at least part of the medical profession to regulate and improve the quality of medical care.

Finally, there is a strong social ethic in our culture to value doing a good job in and of itself. This principle has deep historical roots in the Judeo-Christian tradition; its origins probably stem from the individual and species survival value of performing tasks well. In health care, of course, there is a direct link between both individual and species survival and doing a good job in personal and community health services.

Can the Quality of Health Care Be Measured?

The extent to which quality of care be evaluated has been a subject of debate. A former president of the American Medical Association, Russell Roth, said in a presidential address that "good quality in medical care is not something which can be expressed in dollars of cost, hours of time, or for that matter, in decibels of political oratory. Quality of such medical care is not a tangible qualifiable thing" (*American Medical News*, Dec. 10, 1973). He added there are "immense difficulties" inherent in properly identifying high-quality care. On the other hand, many authorities in the field have thought it possible to measure and regulate the quality of discrete instances of care delivery. E. A. Codman has been recognized as the granddaddy of outcome studies (Lewis; Christoffel, 1976a; Brook, 1973b, p. 32; Moore). Emphasizing his faith in their efficacy as measures of quality, he said: "While a layman could not authoritatively inquire into the details of the reasons why, he could insist that the end-result system should be used, that someone must see that it is used, and that an efficiency committee be appointed for the purpose" (Lewis).

Lee and Jones wrote a landmark work on quality determination in 1933, which was built around the concept that "good medical care is the kind of medicine practiced and taught by the recognized leaders of the medical profession at a given time or period of social, cultural, and professional development in a community or population group" (1962, p. 6). In 1951, E. R. Weinerman, reflecting the 1949 statement by the Subcommittee on Medical Care of the American Public Health Association, "The Quality of Medical Care in a National Health Program," said: "The quality of medical care is a composite of all the technical, organizational, and financial aspects of any program for personal health service. Good quality can be defined, consciously planned, and evaluated" (Subcommittee on Medical Care; Weinerman). The APHA's belief in the possibility of measuring quality was amply restated in *A Guide to Medical Care Administration*, Vol. II: *Medical Care Appraisal—Quality and Utilization* (Donabedian, 1969). In their work describing the "tracer method" of quality measurement, David Kessner and his coauthors said: "The question is no longer whether there will be intervention in health services to assure quality, but who will intervene and what methods they will use" (1973). Finally, in a review article, Robert Brook said: "Even though the perfect system for assessment and assurance of quality of care may not yet exist, innumerable simple efforts can be made to improve quality of care. If applied in a systematic manner, many are likely to be successful" (1973a).

Methods of Measuring and Controlling the Quality of Care

The first problem in analyzing quality control in health care is to classify and understand the different methodologies in use. Many review articles (Donabedian, 1966, 1968, 1969; Sanazaro and Williamson; Sheps; Brook, 1973b, pp. 7–16; Blum) have established schemata for classifying the techniques or methodologies used for measuring the quality of medical care delivered by individuals or institutions, a subject to which we shall return. However, before examining the techniques for evaluating the quality of care, it is useful to understand the approaches to quality measurement and control which are actually in use in the U.S. (see Table 13.1). In the early 1970s, M. I. Roemer, Lewis, and Ellwood et al. (ch. 3) began to take this necessary broader view.

The *approaches* are those various methods utilized to ensure quality in the health care delivery system, such as licensing, accreditation, and peer review through hospital medical staff committees. *Techniques* are the ways quality is measured within the

Table 13.1

Approaches, Techniques, and Criteria Used in the Measurement and Control of the Quality of Care

Approaches		Techniques	Criteria
General	Specific		
Licensing	Hospital medical staff review committees	Structure	Explicit
		Process	Implicit
Accreditation	Research studies		
		Outcome	
Certification	Professional Standards Review Organizations		
	Patient satisfaction		
	Malpractice litigation		

various approaches. Techniques are only tools; approaches use the tools to effect control, or at least attempt to do so. Thus techniques are scientific constructs whereas approaches are political ones.

Approaches

The approaches may be divided into two groups—the general and the specific. The general approaches examine an individual's or an institution's ability to meet established evaluative criteria at a particular point in time. Individuals are evaluated in terms of experience, education, and knowledge (usually measured by examination). Institutions are evaluated on the basis of physical structure, administrative and staff organization, minimum services, and personnel qualifications. If the criteria are met at the time of evaluation, it is then predicted that the individual or institution will function well either indefinitely, as in the case of the medical license, or for a given period of time, as in the case of the hospital license. The general approaches used in the United States are licensing, accreditation, and certification (Secretary's Report).

The specific approaches to quality measurement and control, on the other hand, look at discrete instances of provider-patient interaction and evaluate them using one of several available techniques. The major specific approaches in use in the United States are hospital medical staff review committees; research studies;

Professional Standards Review Organizations; patient satisfaction, and its subset, malpractice litigation, an extreme product of patient dissatisfaction.

Techniques

Donabedian has provided the generally accepted classification of the techniques of quality assessment (1969, pp. 2–3) :

> Three major approaches* to the evaluation of quality have been identified. These have been designated as the evaluation of structure, process, and outcome or end results.
>
> Appraisal of structure involves the evaluation of the settings and instrumentalities available and used for the provision of care. While including the physical aspects of facilities and equipment, structural appraisal goes far beyond to encompass the characteristics of the administrative organization and the qualifications of health professionals. . . . Two major assumptions are made when structure is taken as an indicator of quality: First, that better care is more likely to be provided when better qualified staff, improved physical facilities and sounder fiscal and administrative organization are employed. Second, that we know enough to identify what is good in terms of staff, physical structure and formal organization. . . .
>
> Assessment of process is the evaluation of the activities of physicians and other health professionals in the management of patients. The criterion generally used is the degree to which management of patients conforms with the standards and expectations of the respective professions. These standards and expectations may be derived from what is considered to be "ideal," "good," or "acceptable" practice as formulated by recognized leaders in the profession. Such standards may also be inferred from patterns of care observed in actual practice. . . .
>
> When evaluation of process is the basis for judgments concerning quality, a major assumption is that health care is useful in maintaining or promoting health. Furthermore, there is the explicit or implicit assumption that particular elements and aspects of care are known to be specifically related to successful or unsuccessful health outcomes or end results. Assessment of outcomes is the evaluation of end results in terms of health and satisfaction. That this evaluation in many ways provides the final evidence of whether care has been good, bad or indifferent is so because of the broad fundamental social and professional agreement on what results are deemed desirable. Furthermore, it is

* Donabedian uses the word "approaches" in the sense in which the word "techniques" is used in this chapter.

assumed that good results are brought about, at least to a significant degree, by good care.

Thus, the structural approach examines the setting of care;
the process approach examines what goes on between the provi-
der(s) and the patient; the outcome approach examines the
results of the encounter or lack thereof between the patient and
the health care delivery system. In the main, the structural technique is used in the general approaches, while the process and
outcome techniques are used in the specific approaches, sometimes in combination with the structural technique as well.

Explicit criteria. In all three techniques, criteria are used in
the evaluation process. Explicit criteria are written down and the
work under study is checked against them. For example, in a
process study of physician performance, an explicit criterion
might be that in the course of a good physical examination, a
blood pressure measurement is taken. If a medical record is being
used as the medium of evaluation, the evaluator would then check
to see if a blood pressure measurement had been recorded.
Actually, if the evaluation is being made solely on the basis of
what is in the medical record, a blood pressure notation can mean
either that the pressure was taken and recorded, or that it was
not taken and a number put down anyway. The absence of a
blood pressure reading in the record can mean either that it was
not taken, or that it was taken and not recorded. Of these four
possibilities, only the first represents good medical care.

Implicit criteria. Implicit criteria, on the other hand, exist only
in the mind of the evaluator. Nothing specific to look for is written down. Evaluators are picked on the basis of their own credentials and reputations. The assumption is made that since they are
"good" physicians (or dentists, nurses, etc.), they will know
what "good" and "bad" care are and will be able to make valid
and reliable assessments of care as they review it.

Thus, there are two groups of approaches, three sets of techniques, and two categories of criteria. They are organized in various combinations in practice in the United States.

The General Approaches to Quality of Care Assessment and Control

Licensing

Licensing systems exist for both individual and institutional
providers in the United States. Approximately 25 health professions and occupations are licensed by one or more states (Pennell

and Stewart, p. 1) ; approximately 10 types of health facilities
are licensed (Hollis, p. 1). There are certain similarities between
the two types of license as well as several important differences.
Both use structural standards of measurement and both scrupu-
lously avoid investigations of discrete instances of care delivery.
Individual licensing is usually for an indefinite period, whereas
licensure of institutions is usually for a set time period. Both
types involve governmental authority and are backed by the
force of law. The Constitution specifically grants the "police
power" to the states: licensing, having been considered to fall
in this category, is thus a state function (Derbyshire, p. 16).

Individual licensing. Individual licensing is a complex matter
(National Advisory Commission on Health Manpower, Appendix
VII; Secretary's Report, pp. 1–33). It represents a compact
between defined professional groups and state legislatures in
which the profession is granted control over individuals' entrance
into, maintenance of good standing in, and exit from the profession. Most professions generally define the content of their own
work and thus gain a virtual monopoly over the provision to the
public of that body of work. In return, the profession, in theory
at least, guarantees to the several state legislatures that the work
will be of good quality. The States use the criminal justice system
to enforce the agreements. The nature of medicine is such that
"practicing without a license" constitutes assault and battery.

Among the health professions and occupations licensed in all
or most states are chiropractice, dental hygiene, dentistry, allopathic and osteopathic medicine, nursing, optometry, pharmacy,
physical therapy, podiatry, and psychology (Pennell and Stewart, Table A). There are a series of controversial issues relating
to licensure of individuals (Secretary's Report; Cohen, 1973,
1974; Cohen and Miike; Miike; Nolan; Shryock; Spieler; Derbyshire; National Advisory Commission on Health Manpower,
Appendix VII; R. Roemer, 1971 a, b; Egelston).

Licensure can, and apparently often does, lead to elements of
guildism. The licensed group, having an area fenced off for itself,
can become more interested in maintaining the fence than in regulating the work that goes on within its boundaries. The medical
profession in particular has argued that a license, rather than
being a compact with a state government concerning quality, is a
property right; the courts have often upheld this view (Vodicka). If we analyze the membership of the various state licensing
boards for the independent health professions and occupations, it

becomes clear that most are dominated by members of the profession or occupation (Pennell and Stewart). An exception is dental hygiene—most boards licensing dental hygienists are dominated by dentists, and none includes any dental hygienists (Pennell and Stewart, Table 18).

Licensure can lead to rigidity in job descriptions. If they do not change in accordance with changes in preparatory education, in time people will not be properly trained in relation to the licensing laws. The error in this case is usually on the side of overtraining. However, undertraining can also occur when the work content and educational requirements prescribed by licensing laws do not accord with changing health and health care needs.

The rigidities of licensure also limit geographic mobility because of different laws and requirements in different states; inhibit health professionals from moving up the career ladder because most health licensure requirements do not allow credit for education and experience in another health profession or occupation; and discourage innovative and creative use of personnel. Furthermore, until the mid-70s there was virtually no direct public accountability for, or direct public participation in, any health profession or occupation licensing board. By 1976, public members had been added to boards in several states, including California, Michigan, New Jersey, Minnesota, and Washington (*American Medical News,* 1976). It remains to be seen what effects these changes will have. The licensure system rests on the unproven premise that the person who has qualified for a license will tend to deliver good health care over a long period of time. Studies of the work of licensed providers that employ process and/or outcome techniques rather than the structural techniques used in licensure show such a wide variation in quality as to demonstrate that licensing has very little validity as either a predictor or a guarantor of performance. (See the section entitled "Research Studies," below.)

One of the more novel proposals for licensing reform is "institutional licensure" (Miike, 1974). In this approach, institutions would be responsible for the competence of the people they employ. Such a system might produce beneficial results:

> Although licensure of personnel and licensure of facilities are completely separate in our current system of licensure, merger of these two systems into a single regulatory system governing individual and institutional providers of service might be a key to

better regulation of quality and more freedom for innovation in delegation of patient-care tasks among members of the health manpower matrix. . . . The institutional licensure approach, which might result from such a merger, would provide a framework for developing innovations in the use of existing categories of personnel and for undertaking experimental programs to train and use new categories of health professionals (Forgotson and Roemer, p. 352).

The principal affected professions, particularly medicine and nursing, have reacted to this proposal like a neighborhood threatened with a drug-treatment program or a halfway house for discharged mental-hospital patients: "It's a great idea, but not on *my* block, thank you very much." As Miike points out, for this reason, among others, institutional licensure must be considered still very much in the experimental stage.

Ruth Roemer (1971a) considered most of the issues of licensure reform in some detail, as have others (Cohen, 1973, 1974; Spieler; Cohen and Miike; National Commission on Health Manpower). Roemer's most important point is that fundamental reform of the licensure system cannot take place apart from fundamental reform of the health care delivery system. Obviously, neither is a simple task.

Licensing and Physician Dominance

A prime issue in licensure is the degree to which medical licensing laws assure physician dominance of the health care delivery system. Medicine can be defined as that body of knowledge which concerns the processes of human disease, the mechanisms of prevention, treatment, and rehabilitation of disease, the processes by which the human body maintains normal functioning, and the mechanisms of health maintenance. The practice of medicine is the delivery to people of the fruits of that body of knowledge called medicine. Health care delivery systems are not solely concerned with medical practice; they provide for payment for care, construct and operate institutions, provide employment, and carry out educational and research activities; however, the major purpose of all these activities is to make it possible for medical practice to be carried on. Thus, medical practice is the focus, the *raison d' être* of any health care delivery system.

Whoever controls medical practice, therefore, controls the keystone, upon which all the rest depends. For example, insurance companies generally determine their own policies regarding benefits, coverage, premiums, and the like (subject to government regulation in certain instances), but they cannot sell health insurance policies if there is no medical practice to buy. The boards of directors of voluntary hospitals determine hospital size, location, and facilities (again subject to government regulation), but if medical practice is not carried out on their premises, their powers come to nothing. Finally, a local government agency may decide what kind of medical service it wants to offer, but it is dependent upon medical practitioners to supply that service.

In the United States, because of the way the medical licensing laws are written, the physicians have a virtual hammerlock on medical practice. In each state the licensing laws are implemented by Medical Boards, to whom the state legislatures delegate the powers of examination, licensing, and discipline. There is little evidence of accountability, either to the public or the legislature; indeed in most instances Medical Board proceedings are entirely confidential. In most states, physicians dominate the medical boards (Derbyshire, ch. 3; Pennell and Stewart, Table 81). Derbyshire studied the backgrounds of the physician-members of the boards in 1967 and developed this revealing composite picture of a medical board member:

> He is a Caucasian man, a little over 58 years of age (only one woman serves on a board, that of New Hampshire); most likely a general practitioner; if not, a general surgeon or an internist. He is a leader in the medical community and well known to the members of his state medical society. He possesses no singular attributes which qualify him to judge the academic attainments of applicants for licensure, but he is sincere in carrying out his duties and may seek help in formulating his examination questions. He is a graduate of an approved American medical school and is better qualified to carry out the disciplinary duties of his office than the educational and examining functions. (p. 44)

Furthermore, in about one-half of the states, the medical societies have a direct voice in the appointment of members (p. 33) and there is no indication that in other states physicians of whom medical societies would disapprove are appointed (pp. 34-35).

A medical license is generally granted once and is retained for life, barring practice of extremely poor quality, "moral turpitude," or some similar offense. Physicians in the United States rarely lose their licenses (Derbyshire, ch. 6). In the period 1963–1967, Derbyshire found that nationally 938 disciplinary

actions were undertaken by state medical boards. Of these, 334
involved revocation of license, while the rest involved probation,
suspension, and reprimand. Nearly 50% of these actions were
related to narcotics addiction; only seven involved "gross malpractice." For the period 1971–1974, there were an average of 72
revocations annually, fewer than 2% for incompetency (*New
York Times*, Jan. 29, 1976).

Discounting the possibility that this was all the disciplinary
action needed, there are several reasons to account for this relatively low level of activity. One is the professional dominance of
medical licensing boards, noted above, and the possible
"reluctance to enforce sanctions against fellow practitioners
(perhaps in part because of close professional and social interre-
lationships)" (Ellwood et al., pp. 30-31). A lack of graduated
means of discipline is another problem: only 19 states provide for
probation and only 6 for reprimand, while all states give their
medical boards revocation authority and 48 give suspension
authority (Ellwood et al., p. 31). Moreover, some medical boards
may be reluctant to act because they do not want to get involved
in litigation. Physicians who have had their licenses revoked or
suspended have been known to successfully sue medical boards on
the grounds of deprivation of livelihood without due process—
taking the position that the license is a property right (Derbyshire, ch. 7).

Thus, through the licensing laws physicians independently control medical practice, the core of the health care delivery system.
In addition, of course, they exert control through the mechanism
of fee-for-service private practice, under which they function as
independent contractors to their patients, regardless of what
relationships patients may have to other components of the
system, be they hospitals or third-party payors. Because of the
power it gives physicians, medical licensure, far from being an
obscure influence on the health care delivery system, is in fact an
extremely important determinant of the shape of that system.

Licensure of institutions. As of 1968, 11 types of medical or
residential-care facilities were subject to licensure in the U.S.
(Hollis, pp. 1–20). All or most states required licensing of psychiatric, short- and long-stay hospitals, hospitals and homes for
the mentally retarded, nursing and other homes for the aged, and
homes for unwed mothers and for dependent children (Hollis,
Table A). State health departments were most commonly responsible, with social welfare, mental health, and occasionally other

departments involved as well (Hollis, Table B). Licensing of major health care facilities did not become common until the 1940s (Hollis, Table C). The evaluation techniques are almost entirely structural (Hollis, pp. 7–8). Licenses are usually granted on an annual or biennial basis. Although the statutory boards involved in institutional licensing usually include representatives from the health care field, they are much less likely to be completely dominated by providers from the type of institution being regulated than are statutory boards in individual licensing (Hollis, Table H). However, in institutional licensing, unlike individual licensing, the state departments usually have more control over the actual licensing process than do the statutory boards.

Accreditation

Accreditation is another popular general approach to quality measurement and control in the United States (Secretary's Report, pp. 9–15). Unlike licensing, accreditation is a voluntary system used only in institutions. Groups of like institutions or organizations with mutual interests get together, set up an organization, establish standards and an examination program, and proceed to inspect and "accredit" (or not accredit) themselves, or the institutions in which they have an interest, on a periodic basis. Certain types of institutions that deliver care, and most of those that educate health care personnel, are subject to accreditation. There is a national voluntary agency originally called the National Commission on Accrediting (Pennell, p. 67), now called the Council on Postsecondary Accreditation, which recognizes accrediting bodies for educational institutions. In cases in which such accreditation is necessary to qualify for federal funds, the accrediting body must be recognized by the Office of Education of the USDHEW as well.

In general, accreditation involves the use of structural techniques of quality assessment. Institutions are evaluated on the basis of their physical and organizational structures and the qualifications of their personnel, who themselves are evaluated, mostly by structural techniques. For example, in accrediting health personnel educational institutions, curricula are closely examined for organization and content on paper. However, the teaching process is rarely, if ever, evaluated.

The basic principles of accreditation are similar to those of licensure in that it is assumed that if the institution meets certain standards of physical and organizational structure at one point in time, then: (1) good quality health care, or health personnel education, is being delivered at that point in time and (2) it can be predicted that the care will continue to be of good quality for a discrete period of time. The latter provision applies to most institutional licensing.

Accreditation is not a legal procedure, but there are strong legal incentives for accrediting certain kinds of institutions. For example, the Medicare law restricts payments which may be made to unaccredited hospitals, and state medical boards will not grant licenses to graduates of unaccredited medical schools without requiring such persons (that is, most foreign medical graduates) to meet conditions not required for graduates of accredited medical schools.

One organization that carries out institutional accreditation is the Joint Commission on the Accreditation of Hospitals. It had its origins in a program for hospital evaluation established by the American College of Surgeons in 1918 (Schlicke; Joint Commission on Accreditation of Hospitals, p. 1). In 1951, the JCAH was formed under the joint sponsorship of the American College of Surgeons, the American College of Physicians, the American Hospital Association, the American Medical Association, and the Canadian Medical Association. In 1959, the Canadians set up their own hospital accreditation program. By 1974, 5,285 of the 7,174 hospitals registered with the American Hospital Association were accredited (American Hospital Association, *1975 Ed.*, Tables 1, 9).

The JCAH uses structural standards in its evaluations. The Preamble to the JCAH *Manual for Hospitals* states explicitly that "The new standards are free of all direct demands upon the physicians' clinical judgment and decision. Current standards relate entirely to the supporting elements of hospital life and the environment of medical practice" (Joint Commission on Accreditation of Hospitals, p. 21). Thus the JCAH intentionally avoids evaluations using the process and/or outcome methods, which do concern themselves with physicians' actions. It sets standards for the governing body and management; for medical staff organization and functioning; for the various hospital services—nursing, anesthesia, outpatients, medical records, laboratory, radiology, and the like—and for physical plant design, structure, and functioning. Rather than dealing with discrete instances of care delivery, the standards focus on organization, equipment, quality (as determined by criteria for education and experience) and quantity of staff, and the like (Joint Commission on the Accreditation of Hospitals, pp. 23–178).

Beginning in the early 1970s, the JCAH came under increasingly heavy criticism, particularly from consumer groups (Consumer Commission on the Accreditation of Health Services, 1974a, b, 1975a), which questioned the ability of the JCAH, "sponsored by the industry," to inspect hospitals adequately and to protect the public interest. The Medicare Law was criticized for delegating government inspectorial functions to a private agency. Controversy exploded on this point in 1975, when inspection teams sponsored by the Social Security Administration checked JCAH hospital inspections under Medicare, in a so-called "validation survey," and found those inspections wanting (Bird; Phillips and Kessler; Consumer Commission on the Accreditation of Health Services, 1975a). The furor continued into 1976, centering on questions of the JCAH role, confidentiality, the powers of the Secretary of the USDHEW, and the actions of Congress.

Other, quieter criticisms concerned the JCAH's use of structural standards only. It has indeed never been shown that there is any relationship between retrospective measurements of the quality of medical care undertaken using structural techniques and those undertaken using process and/or outcome techniques. In fact, the structural technique has fallen into such disfavor that it is not even considered by several prominent contemporary academic investigators of methodological problems in medical care evaluation (Kessner et al., 1973; Brook, 1973a, b), who concern themselves with the evaluation of process and outcome techniques only. The evaluation of structure is considered too indefinite to be useful (Donabedian, 1969); however, such evaluation is not entirely worthless: "While the presence of various input measures in no way assures good care, the converse—good care is unlikely where such inputs are lacking—probably makes sense" (Christoffel, 1976b).

When the Secretary of the USDHEW released the results of the validation surveys—which seriously questioned the JCAH's way of doing business—the Commission sued (*Hospital Week*, June 6, 1975). In response to the criticism of the use of structural standards, they did try to change, however. In the early 1970s the JCAH developed the "Performance Evaluation Procedure for Auditing and Improving Patient Care," or the PEP (Fitzgibbon; Jacobs et al.), The JCAH described it as an "outcome-oriented [technique]," and beginning on July 1, 1975, PEP or an acceptable equivalent became a requirement for accreditation. In the Donabedian definition, PEP is probably more of a process technique, but nonetheless it definitely represents a step forward for the JCAH. The Commission still does not involve itself in the process or outcome evaluation of discrete instances of patient care, but rather requires hospitals to show that they have engaged in this type of audit. In that sense, it is still a structural standard, but it is of a different order than the Commission's usual standards. The PEP has been explained by the Commission's staff in great detail (Jacobs and Christoffel; Jacobs et al.). A periodical published by the Commission, *Quality Review Bulletin*, keeps hospitals current on auditing techniques. By 1976, it was estimated that 2,500 hospitals were using the PEP in some form (Christoffel, 1976b). It is a prime example of moving from the general to the specific.

Accreditation of health sciences educational institutions operates in a different fashion. Medical schools, for example, are accredited in a sequential process, first separately, by the Council on Medical Education of the American Medical Association and the Executive Council of the Association of American Medical Colleges, and then by the Liaison Committee on Medical Education, on which the AMA and the AAMC are equally represented (National Commission on Accrediting; Liaison Committee on Medical Education, 1973). Schools are accredited for seven-year periods, based primarily on a three- to four-day visit by a four-person team. The standards to be met are stated in a 3,000-word document entitled "Functions and Structure of a Medical School" (Liaison Committee on Medical Education, 1973). Compared with the lengthy and detailed JCAH standards, the LCME standards seem vague, general, and incredibly brief, although this is not necessarily bad. The requirements for new medical schools seem much more rigorous than those for existing, previously accredited schools (Liaison Committee on Medical Education, 1972, 1974). In any event, medical school accreditation shows an extreme reliance on structural standards. There are no examinations of instances of patient care or even of the educational process. The JCAH Accreditation Manual is full of explicit criteria. The LCME consciously shies away from them for the most part, being content with some general guidelines for the surveyors' implicit criteria.

Medical school accreditation in the United States receives virtually no publicity, even though it may well be more critical for the development of American medicine as a whole than hospital accreditation or physician licensing, because of the commanding position of the physicians, who happen to be selected exclusively by medical school admissions committees. There is no trace of public accountability in medical school accreditation. It is invisible, and totally under the control of the largest organizations of physicians and the medical schools. From the time of the Flexner Report (1910) until the mid-1960s, the medical school accreditation process was a principal weapon used by the American Medical Association in its struggle to keep down the number of physicians (Rayack). Because of its isolation from public scrutiny and its total reliance on structural criteria, serious questions must be raised about the validity and reliability of accreditation as a measure of the quality and relevance of medical education in the United States.

Certification

Certification is the third general approach to quality control found in the United States health care delivery system (Secretary's Report, pp. 15–20; Bureau of Health Manpower Education; Pennell, pp. 70–76).* Certification combines features of licensing and accreditation. Applied to individuals, it uses standards of education, experience, and achievement on examination to determine qualification. However, it is a voluntary system undertaken by health care provider professions and occupations and is neither directly sanctioned nor backed up by the force of law. Nevertheless, like accreditation, there are incentives for individuals to become certified. For example, speech therapy is a health profession licensed in some, but not all, states. The American Speech and Hearing Association has a national certification program, however, and many school districts will hire only speech therapists who are certified by ASHA.

---

* Confusion may arise in the terminology here. Some occupations use "registration" in the sense in which we use "certification," while some states use the term "registration" instead of "licensing" in dealing with certain health occupations. In studying a particular state, one should determine exactly how that state uses the various terms. In nursing, "registration" always means licensing.

One variety of certification is used to designate specialists among physicians.* By the 1950s, the majority of medical school graduates in the United States were choosing to become specialists—that is, to devote themselves to one particular field of medical work like orthopedics, dermatology, or psychiatry. The average length of training beyond the B.A. or B.S. degree (ordinarily a prerequisite for admission to medical school), was around eight years: four years of medical school, a first postgraduate year of hospital work called the "internship," and then subsequent postgraduate years of hospital work in specialty training called "residencies," followed in certain specialties by additional "fellowship" time, ranging in all from two to five years or even more in such technically demanding subspecialties as neurosurgery.

One is eligible for licensing by a state medical board after the internship. However, a physician is not designated competent in a specialty until after he or she has completed the residency/fellowship and passed additional examinations. More than 20 "specialty boards"—private voluntary certifying authorities, originally self-appointed—are in charge of these designations. Specialty boards derive their power from the fact that many hospitals will not appoint a physician to their staffs with admitting privileges (the authority to admit and take care of their own patients in the hospital) in a particular specialty unless he is certified by the appropriate board. (The most frequent exceptions to this rule are found in smaller hospitals which still allow general practitioners to practice adult and pediatric medicine, surgery, and obstetrics. In certain cases, hospitals limit this sort of privilege to grandfathers.) The specialty boards themselves are approved by the American Medical Association through its Council on Medical Education, and the organization of the boards themselves, the Advisory (now American) Board of Medical Specialties.

Medical specialty boards rely entirely on structural techniques of evaluation. Most specialty boards, like licensing boards, certify once, for life. As of 1976, only the American Board of Family Practice required periodic recertification for all of its diplomates (every six years), and the American Board of Surgery was planning to introduce such a requirement for new applicants. As with

---

* The history of medical specialization in the United States has been treated by Stevens (1971), and its status in the mid-70s has been discussed in great detail by Herbert Lerner.

all approaches that use structural techniques, data are lacking relating level of quality at the time of certification with the quality of the individual's output at later times; thus the utility and validity of specialty certification as it is now carried out must be carefully questioned.

The Specific Approaches to Quality of Care Assessment and Control
Hospital Medical Staff Review Committees

The most common specific approach in the United States is the institution of hospital medical staff review committees. The JCAH requires that the hospital medical staff be organized to provide for committees to review at least the following: the quality of physician care; the products of surgical operations; deaths; the utilization of hospital services, in particular length of stay; the use of medical consultation services; and the general operations of all hospital divisions, whether direct patient care or support (Joint Commission on the Accreditation of Hospitals, pp. 43-44).

The committees dealing directly with physician services all evaluate individual instances of care delivery. They are usually concerned with physician performance in a particular case, although they may become involved with the work of other hospital staff as well.

The Tissue Committee is concerned with the products of surgery and deals with such issues as the technique and necessity of surgical operations. A Medical Records Committee may look at the quality of the records themselves as an indication of the quality of the work, or they can evaluate the work itself, as it is reflected in the record. Usually they do both.

Utilization review was mandated by the original Medicare law as a cost-control measure. Norms were supposed to be established for acceptable lengths of hospital stay for most common conditions. If a patient stayed longer than the norm, the case was to be reviewed and the admitting physician was to justify the excess. If the committee decided that the excess stay was not medically justified, Medicare would not pay for the extra days. Little is known in detail about how the system functioned nationally (Ellwood, et al., p. 31). However, it seemed not to work well as originally designed, and it was recast in the 1972 amendments to the Social Security Act as part of the responsibilities of the Professional Standards Review Organizations (see below).

Although hospital medical staff review committees, being required for accreditation, are the most prevalent specific approach to quality measurement and control, little is actually known about how they work or what they do. They have never been comprehensively studied.

An important aid to the work of many hospital medical staff review committees is the Professional Activity Study of the Commission on Professional and Hospital Activities (Kuehn), a process-oriented, computerized system providing information useful in medical auditing. It is carried on by an outside firm, under contract, from data collected by the hospital. A variety of medical staff committees can use the material in their work.

Research Studies

Over the years, a large number of research studies have been carried out in the problem area of measuring and controlling the quality of particular instances of medical care delivery.* Certain studies can be considered landmarks. In one of the earlier ones, Lee and Jones attempted to describe what "good medical care" was at the time, using, in essence, process criteria. In 1953–54, a study of general practice in North Carolina used both structural and process techniques and explicit criteria, in a direct observation method. It was found that: "Many physicians were performing at a high level of professional competence. Of greater importance is the fact that other physicians were performing at a lower level . . . " (Peterson, et al., p. 143). Of the various parameters measured, only the length of postgraduate hospital training in internal medicine was consistently related to the quality of a physician's clinical work. Academic performance, for example, was related to quality of clinical work only for physicians aged 35 and less (Peterson, et al., p. 55). Paul Lembcke was one of the

---

* There have been a number of reviews of the literature. Mindel Sheps considered a large series of primarily clinical evaluations. Her review included one of the earliest attempts to categorize the techniques of quality evaluation. Anderson and Altman produced an annotated bibliography covering the period 1955–61. Avedis Donabedian produced three major reviews in the late 1960s (1966, 1968, 1969). In the early 1970s, a large literature review was undertaken by Brook (1973b, ch. III). A major review of the state of the art in the early 70s was held under the aegis of the Graduate Program in Hospital Administration of the University of Chicago in 1973 (Scheye). Christoffel published a comprehensive bibliography in the mid-70s (1976c).

pioneers in developing the hospital medical audit, using analysis of clinical records (1956). As an example, he evaluated major female pelvic surgery in several hospitals and found that the introduction of auditing techniques reduced both the population hysterectomy rate and the proportion of unnecessary hysterectomies.

In the period 1957–1961, a study of 406 admissions of members of the Teamsters Unions and their families to hospitals in New York City used review of medical records, process and outcome techniques, and implicit criteria (Trussell et al.). The study found that 88% of admissions were justifiable (Trussell et al., p. 21). However, only 57% of the patients received "good or excellent medical care," while a fifth received fair, a fifth poor care (Trussell et al., p. 25). A second study by this group in 1962, using a slightly different evaluation technique, arrived at similar conclusions (Morehead et al., 1964). Some observers consider that implicit criteria have limited applicability since they rely entirely on the internal judgments of the evaluators (Koran).

An important early approach to the use of the computer in aiding the medical audit was developed by Shindell and London. In the late 60s and early 70s, a series of studies of quality of medical care in Neighborhood Health Centers, primarily using process techniques (Morehead; Morehead et al., 1971; Morehead and Donaldson), showed that such auditing methods could be widely applied; the quality of care in Neighborhood Health Centers was found to be reasonably good compared to that found in other organized ambulatory care settings.

In the early 1970s, a new approach to quality evaluation called the Tracer Method emerged (Kessner et al., 1973; Kessner and Kalk). According to the researchers, "The tracer method measures both process and outcome of care, which we consider important in any evaluation scheme. It is impossible to pinpoint the strengths and weaknesses without knowing the outcome, but outcome alone can be misleading if the patient receives unnecessary diagnostic tests or inappropriate therapy" (Kessner et al., 1973, p. 190). A tracer is a particular disease process with the following characteristics (Kessner et al., 1973, pp. 15-17) :

1. A tracer should have a definite functional impact. . . .
2. A tracer should be relatively well defined and easy to diagnose. . . .
3. Prevalence rates should be high enough to permit the collection of adequate data from a limited population sample. . . .

4. The natural history of the condition should vary with utilization and effectiveness of medical care. . . .
5. The technics of medical management of the condition should be well defined for at least one of the following processes: prevention, diagnosis, treatment or rehabilitation. . . .
6. The effects of nonmedical factors on the tracer should be understood. . . .

The tracer method is best suited either to the evaluation of health care received by a population group or delivered by an institution, rather than that given by an individual practitioner, who probably would not have a high enough volume of patients having tracer conditions to make evaluation meaningful. The tracer method has been applied to two different pediatric population groups in Washington, D.C. (Kessner and Kalk, 1973, pp. 15-17). The results were not encouraging: "Inappropriate or ineffective treatment for specific tracer conditions was documented in a large proportion of the children" (Kessner et al., 1974, p. 4).

At the same time Kessner was breaking new ground in developing a quality measurement method combining the process and outcome techniques, Robert Brook was carrying out another landmark study, comparing different process and outcome evaluations of the same medical care episodes (Brook, 1973b; Brook and Appel). Brook and Appel summarized their work as follows:

> To evaluate the procedures used to assess quality of care, five peer-review methods were compared. These methods involved judgments based on two kinds of data: what physicians did for the patients (process); and what happened to the patients (outcome). Criteria used to make judgments were either predetermined by group consensus (explicit), or selected subjectively by individual reviewers (implicit). The care of 296 patients with urinary-tract infection, hypertension or ulcerated gastric or duodenal lesions was reviewed with use of the five methods. Depending on the method, from 1.4 to 63.2 per cent of patients were judged to have received adequate care. Judgment of process using explicit criteria yielded the fewest acceptable cases (1.4 per cent). The largest differences found were between methods using different sources of data. Thus, medical care, judged with implicit criteria, was rated adequate for 23.3 percent of patients when process, and 63.2 percent when outcome was used. (p. 1323)

In his major publication on his study, Brook (1973b, p. 60) concluded that although serious methodologic problems remain in quality of care assessment, it is still nevertheless true that as many as 25% of the patients would have had better outcomes if the medical processes had been better. "It is, therefore, recommended that simple routine assessments of quality of care which employ carefully selected outcomes and processes should begin even while awaiting definitive methodologic research. Such studies using outcome measurements as a means to identify high priority areas could have a major impact on the health of the American people without dramatically increasing the cost of such care."

In 1976, Rutstein et al. described an approach to quality evaluation based on epidemiology. They called it the "sentinel method," summarizing it as follows:

> We outline the implementation of a new method of measuring the quality of medical care that counts cases of unnecessary disease and disability and unnecessary untimely deaths. First of all, conditions are listed in which the occurrence of a single case of disease or disability or a single untimely death would justify asking, "Why did it happen?" Secondly, we have selected conditions in which critical increases in rates of disease, disability, or untimely death could serve as indexes of the quality of care. Finally, broad categories of illness are noted in which redefinition and intensive study might reveal characteristics that could serve as indexes of health. . . . These indexes of outcome can be used to determine the level of health of the general population and the effects of economic, political, and other environmental factors upon it, and to evaluate the quality of medical care provided both within and without the hospital to maintain health and to prevent and treat disease. (p. 582)

This approach uses an outcome technique to look at discrete instances of patient care. Virtually every disease in the Eighth Revision, *International Classification of Diseases Adapted for Use in the United States* (ICDA) was analyzed. The criteria for unnecessary disease, unnecessary disability, and unnecessary untimely death were derived from state-of-the-art epidemiological knowledge. If for any listed disease, an event deemed unnecessary in the light of current knowledge occurs, attention is called to it. The unnecessary event becomes the sentinel. The circumstances surrounding the unnecessary event can than be examined in detail. This approach represents a marriage between clinical medicine and epidemiology, and thus should hold great promise for useful future development.

Thus, research in quality assessment marches on. Meanwhile, we are faced with the problem of taking what we already do know and creating a useful, functioning system. The Performance Evaluation Program of the Joint Commission on Accreditation of Hospitals, now supposed to be in use in every accredited hospital (Jacobs et al.), offers one approach to this problem. Another is the Professional Standards Review Organization approach.

Professional Standards Review Organizations

Historically, the general approaches to quality control in the United States have been widely used, formalized, and institutionalized. The specific approaches, on the other hand, have been used to a very limited extent, and moves to formalize and institutionalize them have been slow to develop. The JCAH in the mid-70s began requiring hospitals to perform process and outcome audits (although it does not evaluate their work). However, the sector in which the bulk of the health care action takes place—private office practice—remained virtually unregulated except for financial audits of high-earning physicians under Medicare/Medicaid. Thus the advent of the so-called Professional Standards Review Organization could be considered a notable event, marking a major step, on the part of the federal government, toward the institutionalization of specific approaches. For the first time a law—with some fairly sharp teeth in it—required peer-review of individual instances of physician delivery of medical care. Although in the beginning evaluations were to be confined to hospital care, there was nothing in the law preventing expansion to office practice.

Professional Standards Review Organizations were established by the 1972 admendments to the Social Security Act (P.L. 92-603). An excellent summary of the basic structure and functions of the PSRO system was offered by the original PSRO Program Manual (Office of Professional Standards Review, pp. 1-5).

102 *Information on the PSRO Program*
The 1972 Amendments to the Social Security Act provide for the creation of Professional Standards Review Organizations (PSROs) designed to involve local practicing physicians in the ongoing review and evaluation of health care services covered under the Medicare, Medicaid, and the Maternal and Child Health programs [of the U.S. Department of Health, Education and Welfare]. The legislation is based on the concepts that health professionals are

the most appropriate individuals to evaluate the quality of medical services and that effective peer review at the local level is the soundest method for assuring the appropriate use of health care resources and facilities. . . .

Until January 1, 1976, only a non-profit professional association representing a substantial proportion of the practicing physicians in an area can qualify as a PSRO. If such an organization does not apply to be a PSRO by that date, the Secretary can designate any other organization that he determines has the professional competence and is otherwise suitable to be a PSRO.

The PSRO is responsible for assuring that health care paid for under Medicare, Medicaid, and Maternal and Child Health Programs is medically necessary and consistent with professionally recognized standards of care. It must also seek to encourage the use of less costly sites and modes of treatment where medically appropriate.

The PSRO is required to review services furnished in and by hospitals and other health care institutions, such as skilled nursing facilities. The review of other types of health care, such as ambulatory care, can be undertaken at the option of the individual PSRO and with the Secretary's approval. The internal review activities of hospitals and other health care institutions are to be utilized by the PSRO in carrying out its functions to the extent these activities are determined to be effective by the PSRO. . . . Fiscal agents are required to abide by the PSRO's determination as to the medical necessity and appropriateness of services in paying Medicare and Medicaid claims. . . .

106   *Summary of PSRO Review Responsibilities*
. . . For review in short-stay general hospitals, the PSRO will at a minimum perform (a) admission certification concurrent with the patient's admission, (b) continued stay review, and (c) medical care evaluation studies. . . . As the capability progresses in its area [it has the responsibility] to develop criteria and standards and select norms for each type of review which it performs*. . . .

* Definitions, as provided in Chapter VII, Sec. 709 of the PSRO Program Manual, are:
Norms—Medical care appraisal norms are numerical or statistical measures of usual observed performance.
Standards—Standards are professionally developed expressions of the range of acceptable variation from a norm or criterion.
Criteria—Medical care criteria are predetermined elements against which aspects of the quality of medical service may be compared. They are developed by professionals relying on professional expertise and on the professional literature.

110   *Hearings, Review and Sanctions ...*
110.20   On the basis of its investigations of situations of possible
abuse identified in its reviews, the PSRO may (after reasonable
notice and opportunity for discussion with the provider or
practitioner) recommend to the Secretary appropriate action
against persons responsible for gross or continued overuse of
services or for inadequate quality of services. . . .

PSROs, to be established nationally in 203 geographic areas
designated by the Secretary of the DHEW, obviously represented
a new game in town. Not only were individual instances of care
to be examined, but penalties could be invoked against transgressors of the law and regulations, although it was not made precisely clear what transgressions were.

The reaction to PSROs clearly demonstrates that one man's
meat is another man's poison. For example, the American Medical Association (1974) felt that the penalties for poor performance by a physician were much too strong, whereas the consumer
advocate organization Health-PAC felt that they were much too
weak (Lander).* We can outline a few of the major points discussed in the extensive literature on the subject.

Peer review itself has certain problems in terms of its efficacy:
even with HEW looking over their shoulders, can physicians
resist guild protectionism any more effectively than they have to
date? (Freidson, pp. 178-183, 363-382). Furthermore, one won-
ders if peer review can effectively deal with patients' complaints
about provider-patient communications: the "my doctor won't
talk to me" syndrome, which seems to concern patients as much
as or more than problems with the technical content of care
(Birch and Wolfe), is not recognized as a problem by most doctors. Finally, PSRO may quickly succumb to what would be a natural tendency to concentrate on economizing rather than on quality control.

Many representatives of organized medicine argue that PSROs
represent "government interference in the practice of medicine"

---

* The literature on the controversy quickly grew to rather large proportions (McCarthy; Nelson, Davidson; Flashner et al.; Welch, 1973,
1974; Brian; *Medical World News*, 1974a, b; McMahon; Fishbein, Bennett; Colock; Greenberg; Slee; Simmons; Ginzburg; Jesse et al.;
Sanazaro). A comprehensive discussion of PSROs is contained in an
early book by Decker and Bonner.

(American Medical Association; Fishbein; *American Medical News*, January 14, 1974, February 25, 1975). This argument has a certain logical fallacy when it comes from organized medicine, as the classification of approaches to quality outlined above indicate. History demonstrates that the medical profession does not like specific approaches to quality control, while it has always lent support to general approaches to quality control, licensing in particular. However, licensing certainly constitutes not only government interference in the practice of medicine, but outright suppression of the rights of the unlicensed. Government, through the force of law and the criminal justice system, gives the medical profession a monopoly over that which it defines as the practice of medicine and prevents anyone else from competing. In return, the profession provides a structure-based approach to quality, operated independently. The highest form of governmental interference—a refusal to allow those who have not met organized medicine's requirements to practice—receives the profession's strongest support; that being true, the profession cannot logically attack PSROs simply on the grounds of "government interference in the practice of medicine."

A more serious hurdle to be faced by PSRO as an institution is that it is being called upon to do a massive job in quality control for which not all theoretical and technological problems have been solved, to say the least (Brook, 1973b; Brook and Williams; Bellin). The will was legislated but the way is not yet clearly demarcated. By late 1975, only 65 of the 203 PSRO areas designated by the secretary of Health, Education, and Welfare had operating PSROs, with another 58 in planning phase (Washington Report on Medicine and Health, Nov. 24, 1975, p. 2). However, a change in the method of financing PSROs was passed by Congress in December 1975. Until that time, PSROs were entirely dependent upon annual congressional appropriations. From 1976 onwards, PSROs have been able to bill hospitals for their services, the hospitals being reimbursed through Medicare/Medicaid (Knaus), a system which will ensure support independent of congressional action. This change should prove beneficial to the growth and development of PSROs. Another important dimension of PSRO development is the relationship or lack thereof with the JCAH's PEPs. If methodologies, forms, and committees meld positively, both will be helped; if they become competing entities, both will be harmed, perhaps irrevocably.

In conclusion, PSROs represent a distinct departure from the American tradition of quality control. For the first time, a specific approach to quality control has been legally mandated. It still remains to be seen how effective it will become.

Patient Satisfaction and Malpractice Litigation

Patient satisfaction is one specific approach to quality of care measurement and control that has received little attention. A review has pointed out that although little is known about patient satisfaction, in general patients appear to be less critical of the technical content of care than they are of attitudinal and situational components (Lebow), a conclusion confirmed in one of the largest-scale studies of patient satisfaction carried out by the mid-70s (Birch and Wolfe).

One gauge of patient satisfaction is the extent of medical malpractice litigation. By the mid-70s, malpractice litigation had become a matter of major concern in the United States. In 1973, a major commission reported on the matter (USDHEW, 1973), and its many findings and recommendations created a great deal of controversy (Welch, 1975). During the 1970s, the volume of suits increased, the magnitude of settlements rose, and insurance premiums threatened to rise out of sight (Curran, 1975a). The problem is not entirely new. As Curran himself pointed out, in the 1940s there had been complaints about "a plague of malpractice suits." Katz refers to physicians' "alarm at the increase in [malpractice] claims" in the 1840s! Nevertheless, by 1975 the situation had seriously worsened. Insurance companies stopped writing malpractice policies in several states, often after requests for premium increases of 300% or more were denied by state insurance commissioners. In several states, medical societies set up their own insurance companies. Hospitals saw their rates skyrocket: the annual premium for the Massachusetts General Hospital increased 10 times between 1969 and 1975 (Katz). In California, physicians struck in the spring of 1975, seeking to force legislative changes (Phillips), as they did or threatened to do elsewhere (Curran, 1975b).

The wave of legislative remedies became a flood during that summer. Curran (1975b) states: "The thrust of most of the enacted bills can be classified into three major categories: insurance coverage changes; legal-system reforms; and the strengthening of medical disciplinary mechanisms." Most significant legislative changes, however, gored one ox or another, and, as is well known, in the United States gored oxen often go to court seeking a remedy. As a result, the whole legal picture remained quite unsettled.

It is useful to examine some of the causes of the increase in malpractice litigation. First of all, some care provided by physicians in this country is of poor or doubtful quality. Some, but not all, of this poor care involves negligence. Second, as we have seen, physicians have not shown themselves to be particularly competent or capable of policing their own ranks (*Medical World News*, March 15, 1974). Third, some observers think that the incidence of malpractice litigation is related to the deterioration of the doctor-patient relationship. A medical writer in the *Dallas Morning News* wrote a "Message to Doctor and Hospitals." In part she said: "Most of all, doctors and nurses . . . please listen to me . . . You treat me like a human being, and I wouldn't sue you even if you sew up a scalpel in my stomach (*American Medical News*, Aug. 25, 1974).

The role of the profit-making companies that write malpractice insurance should also be considered. Although companies are getting out of the business right and left, it apparently has been profitable (*New York Times*, June 11, 1975). Retention of premiums for expenses and profits, after paying out settlements, was running as high as 50% (*The Lancet*, Feb. 8, 1975). Companies also make profits by investing premiums while they have them. Apparently, the companies were looking at the rapidly rising level of awards made by the courts, and also, it was reported, were having problems with their own investments. Thus, they were asking for huge rate increases, and, if refused, dropped out. As far as is known, however, no insurance company ever saw fit to try to institute reform of quality control and the whole malpractice problem.

Patients, faced either with a true disaster, like total paralysis resulting from negligence during anesthesia, or a medical profession unresponsive to complaints of a not-so-catastrophic nature, have, as a last resort, only the malpractice suit route. The contingency fee system—whereby a lawyer takes on a case on the basis that he will get a percentage of any settlement and nothing if the suit fails—makes access to legal assistance relatively easy.

The problems, then, are evident; solutions, involving as they do the interests of both the legal and medical professions, health care institutions, the commercial insurance industry, state governments, and aggrieved and injured patients (Consumer Commission on the Accreditation of Health Services, May–June, 1975), are difficult to find. Among proposed measures are: changes in tort (negligence) law; modification of the contingency fee system for lawyers; no-fault insurance; shorter statutes of limitations; upper limits on judgments for "pain and suffering"; voluntary arbitration; better regulation and improved quality control of physicians and hospitals; and better controls over elective surgery (Special Advisory Panel on Medical Malpractice).

Some Remaining Problems

A number of serious problems remain in quality measurement and control. One encounters methodologic problems in both process and outcome techniques (Brook, 1973a; Brook and Appel). Physicians cannot be sure that their clinical assessments are valid, even when undertaken (Koran, 1975). Moreover, any evaluation of the quality of care that relates to health must take into account that health care is only one factor in the determination of health status (Blum; Lewis; Brook and Williams). (See also Chapters 2 and 15.)

Regardless of the direction of the academic discussion of process versus outcome, the structural technique for quality measurement and control is the only one widely and consistently applied in the United States. It is the basis for licensing, accreditation, and certification, the only approaches that meet with broad provider acceptance. As noted above, experts in the field reject structural techniques as ineffective, but the governmental and medical establishments continue to rely on them.The structure/process-outcome gap leads one to recognize the chasm that exists between the academic researchers in the quality field and those professionals who are charged with implementing the quality control measures on the books. Not only do they generally not talk to each other, but they sometimes don't even speak the same language. In a study of the work of the New York State Health Department in implementing quality control programs enacted by law, it was found that certain high officials involved were unfamiliar even with the "structure-process-outcome" vocabulary, much less the literature (Jonas). At one time the Health Department had a Bureau of Medical Review which was supposed to concern itself with broad methodological problems, but it was closed down in an economy drive. It is not known what the Bureau did, but as one measure of its success and influence, the Health Department had no summary material on its work available (Jonas, p. 114). At the same time, there is a noticeable lack in the academic literature of any consideration of the real problems encountered by professionals in the field, whether they are with governmental or voluntary agencies, when they attempt to implement quality control measures. The two groups virtually ignore each other, with sad results.

The limitations of peer review must be carefully considered (Ellwood et al., p. 54; McCarthy, pp. 11ff.). Peer review is central to most approaches, both general and specific, in regular use today, with the possible exception of the licensing of institutions. Consumer involvement is a possible option (Lewis, 1974); the Consumer Commission on the Accreditation of Health Services thinks that quality measurement and control without consumer involvement is virtually worthless (1973).

Finally one must recognize that the public at large is generally not concerned with quality measurement and control. Most people never seem to question the technical competence of their physicians, although they are concerned with other aspects of their performance (Birch and Wolfe). Patient complaints about health services are more likely to focus on provider attitudes, waiting time, the physical environment of care, availability and accessibility, and, of course, costs. Creating public awareness of the technical failings of medical care, and then translating such awareness into action, is the greatest challenge faced by those concerned with the quality of health care.

References

American Hospital Association. *Hospital Statistics, 1975 Edition.* Chicago, Ill., 1974.

American Medical Association. *PSRO Deleterious Effects: Information Kit.* Chicago, May, 1974.

American Medical News. "Peers' Role Stressed by AMA President." December 10, 1973, p. 3.

———. "PSRO Prompts Surgeon to Retire." January 14, 1974.

———. "In the Hospital, I Am a Bundle of Fears." August 25, 1974.

———. "PSRO Law Assailed by Indiana Legislature." February 25, 1975.

———. "MD-Public Meeting Favorable, So Far." January 19, 1976, p. 13.

Anderson, A. J., and Altman, I. *Methodology in Evaluating the Quality of Medical Care.* Pittsburgh, Pa: University of Pittsburgh Press, 1962.

Bellin, L. E. "PSRO—Quality Control or Gimmickry?" *Medical Care,* *12,* 1012, 1974.

Bennett, W. F. "Education Is PSRO Goal." *Hospitals, J.A.H.A.,* March 1, 1974, p. 53.

Birch, J. S., and Wolfe, S. "Consumers Assess Alternative Kinds of Health Service." Delivered at Annual Meeting, American Public Health Association, November 20, 1975, Chicago, Illinois.

Bird, D. "Substandard Care Is Found in the Majority of 105 Hospitals in Federal Spot Check." *The New York Times,* March 23, 1975.

Blum, H. L. "Evaluating Health Care." *Medical Care, 12,* 999, 1974.

Brian, E. "Foundation for Medical Care Control of Hospital Utilization: CHAP—A PSRO Prototype." *New England Journal of Medicine, 288,* 878, 1973.

Brook, R. H. "Critical Issues in the Assessment of Quality of Care and Their Relationship to HMO's." *Journal of Medical Education, 48,* 114, April, 1973. Part 2(a).

Brook, R. H. *Quality of Care Assessment: A Comparison of Five Methods of Peer Review.* National Center for Health Services Research and Development. Washington, D.C.: USDHEW, 1973 (b).

Brook, R. H., and Appel, F. A. "Quality of Care Assessment: Choosing a Method for Peer Review." *New England Journal of Medicine, 288,* 1323, 1973.

Brook, R. H., and Williams, K. N. "Quality of Health Care for the Disadvantaged." *Journal of Community Health, 1,* 132, 1975.

Brown, C. A. "The Division of Laborers: Allied Health Professions." *International Journal of Health Services, 3,* 435, 1973.

Bureau of Health Manpower Education. *Certification in Allied Health Professions: 1971 Conference Proceedings.* Bethesda, Md.: USDHEW 1973, Pub. No. (NIH) 73–246.

Christoffel, T. "Medical Care Evaluation: An Old New Idea." *Journal of Medical Education, 51,* 83, 1976 (a).

Christoffel, T. Personal communication, March 15, 1976 (b).

Christoffel, T. "A Selected Bibliography of Literature of Quality Patient Care." *Quality Review Bulletin,* Jan./Feb., 1976, p. 30 (c).

Cohen, H. S. "Professional Licensure, Organization Behavior and the Public Interest." *Health and Society, 51,* 73, 1973.

Cohen, H. S. "Manpower and Social Controls." *Hospitals, J.A.H.A.,* April, 1974, p. 105.

Cohen, H.S., and Miike, L. H. "Toward a More Responsive System of Professional Licensure." *International Journal of Health Services, 4,* 265, 1974.

Colock, B. P. "PSRO's." *New England Journal of Medicine, 290,* 1318, 1974.

Consumer Commission on the Accreditation of Health Services. "A Message about the Commission." *Health Perspectives, 1,* April, 1973.

――――. "Consumer Experiences in Hospital Accreditation." *Quarterly,* Spring, 1974 (a).

――――. "JCAH Accreditation—The Lincoln Experience." *Quarterly,* Summer, 1974 (b).

――――. "Hospital Accreditation—Where Do We Go from Here?" *Health Perspectives,* March–April, 1975 (a).

――――. "Malpractice! A Consumer View." *Health Perspectives,* May–June, 1975 (b).

Curran, W. J. "Malpractice Insurance: A Genuine National Crisis." *New England Journal of Medicine, 292,* 1223, 1975 (a).

Curran, W. J. "Malpractice Crisis: The Flood of Legislation." *The New England Journal of Medicine, 293,* 1182, 1975 (b).

Davidson, S. M. "Professional Standards Review Organizations: A Critique." *Journal of the American Medical Association, 226,* 1106, 1973.

Decker, B., and Bonner, P. *PSRO: Organization for Regional Peer Review.* Cambridge, Mass.: Ballinger Publishing Co., 1973.

Derbyshire, R. C. *Medical Licensure and Discipline in the United States.* Baltimore, Md.: Johns Hopkins Press, 1969.

Donabedian, A. "Evaluating the Quality of Medical Care." *Milbank Memorial Fund Quarterly, 44,* 166, 1966.

Donabedian, A. "Promoting Quality through Evaluating the Process of Patient Care." *Medical Care, 6,* 181, 1968.

Donabedian, A. *A Guide to Medical Care Administration.* II: *Medical Care Appraisal—Quality and Utilization.* New York: American Public Health Association, 1969.

Egelston, E. M. "Licensure—Effects on Career Mobility," *American Journal of Public Health, 62,* 50, 1972.

Ellwood, P. M., Jr., et al. *Assuring the Quality of Health Care.* Minneapolis, Minn.: Interstudy, 1973.

Fishbein, M. "On PSRO's and Government Interference with Medicine." *Medical World News,* February 8, 1974, p. 88.

Fitzgibbon, A. "Future of the J.C.A.H., Part II, Joint Commission's Strengths Emerge amid wide Criticism." *Hospital Tribune,* May 19, 1975.

Flashner, B. A. et al. "Professional Standards Review Organizations." *Journal of the American Medical Association, 223,* 1473, 1973.

Forgotson, E. H., and Roemer, R. "Government Licensure and Voluntary Standards for Health Personnel and Facilities: Their Power and Limitation Is Assuring High Quality Care." *Medical Care, 6,* 345, 1968.

Freidson, E. *Profession of Medicine*. New York: Dodd, Mead, 1975.
Ginzburg, E. "Notes on Evaluating the Quality of Medical Care." *New England Journal of Medicine, 292,* 366, 1975.
Greenberg, D. S. "Medicine and Public Affairs." *New England Journal of Medicine, 290,* 1493, 1974.
Hollis, G. *State Licensing of Health Facilities*. Washington, D.C.: National Center for Health Statistics, USDHEW, 1968.
Hospital Week. "The Joint Commission on Accreditation of Hospitals Filed Suit." June 6, 1975.
Jacobs, C. M., and Christoffel, T. M. *The Rationale for Outcome Audit*. Chicago, Ill.: Quality Review Center, Joint Commission on Accreditation of Hospitals, 1975.
Jacobs, C. M. et al. *Measuring the Quality of Patient Care*. Cambridge, Mass.: Ballinger, 1976.
Jesse, W. F. et al. "PSRO: An Educational Force for Improving Quality of Care." *New England Journal of Medicine, 292,* 668, 1975.
Joint Commission on Accreditation of Hospitals. *Accreditation Manual for Hospitals, 1970, Updated 1973*. Chicago, Ill., 1973.
Jonas, S. *Aspects of Ambulatory Care Quality Control in New York State: Implications for National Health Insurance*. New York: Springer Publishing Co., in press.
Jonas, S., and Sidel, V. W. "The Delivery of Health Care." In Tice's *Practice of Medicine*, Vol. I, Chapter 21. Harper and Row, Hagerstown, Md., 1973.
Katz, B. F. "The Medical Malpractice Crisis—Its Cause and Effects." Presented at the Annual Meeting, American Public Health Association, November 19, 1975, Chicago, Illinois.
Kessner, D. M., and Kalk, C. E. *Contrasts in Health Status, 2: A Strategy for Evaluating Health Services*. Washington, D.C.: Institute of Medicine, 1973.
Kessner, D. M. et al. "Assessing Health Quality—The Case for Tracers." *New England Journal of Medicine, 288,* 189, 1973.
Kessner, D. M. et al. *Contrasts in Health Status, 3: Assessment of Medical Care for Children*. Washington, D.C., Institute of Medicine, 1974.
Knaus, W. A. "Eleventh Hour Reprieve for PSRO." *American Medical News-Impact*, February 23, 1976, p. 4.
Koran, L. M. "The Reliability of Clinical Methods, Data and Judgments." *New England Journal of Medicine, 293,* 642, 695, 1975.
Kuehn, H. R. "The Commission on Professional and Hospital Activities." *Bulletin, American College of Surgeons*, October, 1973.
Lander, L. "PSRO's: A Little Toe in the Door." *Health/PAC Bulletin*, July/August, 1974, p. 1.
Lebow, J. L. "Consumer Assessments of the Quality of Medical Care." *Medical Care, 12,* 328, 1974.

Lee, R. I., and Jones, L. W. *The Fundamentals of Good Medical Care.* Chicago, Ill.: University of Chicago Press, 1933. Reprinted, Hamden, Conn.: Archon Books, 1962.

Lembcke, P. A. "Medical Auditing by Scientific Methods." *Journal of the American Medical Association, 162,* 646, 1956.

Lerner, H. J. *Manpower Issues and Voluntary Regulation in the Medical Specialty System.* New York: Prodist, 1974.

Lewis, C. E. "The State of the Art of Quality Assessment—1973." *Medical Care, 12,* 999, 1974.

Liaison Committee on Medical Education. *Information to Be Supplied by Developing Medical Schools.* Chicago, Ill., 1972.

————. *Functions and Structure of a Medical School.* Chicago, Ill., 1973.

————. *Provisions Leading to Provisional Accreditation of New Medical Schools.* Chicago, Ill., 1974.

McCarthy, C. M. "Public Policy and Peer Review: A Study of the Implications of the PSRO Amendment and Its Impact in Nassau and Suffolk Counties in New York." Master of Science thesis, State University of New York at Stony Brook, 1974.

McMahon, J. A. "PSRO's—Implications for Hospitals." *Hospitals, J.A.H.A.,* January 1, 1974, p. 53.

Medical World News. "How Well Does Medicine Police Itself?" March 15, 1974, p. 62 (a).

————. "NMA Blasts PSRO as Discriminatory." September 6, 1974, p. 16 (b).

Miike, L. H. "Institutional Licensure: An Experimental Model, Not a Solution." *Medical Care, 12,* 214, 1974.

Moore, F. D. "Surgical Biology and Applied Sociology: Cannon and Codman Fifty Years Later." *Harvard Medical Alumni Bulletin,* January-February, 1975, p. 12.

Morehead, M. A. "Evaluating Quality of Medical Care in the Neighborhood Health Center Program of the Office of Economic Opportunity." *Medical Care, 8,* 118, 1970.

Morehead, M. A. et al. *A Study of the Quality of Hospital Care Secured by a Sample of Teamster Family Members in New York City.* New York: Columbia University School of Public Health and Administrative Medicine, 1964.

Morehead, M. A. et al. "Comparisons between OEO Neighborhood Health Centers and Other Health Care Providers of Ratings of the Quality of Health Care." *American Journal of Public Health, 61,* 1294, 1971.

Morehead, M. A., and Donaldson, R. "Quality of Clinical Management of Disease in Comprehensive Neighborhood Health Centers." *Medical Care, 12,* 301, 1974.

National Advisory Commission on Health Manpower. *Report,* Vol. II. Washington, D.C.: GPO. November, 1967.

National Commission on Accrediting. *Accreditation in Medicine.* Washington, D.C., November, 1970.

Nelson, A. R. "The Utah Professional Review Organization." *Viewpoint,* Health Insurance Council, January, 1973.

New York Times. "State Malpractice Insurers Found to be Profit-Making." June 11, 1975.

———. "Few Doctors Ever Report Colleagues' Incompetence." January 29, 1976.

Nolan, P. "A Matter of License." *Physicians Forum,* Fall, 1975, p. 1.

Office of Professional Standards Review. *PSRO Program Manual.* Washington, D.C.: USDHEW, 1974.

Pennell, M. Y. "Accreditation, Certification and Licensure." In McTernan, E. T., and Hawkins, R. O., eds., *Educating Personnel for the Allied Health Professions and Services,* Ch. 7. St. Louis, Mo.: Mosby, 1972.

Pennell, M. Y., and Stewart, P. A. *State Licensing of Health Occupations.* Washington, D.C.: USDHEW, 1968.

Peterson, O. L. et al. "An Analytical Study of North Carolina General Practice." *The Journal of Medical Education, 31,* December, 1956, Part 2.

Phillips, D. F. "The California Physician's Strike." *Hospitals, J.A.H.A.,* August 1, 1975, p. 49.

Phillips, D. F., and Kessler, M. S. "Criticism of the Medicare Validation Survey." *Hospitals, J.A.H.A.,* September 1, 1975, p. 61.

P. L. 92–603. 1972 Amendments to the Social Security Act.

Rayack, E. "The American Medical Association and the Supply of Physicians: A Study of the Internal Contradictions in the Concept of Professionalism." *Medical Care, 2,* 244, 1964; *3,* 17, 1965.

Roemer, M. I. "Controlling and Promoting Quality in Medical Care." In Havighurst, C. C., and Weistart, J. C., eds. *Health Care from the Library of Law and Contemporary Problems.* Dobbs Ferry, N.Y.: Oceania Publications, 1972.

Roemer, R. "Legal Regulation of Health Manpower in the 1970's." *HSMHA Health Reports, 86,* 1053, 1971 (a).

Roemer, R. "Licensing and Regulation of Medical and Medical-related Practitioners in Health Service Teams." *Medical Care, 9,* 42 1971 (b).

Rutstein, D. D. et al. "Measuring the Quality of Medical Care: A Clinical Method." *New England Journal of Medicine, 294,* 582, 1976.

Sanazaro, P. J. "Private Initiative in PSRO." *New England Journal of Medicine, 293,* 1023, 1975.

Sanazaro, P. J., and Williamson, J. W. "End Results of Patient Care: A Provisional Classification Based on Reports by Internists." *Medical Care, 6,* 123, 1968.

Scheye, E., ed. "The Hospital's Role in Assessing the Quality of Medical Care." Proceedings of the Fifteenth Annual Symposium on Hospital Affairs, May, 1973, Graduate Program in Hospital

Administration and Center for Health Administration Studies, Graduate School of Business, University of Chicago.

Schlicke, C. P. "American Surgery's Noblest Experiment." *Archives of Surgery, 106,* 379, 1973.

Secretary's Report on Licensure and Related Health Personnel Credentialing. Washington, D.C.: USDHEW, Pub. No. (HSM) 72–11, 1971.

Sheps, M. "Approaches to the Quality of Hospital Care." *Public Health Reports, 70,* 877, 1955.

Shindell, S., and London, M. *A Method of Hospital Utilization Review.* Pittsburgh, Pa.: University of Pittsburgh Press, 1966.

Shryock, R. H. *Medical Licensing in America, 1650–1965.* Baltimore, Md.: Johns Hopkins Press, 1967.

Simmons, H. E. "PSRO Today: The Program's Viewpoint." *New England Journal of Medicine, 292,* 365, 1975.

Slee, V. N. "PSRO and the Hospital's Quality Control." *Annals of Internal Medicine, 81,* 97, 1974.

Special Advisory Panel on Medical Malpractice. State of New York, *Report.* January, 1976.

Spieler, E. "Division of Laborers." *Health-PAC Bulletin,* November, 1972, p. 3.

Stevens, R. *American Medicine and the Public Interest.* New Haven, Conn.: Yale University Press, 1971.

Subcommittee on Medical Care. "The Quality of Medical Care in National Health Program." *American Journal of Public Health, 39,* 898, 1949.

The Lancet. "Keeping Calm on Malpraxis Insurance." February 8, 1975, p. 325.

Trussell, R. E. et al. *The Quantity, Quality and Costs of Medical and Hospital Care Secured by a Sample of Teamster Families in the New York Area.* New York: Columbia University School of Public Health and Administrative Medicine, 1962.

USDHEW. *Report of the Secretary's Commission on Medical Malpractice.* Washington, D.C., 1973.

Vodicka, B. E. "Medical Discipline. Part VI. The Offenses." *Journal of the American Medical Association, 235,* 302, 1976.

Washington Report on Medicine and Health. "High Court Affirms PSRO's as HEW Ponders Deadline." November 24, 1975.

Weinerman, E. R. "The Quality of Medical Care." *The Annals of the American Academy of Political and Social Science,* January 1, 1951, p. 185.

Welch, C. E. "Professional Standards Review Organizations—Problems and Prospects." *New England Journal of Medicine, 289,* 291, 1973.

Welch, C. E. "PSRO's—Pros and Cons." *New England Journal of Medicine, 290,* 1319, 1974.

Welch, C. E. "Medical Malpractice." *New England Journal of Medicine, 292,* 1372, 1975.

14

Biomedical and Health Services Research: Policy Issues and Financial Support

David Banta

Introduction

The effectiveness of health care services in preventing, diagnosing, and treating disease depends in large measure on the state of knowledge and the success with which knowledge is being applied. As scientific knowledge grows mainly through research, research plays a critical part in determining the future health of the population.

The 1975 Forward Plan for Health of the USDHEW identified four areas where most research is now concentrated:

—normal biological structure and process, and the alteration in structure and process that we call disease
—exogenous environmental threats to health and well-being
—human behavior as it relates to health in individual life styles and public and professional health practices, in choosing known beneficial behavior and avoiding known health hazards
—modes of organizing and delivering health services in order to improve health status and satisfy consumers and providers as well. (DHEW, p. 61)

National health research and development (R & D) expenditures are estimated to have been about $4.7 billion in 1975, about 3.9% of the national health expenditure (NIH, 1976, p. 1).* By

* Research expenditure estimates from the National Institutes of Health, which we use in this chapter, are not consistent with those from the Social Security Administration (see Chapter 9). At least part of the discrepancy is due to the fact that the SSA includes research expenditures of drug companies in the "Drugs and Drug Sundries" category of expenditure (Mueller and Gibson, Table 2). Furthermore, the SSA includes private research expenditures under "service expenditures," because otherwise they would be counted twice.

1974, 68% of the total national health expenditure for research was governmental, and most of this was federal (Table 14-1). The private sector also invested heavily in health research, with industry contributing an estimated $1.2 billion and other private sources accounting for $227 million. These funds were used by a wide variety of institutions. Private nonprofit institutions performed slightly more than half of the research, with industry being the next largest performer. The federal government performed considerable research "in-house," expending $668 million directly in 1974. However, the predominant institution in health research in the United States is the National Institutes of Health (NIH): of its budget of $1.9 billion, $1.6 billion was spent on health research. Most of the remainder went to research training and construction.

This chapter will focus on current work in the areas of biomedical research and health services research.* Only research work, not research training, will be considered.

* This emphasis should not be taken as a denial of the importance of research on environmental health and human behavior. Major work is now being done in these areas: the total federal effort in environmental R & D is estimated at $1.3 billion in 1976, with $69.6 million supported by the National Cancer Institute of NIH, $31.1 million by the National Institute of Environmental Health Sciences of NIH, $2.5 million by the National Institute of Occupational Safety and Health, and $46 million by the Food and Drug Administration (Federal Council for Science and Technology, p. 114). The federal effort in behavioral science R & D in 1976 is estimated to have cost $1.1 billion, with approximately $250 million invested in health-related research through the Department of Health, Education, and Welfare. Of this total, the Alcohol, Drug Abuse and Mental Health Administration (ADAMHA) spent an estimated $122 million and the National Institute of Child Health and Human Development at NIH spent approximately $96 million (Federal Council for Science and Technology, p. 162).

In our discussion of biomedical and health services research, we will consider the institutions that promote research rather than the content of the research itself. A description of contributions on biological research on human welfare is available (American Biology Council). In the mid-70s the several NIH institutes reviewed their important research findings (House of Representatives, Appendix I). In the area of health services research, various excellent bibliographies are available (Flook and Sanazaro; Georgopoulos; White and Vlasak; Williamson and Tenney).

Table 14.1

National Support for Health R & D, Even Years 1960–1974 (in millions of dollars)

Sector	1960	1962	1964	1966	1968	1970	1972	1974
Total (of A or B)	$932	$1,372	$1,730	$2,147	$2,600	$2,856	$3,515	$4,452
A. By Source of Funds								
Government	558	901	1,180	1,471	1,754	1,868	2,387	3,038
Federal	448	782	1,049	1,316	1,582	1,667	2,147	2,754
State	110	119	131	155	172	201	240	284
Industry	253	336	400	510	661	795	925	1,187
Private nonprofit	121	135	150	166	185	193	203	227
Foundations	40	40	43	44	49	47	53	54
Voluntary health agencies	36	38	42	47	57	61	63	84
Other	45	57	65	75	79	85	87	89
B. By Performer								
Government	155	236	308	398	482	575	716	814
Federal	138	215	272	345	403	489	609	668
State and local	17	21	36	53	79	86	107	146
Industry	257	354	438	560	725	828	964	1,230
Private nonprofit	494	736	928	1,122	1,307	1,366	1,719	2,217
Higher education	375	571	713	865	1,030	1,075	1,366	1,740
Other	119	165	215	257	277	291	353	477
Foreign	26	46	56	67	86	87	116	191

Source: *Basic Data Relating to the National Institutes of Health* (Washington, D.C.: National Institutes of Health, 1976), Table 1.
Note: Source and performer data were revised in 1975 to accommodate new figures on state and voluntary health agencies.

Biomedical Research And Development

The USDHEW 1975 Forward Plan for Health describes the following spectrum of activities in biomedical research and technology development:

1. Basic research—activity and pursuit of new fundamental knowledge in the biological sciences and related fields with a high level of uncertainty;
2. Applied research and development—activity drawing upon basic information to create solutions to problems in prevention, treatment, or cure of disease;
3. Clinical investigation—studies in man to increase knowledge in such areas as etiology, pathophysiology, and epidemiology of disease;
4. Clinical trials—research activities to test and evaluate prophylactic, diagnostic, and therapeutic agents in human beings under varying degrees of control in a more defined population;

Table 14.2

Federal Expenditures for Health Research by Agency, 1975 (in millions of dollars)

Agency	Expenditure
Department of Health, Education, and Welfare (total)	$1,867
Health Services Administration	9
Health Resources Administration	58
Alcohol, Drug Abuse, and Mental Health Administration	114
Center for Disease Control	42
National Institutes of Health	1,598
Food and Drug Administration	27
Assistant Secretary for Health	4
Social Security Administration	—
Social and Rehabilitation Service	2
Other HEW	13
Department of Defense	104
Veterans' Administration	93
Department of Housing and Urban Development	—
Department of Agriculture	47
Environmental Protection Agency	20
National Aeronautics and Space Administration	59
Energy Research and Development Administration	143
Department of Labor	1
Department of State	—
National Science Foundation	44
Department of the Interior	35
Department of Transportation	15
Department of Justice	—
Other agencies	31
Agency contributions to employee health funds	—
Total outlays for health, 1975	2,459

Source: *Special Analysis, Budget of the United States Government, 1977* (Washington, D.C.: Government Printing Office, 1976), p. 215.
Note: Because obligations and expenditures are calculated separately, the figures in this table differ somewhat from those in Table 14.5.

5. Demonstration programs—activities to show the efficiency of verified clinical techniques or procedures in a practical clinical setting in a specific region population group, etc.;
6. Control programs—activities to prevent or control disease that span major categories of effort from prevention to demonstration of improved treatment;
7. Education programs—activities to disseminate and communicate to the health professions and the public new and existing information and techniques of therapy and prevention, as well as information concerning the magnitude of disease problems;
8. Health care, per se. (DHEW, p. 74)

Although this framework is attractive and easy to understand, it is important to recognize that these activities do not occur in a well-ordered sequence in the real world. The process is much more complex and much less systematic than this description implies (Office of Technology Assessment). Many programs of biomedical R & D do not fit neatly into one of these categories, and many new applications skip steps in the process. In particular, the difference between basic and applied research is not always clear. Indeed, important basic scientific information often results from applied research activities which, according to the scheme, should be merely following up on basic research (Comroe and Dripps).

The National Institutes of Health

As was mentioned earlier, NIH is the predominant institution in the United States supporting biomedical R & D. NIH is recognized nationally and internationally for excellence in biomedical research. It consists of research institutes (Table 14.3), several support divisions, and the National Library of Medicine. It had obligations of more than $2 billion in fiscal 1975 (Table 14.4). Ten institutes conduct intramural research programs, which consume about 10% of the NIH appropriation, in the NIH's own facilities. Most NIH activities are carried out through research grants and contracts to universities, institutes, and commercial

Table 14.3

Components of the National Institutes of Health, and Year of Founding

Institute	Year Founded
National Cancer Institute	1937
National Heart, Lung, and Blood Institute	1948
National Institute of Allergy and Infectious Diseases	1948
National Institute of Dental Research	1948
National Institute of Neurological and Communicative Disorders and Stroke	1950
National Institute of Arthritis, Metabolism, and Digestive Diseases	1950
National Institute of General Medical Sciences	1958
National Institute of Child Health and Human Development	1962
National Institute of Environmental Health Sciences	1966
National Eye Institute	1968
National Institute on Aging	1974

Note: This table lists the current names of the institutes and the year of establishment of principal responsibility. There have been name changes over time and certain responsibilities have been shifted from one institute to another.

Table 14.4

Distribution of NIH Funds by Category of Expenditure and Institute, Fiscal 1975 (obligations in thousands of dollars)

Function/mechanism	Total	NIAID	NIAMDD	NCI	NICHD	NIDR	NIEHS	NEI	NIGMS	NHLBI	NINCDS	DRR	FIC
Total	$2,056,904	$119,417	$173,564	$699,305	$142,427	$50,019	$35,865	$43,708	$189,533	$327,814	$142,448	$127,131	$5,673
Research:	1,716,165	104,927	154,317	548,256	122,254	41,260	31,021	37,422	130,198	290,903	125,813	124,121	5,673
Regular grants	808,404	64,587	114,632	130,611	78,384	17,436	12,863	29,173	100,939	178,198	81,581	0	0
Centers, resources & other grants	259,001	2,400	3,611	136,337	5,608	7,744	5,270	0	20,257	775	5,891	70,608	500
Animal resources	17,246	0	0	0	0	0	0	0	0	0	0	17,246	0
Biotechnology research	11,076	0	0	0	0	0	0	0	0	0	0	11,076	0
General clinical research centers	42,286	0	0	0	0	0	0	0	0	0	0	42,286	0
Special research centers	125,976	0	3,611	116,132	0	342	0	0	0	0	5,891	0	0
Other special grants	62,417	2,400	0	20,205	5,608	7,402	5,270	0	20,257	775	0	0	500
Research career program awards	26,939	2,513	4,103	2,806	1,912	591	231	768	7,007	4,778	2,230	0	0
General research support[a]	50,202	0	0	0	0	0	0	0	0	0	0	50,202	0
Research & development contracts	346,924	12,765	6,038	199,585	19,258	5,122	3,178	2,458	1,995	82,322	10,892	3,311	0
Collaborative research & support	59,802	0	0	52,863	0	1,655	0	0	0	0	5,284	0	0
Laboratory and clinical research	158,099	22,662	24,757	26,054	17,092	8,712	9,479	4,578	0	24,830	19,935	0	0
Biometry, epid., and field studies	1,621	0	1,176	0	0	0	0	445	0	0	0	0	0
International center	5,173	0	0	0	0	0	0	0	0	0	0	0	5,173[b]
Research training	154,875	8,283	13,595	23,104	11,743	5,442	3,287	4,212	52,787	19,968	12,020	434	0
Grants	96,854	5,081	8,879	9,736	8,937	2,869	2,226	2,114	35,629	12,533	8,552	298	0
Fellowships	58,021	3,202	4,716	13,368	2,806	2,573	1,061	2,098	17,158	7,435	3,468	136	0
Construction	44,976	0	0	44,976	0	0	0	0	0	0	0	0	0
Cancer control	50,389	0	0	50,389	0	0	0	0	0	0	0	0	0
Management & service[c]	90,499	6,207	5,652	32,580	8,430	3,317	1,557	2,074	6,548	16,943	4,615	2,576	0

Source: Basic Data Relating to the National Institutes of Health (Washington, D.C.: National Institutes of Health, 1976), Table 10.

[a] Includes $7,321 thousand in Minority Biomedical Support Grants.
[b] Contains $2,132 thousand for Fogarty Scholars.
[c] Includes $2,388 thousand in Scientific Evaluation Grants.

firms. Grants to stimulate research in medical and health-related fields are generally provided to support projects proposed and initiated by individual scientific investigators; however, the grants are actually made to nonprofit institutions, such as universities and medical schools, which are required to meet certain performance criteria, including financial accountability and protection of human research subjects. Research grants can be used to pay salaries, to purchase equipment and supplies, and to cover institutional or "indirect" costs.

Contracts, on the other hand, generally support "targeted" or applied research—that is, research done with a specific, practical goal in mind. Contracts are usually initiated by the funding unit, and are much more tightly supervised than grants. Profit-making as well as nonprofit institutions may receive contracts, and in fact much contract money goes to private industry.

During fiscal year 1974, $765 million was distributed as regular grants, $335 million as research and development contracts, and $246 million as grants to research centers or to support such facilities as animal breeding stations or tissue-culture collections. The distribution of NIH monies by category of expenditure is shown in Table 14.5.

NIH grant and contract procedures. The procedures for awarding grants and contracts are organized to take into account the complexities of scientific research and development work. Individuals and institutions generally submit unsolicited grant proposals to NIH (scientists may merely assume that NIH is supporting a certain type of activity, but often make informal inquiries to be sure that their proposal is appropriate.) The proposals are assigned to one of 52 "study sections" of outside scientists organ-

Table 14.5

NIH Extramural Research Obligations in Constant Dollars and Proportional Distribution among Institutes

Obligation	1967	1970	1973	1974	1975	House 1976
NIH total	$100	$88	$118	$146	$160	$161
Cancer	100	89	195	248	275	269
Heart/lung	100	82	129	165	146	151
All other NIH	100	89	96	115	136	140

Source: Assistant Secretary for Planning and Evaluation, "Health Transition Papers" (Washington, D.C.: USDHEW, July 1975).
Note: 1967=100.

ized by discipline or area of research. The study sections assess proposals for scientific merit and award each one a priority score. The proposals are then sent to the institute judged to be interested in the subject of the proposal. Each institute has a national advisory council responsible for determining the order in which proposals are to be funded. These councils are supposed to consider factors such as the importance of the proposed research and the priorities established for the institute's program.

The use of study sections introduces the important element of peer review into the grant awarding process. Since they include lay members as well, the advisory councils are potentially an important mechanism for public accountability. (Similar review procedures are used by other components of the Public Health Service that award grants and contracts, such as the Health Resources Administration and the ADAMHA.) However, peer review has been under attack during the past several years, and, advisory councils having become politicized, these mechanisms are not working as well as they might (House of Representatives; President's Biomedical Research Panel Report). In addition, although the grant system is effective in recognizing the complexities of determining the potential importance of research, it may not always be effective in assuring that important areas of inquiry are pursued.

The contract mechanism is designed to meet that need. When contracts are to be awarded, a Request for Proposal (RFP) is developed by NIH staff based on a perceived need. These RFPs are published and distributed, primarily through a daily government publication called the *Federal Register*. Proposals received are reviewed by special groups of outside scientists assembled for that purpose, in a manner similar to that for grant review. Contracts are usually used for support of research and development when one or more of the following conditions exist:

1. The awarding institute or division has identified a need for certain research work to accomplish its mission and has determined that the work must be done outside its own facilities. The philosophy is that the NIH staff should look at the field of biomedical science and direct funds to those areas that are ready for development or need further development.
2. Funds are to be awarded to profit-making institutions.

Under current regulations, grants cannot be awarded to such organizations.

3. The objective is the acquisition of a specified service or end product.
4. The collaboration of a number of institutions must be obtained and work must be coordinated or carried out in a comparable manner by all so that the data collected can be combined for statistical analysis, such as in clinical trials.

The Mission of the NIH. Classically, the mission of NIH has been to increase knowledge, without a corresponding commitment to knowledge application (House of Representatives). In recent years, four new functions have been stressed (Kupfer and Kretchmer) :

1. Evaluation of the application of research findings, especially through controlled clinical trials and through short-term demonstration and control programs in local communities to evaluate the applicability of new knowledge. NIH is already deeply involved in such activities. For example, in 1975 almost 10% of NIH monies were used to support more than 1,000 clinical trials, 65% of them controlled clinical trials (National Institutes of Health, May 16, 1975).
2. Application of research findings through coordination with other federal agencies, dissemination of information to providers, and education of the public (National Institutes of Health, March 7, 1975).
3. Cooperation with government-wide efforts to resolve special national health problems. Although NIH is not accustomed to working closely with other federal agencies, it has led in the development of a Rubella vaccine, and has been deeply involved in similar efforts.
4. Provision of scientific consultation in the development of new programs to improve the nation's health.

Problems at the NIH. In about 1968, the role and functioning of NIH began to be questioned by critics both inside and outside the institution. The biomedical research community has been concerned about funding levels (Shannon) : extramural research (grants and contracts given to outside institutions) began to fall after 1967, and while the so-called "War on Cancer," initiated in 1971 (Strickland), increased the money available to the National

Cancer Institute, other institutes did not catch up until the mid-1970s. Cancer research now has a larger proportion of NIH resources than it did before 1971, despite the importance of such other disease problems as heart disease (House of Representatives).

Furthermore, during the Nixon Administration, political interference in the operations of NIH became quite alarming (House of Representatives). Two directors of NIH were fired in less than two years. Republican Party membership became almost a requirement for appointment to a national advisory council. Personnel ceilings were imposed so that the total number of personnel at NIH fell after 1968. And a series of impoundments was carried out in an attempt not to spend NIH funds appropriated by the Congress.

These policies led to a series of congressionally mandated investigations in 1975–76. The President's Biomedical Research Panel was established under the Cancer Act Amendments of 1974 to review the biomedical and behavioral research programs supported by NIH and ADAMHA and to recommend policy concerning the content, organization, and operation of these programs. The Panel reported on April 30, 1976 and found little to criticize at NIH, but recommended strengthened advisory structures for the President, the Director of NIH, and the institutes of NIH. Simultaneously, Congressman Paul Rogers, Chairman of the Health Subcommittee of the House Commerce Committee, directed a staff study of NIH headed by the author of this Chapter; this report, while supporting NIH and its programs, suggested the need for certain programmatic changes (to be summarized later in this chapter). Finally, also in 1976, the congressional Office of Technology Assessment examined the impacts of new medical technologies and suggested that NIH should become more involved in technology assessment.

The President's Biomedical Research Panel Report came under fire soon after its release. In Senate hearings on June 17, 1976, Dr. Kerr White criticized the mode of priority setting, which he characterized as being dominated by investigators in academic health sciences centers (1976). He suggested that better methods of priority setting and knowledge application were needed, and particularly stressed the need to validate new medical technology through clinical trials. Dr. Lester Breslow criticized the report for perpetuating the idea that advances in health come only through laboratory and clinical research. He felt that NIH had been reluctant to move beyond discovery of knowledge, and had been especially resistant to demonstration and control programs and to education programs. Senator Edward Kennedy showed considerable concern about the area of knowledge application and technology transfer, and the discussion made clear his intent to see that NIH or some other agency carries such activities out more effectively in the future. The Director of NIH, Dr. Donald Fredrickson, testified the same day to his commitment to improve the "somewhat informal system whereby consensus is reached concerning the validity of the interventions arising from our research."

Thus Congress and the executive branch have identified a series of problems with the present NIH programs:

1. Environmental and behavioral aspects of disease, particularly in the etiology of disease, are not actively pursued. In an era in which chronic diseases of complex etiologies are so important in the U.S. population, a creative blending of laboratory science, clinical acumen, and population studies may offer the best hope for "breakthroughs" (House of Representatives).

2. With the growing involvement of the federal government in health care, NIH has found itself subject to pressures to become more involved in knowledge application and program development and evolution.

3. With increased awareness that new technologies contribute greatly to rising medical care costs, NIH is being asked to help plan the use of new technologies when they are ready for diffusion into the medical care system (Office of Technology Assessment). In particular, clinical trials should be made to test the efficacy of these technologies.

4. NIH, like any other institution, has set ways of doing things which need examination and revision. For example, space and other resources in the intramural program are seldom reallocated.

5. There should be increased public participation in the biomedical research enterprise. The national advisory councils, which offer a mechanism for helping to set priorities as well as for evaluating NIH programs, have seldom been effectively used.

Thus, NIH is an important institution that supports a wide spectrum of biomedical research and development activities, and in general has done its job very well. However, its procedures and policies, like those of most governmental institutions, are being examined with a view to reform, and congressional and administrative assessments may lead to changes along the lines suggested above.

Private Support for Biomedical R & D

Industry provides the major support for private biomedical R & D. The 135 members of the Pharmaceutical Manufacturers Association, which includes some non-drug manufacturers, invested an estimated $932 million in research in fiscal 1974. Companies manufacturing medical supplies and instruments invested an estimated $144 million in that year, and the electronic industry and the non-prescription drug industry invested an estimated $91 million (NIH, 1976). This R & D is conducted largely "in-house," in private research laboratories. A relatively small proportion of this investment is in basic research; drug companies spend an estimated $90 million annually (Silverman and Lee, p. 24). Most of the private money is spent on applied research and technology development, with priorities usually determined by the perceived potential for profit (Mansfield et al., p. 20).

The development of new drugs is based on knowledge of organic chemistry, pharmacology, and human pathophysiology, a body of knowledge created primarily by basic research. A study of 68 pharmaceutical innovations showed that over half were made possible by discoveries made outside of the drug industry (Mansfield et al., p. 185). The targeted work, however, is supported by private funds. Before marketing, drugs must meet standards for safety and efficacy mandated by the Food and Drug Amendments of 1962, which are established and administered by the Food and Drug Administration (Simmons). Tests on human subjects are required, and volunteers, including prisoners, are used. Such testing raises serious ethical questions (Freund; Lasagna).

Medical instruments and devices (e.g., automated clinical laboratory equipment, X-ray equipment, renal dialysis machines, and surgical equipment) are largely developed by the discipline of biomedical engineering, which grew out of a union of mathematics, physics, and the biological sciences (Goodman). The research that makes advances in medical electronics or X-rays possible takes place largely outside the health research community. Such technical advances as the Computed Tomography (CT) Scanner (an advanced X-ray machine) were made by nonmedical people, and some of the earliest publications were made in nonmedical journals. Funding for research and development is largely private, although there is some government funding. In a profit-oriented marketplace, medical equipment manufacturers may develop and produce equipment of questionable utility if it will sell, and may not produce needed innovations of questionable profitability (Utterback).

Finally, the medical community produces innovative procedures, consisting of new techniques, together with drugs and/or equipment (Office of Technology Assessment). An obvious example of a procedure is a new surgical approach requiring not only the surgeon's skill but also specialized equipment and drugs. Procedures are developed in a very complex manner because of their different components. At present, a practitioner or clinical researcher may try out any new procedure on a patient, with only informal constraints such as peer review and the threat of malpractice litigation. These innovations are important, but it has been recognized that human experimentation sometimes occurs without informed consent on the part of patients (Freund). Furthermore, the efficacy of these new procedures is not assured by any formal mechanism. Formal systems to regulate such developments for the protection of the public have been proposed; the National Commission for Protection of Human Subjects, established by statute in 1974, is grappling with some of these issues, as is the Office of Technology Assessment.

Health Services Research*
Content and Uses

Health services research and development is an iterative process which is aimed to influence the delivery of health care (President's Science Advisory Committee). It may be divided into four major components or functions: (1) collection and diffusion of information and statistics; (2) development and evaluation of new health services systems and processes; (3) research and training; and (4) policy analysis. In short, health services research is pragmatic, has no easily defined boundaries, and does not belong to a classical discipline such as medicine or economics.

* This section is modified from D. Banta and P. Bauman, "Health Services Research and Health Policy," *Journal of Community Health, 2,* 1976. It is included with the permission of the publisher.

It encompasses many bodies of knowledge, including epidemiology, biomedical sciences, economics, sociology, engineering, systems analysis, and management science (President's Science Advisory Committee).

Health services research and biomedical research generally complement each other, but they overlap in some areas. Biomedical research seeks the fundamental knowledge necessary to prevent, treat, and control disease, to restore function, and to minimize disability. Health services research strives to make that knowledge more readily available and to define and evaluate the systems by which it can be applied to populations.

Because health services research (HSR) and biomedical research often address similar problems and are often funded together, it is useful to note their differences. Let us take the case of a coronary-care unit (President's Science Advisory Committee). Biomedical research lays the groundwork for treatment, and biomedical engineering designs the diagnostic and therapeutic equipment. Health services research then determines the need and demand for such a service and carries out controlled clinical trials to determine efficacy. Trials are undertaken by biomedical *and* health services researchers, ideally together, with the latter considering primarily cost, staffing, efficiency, size, administrative problems, and acceptability. The health service researchers then plan the location of such units, evaluating their effectiveness, developing methods of quality control, and comparing the performance of different units. This is of course a model of the process, which often works less smoothly and systematically in practice.

The impact of health services research, unlike biomedical research, is ambiguous. Who should respond to the findings of such research? Two levels of potential impact have been identified: provider-consumer interaction and government decision-making. This view considers that the traditional model of the authoritarian medical professional and the care-seeking, naive patient is not conducive to change (White and Murnaghan). It has further been said that health services research poses a threat to professional autonomy; for this reason, the outcomes of health services research often fail to affect health care (Mechanic, p. 60). Since the profession will ignore such research, Mechanic argues that researchers must aim to influence governmental, especially federal, policy-making.

Governmental health policy is set by both Congress and the

executive.* As the government functions, the consumers of health services research comprise the advisers of policy makers: that is, staff to committees or individuals in Congress, staff to the Secretary of the USDHEW and other HEW officials, staff in the Office of Management and Budget (OMB), and staff to White House officials. In the mid-70s, staff in the executive branch had a predominantly economic orientation, while physicians and lawyers predominated in the Congress (Ellwood). The communication barriers between these "two cultures" of consumers and producers are considerable.

These staff people, who continually search for data to help the decision-making process, value health services research. Of course, there is a vast difference between raw data—which is difficult for executive and congressional staff to interpret, since they are not prepared by their professional education to do so—and analysis of data that reveals an array of policy opportunities. The use of data takes different forms in the two branches of government. The executive is interested in generating policy; thus courses of action are advocated based on available data. The Congress, however, is accustomed to reacting to executive branch proposals, so it tends to seek data that prove or disprove a particular point, that justify its positions.

Of course, there are limits to the use of data. In the first place, many decisions made in the government are appropriately political, being determined by what the people or influential subsets of the people want. Second, as has been pointed out in Chapters 10 and 11, the federal health policy process is fragmented among three branches, and, within branches, among many congressional committees and numerous executive departments and agencies. This fragmentation means that incrementalism—moving by small steps—rather than coherent, rational health policy development, is likely to remain the predominant method of policy-making in the United States. However, this long-range approach allows

---

* Policy has been defined as "any set of values, opinions and actions which moves decision-making . . . in certain directions" (Anderson, 1966). Titmus (1974) expanded on this formulation: ". . . policy can be taken to refer to the principles that govern action directed towards given ends. The concept denotes action about means as well as ends, and it, therefore, implies change: changing situations, systems, practices, behavior. . . . The concept of policy is only meaningful if we . . . believe it can affect change."

more opportunity for application of data, information, and technical feedback, and we may assume that health services research will grow in importance.

Financial Support for Health Services Research

Amount of funding available. There is no overall survey information available about the total amount of funding for HSR, but government officials estimate expenditures in excess of $100 million annually in the United States from all sources. Most funding is federal, but private organizations, including service institutions, also carry out research, and industry engages in activities that might be termed HSR.

National Center for Health Services Research. Given the complexity of the federal policy-making process and structures, it is not surprising that federal support for health services research exists in a variety of agencies and programs in the executive branch. The most visible agency—the National Center for Health Services Research (NCHSR)—was established in 1968 to serve as a focal point for investigations of the health care delivery system. Yearly appropriations for the Center grew steadily until 1972, and then began to decline: the appropriation fell from $56 million in 1972 to $38 million in 1974 (National Center for Health Services Research, Forward Plan) to $26 million in the fiscal year 1976 HEW appropriation.

This reduction is often interpreted as reflecting a lack of interest in HSR on the part of Congress and the Administration. In reality, the loci of funding have shifted, and it is far from clear that actual total expenditures by the federal government for HSR have fallen. The National Center has not competed well for funding; its dwindling appropriations reflect in part a failure to project a strong image and to make a convincing case for the Center's success in translating research into improved health care delivery systems.

Other HEW funding. The difficulty of determining federal expenditures for HSR is indicated by the fact that the Office of Management and Budget (OMB) lists nine sources that dispense health research funds within the DHEW, and eight departments besides HEW that fund health research (see Table 14-1). Some of these funds undoubtedly were used to support health services research, as well as biomedical research.

Within HEW, almost 10% of the appropriation for NIH supports clinical trials, as already mentioned. Furthermore, the cancer and heart programs, among others, include demonstration and control programs, many functions of which are germane to health services research. For example, a recent research paper commissioned by the National Cancer Institute analyzed and made recommendations about improving the geographic siting of cancer centers (Ellwein and Kalberer).

In addition, two major federal sources of funding for health services research are not reflected in the OMB analysis. Under Section 513 of the Public Health Service Act, the Secretary of HEW is authorized to spend up to 1% of health program appropriations—about $35 million at present—to evaluate those programs. Most of these monies are spent for contract research and evaluation, which is carried out by private, profit-making firms.

According to HEW and congressional staff, these studies are of dubious value because of their inferior quality, inappropriate timing, and consideration of issues irrelevant to decision-making. Campbell (1975) feels that such evaluation funding has been a failure, since the findings do little to improve the programs being evaluated.

Another major source of federal funds for HSR is the Social Security Administration, whose Office of Research and Statistics (ORS) was established under the 1935 Act. A recent publication describes some of the activities of the Office (Rice). The Social Security Amendments of 1972 (Public Law 92-603) gave further impetus to health service research activities, directing the Secretary of HEW to carry out studies and demonstration projects with regard to such issues as prospective payment systems, physician services and their reimbursement, and utilization of and payment for ambulatory care services (Social Security Administration). About $9 million was spent for these purposes in 1975, and the sums have been rapidly increasing.

There are multiple sources of funding for HSR, but problems do accrue, especially those of information collection and transfer. It is also easy to make the case that the field is underfunded, even using the most optimistic estimates of its resources, relative to overall expenditures for health care delivery (White, 1967).

Problems in Health Services Research

The greatest problem of health services research may well lie in what has been referred to as "disciplinary research" (Williams and Wysong). HSR is in fact not a scientific discipline; rather, it is a pragmatically oriented, problem-solving activity. The objective of disciplinary research, on the other hand, is to advance the state of knowledge in a particular field, testing hypotheses derived from a theoretical framework. Disciplinary research has been said to reinforce the *status quo*, whereas an "external" or problem-solving orientation is an impetus to change or innovation (Gordon and Morse).

The difference between disciplinary and problem-oriented research has been defined as follows:

> The first might be termed the scientifically selfish approach. The health services are viewed as yet another area in which the social scientist can test the appropriateness and universality of concepts he has forged or in which he can test the validity and applicability of his hypotheses of relationships. The second attitude is the professionally helpful approach. The social scientist can apply himself to the problems with which the health professions are struggling and put his knowledge and research skills to use in solving them. (Burns, p. 224)

While recognizing that interdisciplinary problem-solving is desirable, Pflanz nevertheless advocates autonomy of the social science disciplines when they function within the medical system. The balance of power and of professional values resides so heavily within the medical establishment that autonomy for the social scientist, with attendant self-esteem, is a necessary antidote to cooptation. He concludes: "Rarely is cooperation realized in such a way that each contributes his talent and knowledge while trying to grasp the thought and operational processes of the other discipline" (p. 11).

In short, interdisciplinary research is rare and difficult to achieve, though it deserves to be nurtured. The slow development of interdisciplinary activity, however, should not justify ongoing broad support for disciplinary research that is easier to undertake and that rests on an established academic base. Problems in the health care system are too pressing for policy-makers to rely on abstract disciplinary research to produce needed answers and choices; a more pragmatic approach is essential. The best environment must be that in which well-grounded disciplinarians function in interdisciplinary settings. Variables of interest to a sociologist may not be amenable to manipulation and control in the context of an operating program (Scott and Shore); to be policy-relevant, research must ask appropriate questions that policy decisions can attempt to answer.

Eichhorn and Bice summarize the conflict:

> Health services research conducted by university-based discipli-
> narians has had little impact on policy formulation. . . . Academics
> argue that managers and government officials cannot state objec-
> tives with sufficient clarity to make research possible. . . . On the
> other hand, academics are considered to be cavalier about dead-
> lines, speciously precise about experimental conditions, and gener-
> ally disinterested in the relevance of their findings to policy. Con-
> sequently, leaders . . . [in] government question the value of
> social science research as an aid to decision-making, while aca-
> demics grow wary of the intentions of decision-makers and feel
> misused and misunderstood. (p. 147)

One must also raise questions about the quality of health services research. Recent analyses of studies on policy-relevant topics
have criticized methodology and findings, leading one to ask if
reliable research findings are available to assist policy-makers
(Cohen et al.; Kimball and Yett).

Conclusion

Health research will never provide the answers to all our health
problems. It is clear that, whatever researchers recommend,
many important policies will be formulated or modified on political grounds—that is, on the basis of the fundamental values and
wishes of society, and on changes in these values transmitted
through the political process of a democracy. Moreover, health
services researchers and governmental consumers may both
expect too much. As one writer noted, ". . . research will seldom,
if ever, give cut and dried answers to cut and dried problems in a
cut and dried area. It may do no more than supply the information for an informed guess, or set another set of questions
demanding study in an entirely different area" (Beddard, p. 15).

Nevertheless, many decisions or changes can be influenced by
sound information and analysis, and there is a great demand for
high quality health services research. It may then be asked
whether it is available, and how it may be improved.

Systematic research may well depend on the emergence of
a public policy consensus providing a framework for that research
(Anderson). Despite the difficulties of the policy making process
in a democracy such as the United States, it does appear that the

broad outlines of a consensus have begun to emerge in this country in response to the problems of costs, access, and quality of medical care, all of which are therefore essential areas for health service research activity. The critical task is to develop and test methodology for interdisciplinary, targeted problem-solving.

This author believes that Britain provides a fruitful example of how health research could evolve in this country. In 1971, after Lord Rothschild proposed that more explicit priorities be developed in government-funded research and development, an organizational structure was established. This structure addresses the need that had been identified for a three-pronged organization to bring together the Department of Health and Social Security for England and Wales and its planning process; practitioners and research workers in the field; and a strong expert advisory team led by a Chief Scientist. Research liaison groups have since been set up in different subject areas to meet this need and to present advice on research objectives (Beddard). An alternative but similar structure has been proposed for the U.S., linking those responsible for planning and funding research, those responsible for doing the research, and those responsible for making policy decisions concerning specific problems (Williams and Wysong).

The National Center for Health Services Research has already taken steps in this direction (National Center for Health Services Research, Forward Plan). It may be hoped that interdisciplinary research will be nurtured within health services centers and by means of the intramural research program mandated by Congress in the 1974 Act (Public Law 93-353).

More important, the National Center has changed its orientation. Initially, the center made grants to support studies on fundamental questions in health services. That approach—which did *not* ask for policy-relevant research—probably explains in large part the irrelevance of the Center and its subsequent loss of congressional support. The Center is currently attempting to focus its resources on issues of social utility. It has defined seven program areas of special significance: quality of care, inflation and productivity, health care and the disadvantaged, health manpower, health insurance, planning and regulation, and emergency medical services. These steps represent principles and objectives stated in the British approach.

The central problem, then, is how to improve the image, substance, and process of health services research without fostering unrealistic expectations that technical information can solve broad political and moral problems. The links between the governmental and research communities must be explicitly forged if the questions asked are to be relevant and the answers found translated into actual policy.

References

Aday, L., and Eichhorn, R. *The Utilization of Health Services: Indices and Correlates.* DHEW Pub. No. HSM 73–30003. Washington, D.C.: The National Center for Health Services Research and Development, 1972.

American Biology Council. "Contributions of the Biological Sciences to Human Welfare." *Federation Proceedings,* November-December, 1972, Part 2.

Anderson, O. "Influence of Social and Economic Research on Public Policy in the Health Field, A Review." *Milbank Memorial Fund Quarterly, 44,* 11, 1966.

Assistant Secretary for Planning and Evaluation. *Health Transition Papers.* Washington, D.C: USDHEW, 1975.

Banta, D., and Bauman, P. "Health Services Research and Health Policy." *Journal of Community Health,* 2, 1976.

Beddard, F. "The DHSS." In McLachlan, G., Ed., *Positions, Movements and Directions in Health Services Research,* pp. 7–15. London: Nuffield Provincial Hospitals Trust, 1974.

Breslow, L. Statement before the Subcommittee on Health, Committee on Labor and Public Welfare. United States Senate, Washington, D.C., June 17, 1976.

Burns, E. "Comments on the Health Services Research Papers Conferences." *Milbank Memorial Fund Quarterly, 44,* 224, 1966.

Campbell, D. "Assessing the Impact of Planned Social Change." In Lyons, G., Ed., *Social Research and Social Priorities,* pp. 3–43. Hanover, N.H.: The University Press of New England, 1975.

Cohen, E. et al. *An Evaluation of Policy Related Research on New and Expanded Roles of Health Workers.* Prepared with the Support of Research Applied to National Needs. Washington, D.C.: National Science Foundation, 1974.

Comroe, J., and Dripps, R. "Scientific Basis for the Support of Biomedical Science." *Science, 192,* 105, 1976.

Department of Health, Education, and Welfare. *Forward Plan for Health, FY 1977–81.* Washington, D.C., 1975.

Eichhorn, R., and Bice, T. "Academic Disciplines and Health Services Research." In Flook, E., and Sanazaro, P., Eds., *Health Services Research and R & D in Perspective*, pp. 136–149. Ann Arbor, Mich.: Health Administration Press, 1973.

Ellwein, L., and Kalberer, J. "Optimal Locations of Cancer Centers on the Basis of Population Access." *Federal Proceedings, 34*, 1411, 1975.

Ellwood, P. "Uses of Data in Health Policy Formulation." Presented at the Annual Meeting of the Association of Teachers of Preventive Medicine, November 16, 1975, Chicago, Illinois.

Falcone, D., and Jaeger, B. "The Policy Effectiveness of Health Services Research." Presented at the Medical Care Section, American Public Health Association Meeting, November 19, 1975, Chicago, Illinois.

Federal Council for Science and Technology. *Report on the Federal R & D Program FY 1976*. Washington, D.C.: Government Printing Office, 1976.

Flook, E., and Sanazaro, P., Eds. *Health Services Research and R & D In Perspective*. Ann Arbor, Mich.: Health Administration Press, 1973.

Fredrickson, D. *Statement Before the Subcommittee on Health*, Committee on Labor and Public Welfare. United States Senate, Washington, D.C., June 17, 1976.

Freund, P. "Introduction." In Freund, P., Ed., *Experimentation with Human Subjects*, pp. xii-xviii. New York: George Braziller, 1969.

General Accounting Office. *Federal Efforts to Protect the Public From Cancer-Causing Chemicals Are Not Very Effective*. Washington, D.C., June 16, 1976.

Georgopoulos, B. *Organizational Research on Health Institutions*. Ann Arbor, Mich.: The Institute for Social Research, 1972.

Goodman, L. "The Intersection of Technology with Medicine." In *Engineering and Medicine*, pp. 14–22. Washington, D.C.: National Academy of Engineering, 1970.

Gordon, G., and Morse, E. "Evaluation Research." *Annual Review of Sociology, 1*, 339, 1975.

House of Representatives. *Investigation of the National Institutes of Health*. Prepared by the Staff for the Use of the Committee on Interstate and Foreign Commerce and its Subcommittee on Health and the Environment. Washington, D.C., Government Printing Office, 1976.

Katz, J., and Capron, A. *Catastrophic Diseases: Who Decides What?* New York: Russell Sage Foundation, 1975.

Kimball, L., and Yett, D. *An Evaluation of Policy Related Research on the Effects of Alternative Health Care Reimbursement Systems*. Prepared with the Support of Research Applied to National Needs. Washington, D.C.: National Science Foundation, 1975.

Kupfer, C., and Kretchmer, N. "New Missions Statement for NIH." NIH Memorandum, April 2, 1975.

Lasagna, L. "Special Subjects in Human Experimentation." In Freund, P., Ed., *Experimentation with Human Subjects*, pp. 262–275. New York: George Braziller, 1969.

Mansfield, E., Rapoport, J., Schnee, J., Wagner, S., and Hamburger, M. *Research and Innovation in the Modern Corporation.* New York: W. W. Norton, 1971.

Mechanic, D. *Politics, Medicine, and Social Science.* New York: John Wiley, 1974.

Mueller, M., and Gibson, R. "National Health Expenditures, Fiscal Year 1975." *Social Security Bulletin, 39,* Feb., 1976, p. 3.

National Center for Health Services Research. *Forward Plan, FY 1977–1981.* Washington, D.C.: USDHEW, 1975.

National Institutes of Health. "A Review of Present Practices of NIH in Disseminating Research Findings." Staff Paper, March 7, 1975.

———. "NIH Support of Clinical Trials." Staff Paper to the Director, May 16, 1975.

———. *Basic Data Relating to the National Institutes of Health.* Washington, D.C., 1976.

Office of Management and Budget. *Special Analyses, Budget of the United States Government, 1977.* Washington, D.C.: Government Printing Office, 1976.

Office of Technology Assessment, U.S. Congress. *Development of Medical Technology: Opportunities for Assessment.* Washington, D.C.: GPO, 1974.

Peltzman, S. *Regulation of Pharmaceutical Innovation, The 1962 Amendments.* Washington, D.C.: American Enterprise Institute for Public Policy Research, 1974.

Pflanz, M. "Relations between Social Scientists, Physicians and Medical Organizations in Health Research." *Social Science and Medicine, 9, 7,* 1975.

President's Biomedical Research Panel. "Federal Funding for Health and Health-Related Research." Staff Paper for the Panel, 1975.

———. *Report.* USDHEW Pub. No. OS 76–500. Washington, D.C.: Government Printing Office, 1976.

President's Science Advisory Committee (PSAC). *Improving Health Care through Research and Development.* Report of the Panel on Health Services Research and Development. Washington, D.C., Government Printing Office, 1972.

Rand Corporation. "Policy Analysis for Federal Biomedical Research." In Appendix B, *Report of the President's Biomedical Research Panel,* pp. 73–109. Washington, D.C.: USDHEW, 1976.

Rice, D. "Health Care Research in Social Security." *Milbank Memorial Fund Quarterly, 52,* 225, 1974.

Rothschild, Lord. "The Organization and Management of Government R & D." In *A Framework for Government Research and Development*, pp. 1–24. London: Her Majesty's Stationery Office, 1971.

Scott, R., and Shore, A. "Sociology and Policy Analysis." *American Sociologist, 9*, 51, 1974.

Shannon, J. "Federal and Academic Relationships, The Biomedical Science of 1974." *Proceedings of the National Academy of Science, 71*, 3309, 1974.

Silverman, M., and Lee, P. *Pills, Profits, and Politics.* Berkeley: University of California Press, 1974.

Simmons, H. "The Drug Regulatory System of the United States Food and Drug Administration: A Defense of Current Requirements for Safety and Efficacy." *International Journal of Health Services, 4*, 95, 1974.

Social Security Administration, Office of Research and Statistics. *Work Plan, Fiscal Years 1976 & 1977.* Washington, D.C.: USDHEW, 1975.

Strickland, S. *Politics, Science and Dread Disease.* Cambridge, Mass.: Harvard University Press, 1972.

Subcommittee on Environmental Carcinogenesis. *Report to the National Cancer Advisory Board.* Washington, D.C.: USDHEW, 1975.

Titmus, R. *Social Policy: An Introduction.* New York: Pantheon Books, 1974.

Utterback, J. "Innovation in Industry and the Diffusion of Technology." *Science, 183*, 620, 1976.

White, K. "Medical Care Research and Health Services Systems." *Journal of Medical Education, 42*, 729, 1967.

White, K. Statement Before the Subcommittee on Health, Committee on Labor and Public Welfare. United States Senate, Washington, D.C., June 17, 1976.

White, K., and Murnaghan, J. "Health Care Policy Formation: Analysis, Information and Research." *International Journal of Health Services, 3*, 81, 1973.

White, P., and Vlasak, G., Eds. *Inter-Organizational Research in Health: Conference Proceedings.* Washington, D.C.: National Center for Health Services Research and Development, 1970.

Williams, S., and Wysong, J. "The Uses of Research in National Health Policy: An Assessment and Agenda." *Medical Care, 13*, 256, 1975.

Williamson, J., and Tenney, J. *Health Services Research Bibliography, 1972–1973.* DHEW Pub. No. HSM 72–3034. Washington, D.C.: National Center for Health Services Research and Development, 1972.

15

National Health Insurance

Steven Jonas

Introduction

The issue of National Health Insurance (NHI) has provoked debate and controversy in the United States since the beginning of the twentieth century.* Since no enacted plan will satisfy everyone, the debate is bound to continue far into the future, even after the first act is finally legislated. If the United States experience follows that of other countries, any NHI program will be amended many times, and each time the legislative debate will be fierce. Some might be distressed to learn that—if the past is any guide—both the content and form of the arguments used by the several sides will remain largely fixed over time, regardless of changed circumstances or new information.

In this chapter, we will briefly consider the history of NHI in the United States; the status of NHI in the 1970s; and the relationship between NHI, sickness, and health.

Historical Background

Otto von Bismarck was known as the "Iron Chancellor," first of Prussia, then, after 1871, of the unified German state. Shortly after the bourgeois revolution of 1848, he said: "The social insecurity of the worker is the real cause of their being a peril to the state" (Sigerist, p. 127). In 1881, Kaiser Wilhelm I, in a speech written by Bismarck, said: ". . . the healing of social evils cannot

---

* The "insurance principle" has been discussed in Chapter 10. "Health insurance" is a misnomer, since the various plans are not "insurance" in the conventional sense, but rather prepayment for health services, spreading the costs over a population at large. Furthermore, almost all "health insurance" does not pay for health, but rather covers costs of care during sickness. Nevertheless, as the term is used by convention, so shall it be used in this chapter.

be sought in the repression of social-democratic excesses exclusively but must equally be sought in the positive promotion of the workers' welfare" (Sigerist, p. 129). Various fragmented accident, workmen's compensation, and sickness schemes, both compulsory and voluntary, had come into existence over the previous half-century. Building on them, Bismarck in 1883 succeeded in ushering a Sickness Insurance Act through the German Reichstag (Parliament) (Sigerist, pp. 121–122, 131). Bismarck had wanted a uniform, national system, excluding the private, profit-making insurance companies (Sigerist, pp. 128–129). However, he settled for one that used the existing network of "sickness societies" (private "health" insurance companies, some profit-making, some not) to establish a program that paid for medical care and provided cash support during periods of sickness and accidental injury for certain categories of workers. Two-thirds of the premiums were to be paid by the employee, one-third by the employer. Thus the first national health insurance scheme was created—not by a radical government, but by a conservative monarchy. By the 1920s, most European industrialized countries, as well as Japan, had some kind of national health insurance system, usually partial and/or voluntary at first, then progressing to comprehensive and compulsory (Fry and Farndale, chs. 2, 3; Douglas-Wilson and McLachlan, pp. 1-123, 211-230). The non-European–English-speaking British Commonwealth countries gradually followed suit after World War II (Lynch and Raphael, chs. 16-20; Fry and Farndale, chs. 5, 8). By the mid-1970s the United States had not yet done so.

The first campaign for a national health insurance program in the United States was undertaken by the American Association for Labor Legislation (AALL), a middle-class, liberal, reform-minded group, founded in 1906 (Anderson, Part 2; Burrow, ch. 7). Proposals for a broad social insurance plan had been included in Teddy Roosevelt's Bull Moose Party platform in 1912 (Burrow, p. 135). In 1916, the AALL put forward a standard bill for compulsory medical care and sickness benefits insurance which it proposed that the several states adopt independently. The program would have covered persons earning below a certain income level and would have used existing insurance carriers, with costs to be shared by employers, employees, and the states (Anderson, pp. 62-65; Burrow, p. 136). At first support was fairly widespread, extending to the American Medical Association and even the National Association of Manufacturers (Burrow, pp. 138–

145). Beginning in 1917, however—when the U.S. entry into World War I was deflating the Reform Movement generally— opposition began to surface from several quarters, including the American Federation of Labor (Anderson, p. 67).

Within the AMA, a battle ensued on the issue (Anderson, ch. 7; Burrow*, pp. 146-151), but, as part of a general takeover of power by the practitioner wing from the academic wing, the conservative faction won out (Harris, July 2, 1966, p. 30). In 1920, the AMA House of Delegates passed the following resolution:

> Resolved, that the American Medical Association declares its opposition to the institution of any plan embodying the system of compulsory contributory insurance against illness, or any other plan of compulsory insurance which provides for medical service to be rendered contributors or their dependents, provided, controlled, or regulated by any state or the Federal government. (Burrow, p. 150)

That remained *in toto* the AMA position until the late 1960s (Harris). Even in the mid-1970s, by which time the AMA had adopted an NHI proposal of its own which ran counter to the bulk of the 1920 resolution, the "noncompulsory" principle was retained (H.R. 6222).

Serious consideration was next given to national health insurance during the development of the Social Security Act of 1935. This consideration was stimulated in part by the final report of the Committee on the Costs of Medical Care (1932). Although it did not recommend NHI per se, concentrating instead on proposals for group practice and health insurance that could be either private or government-operated, compulsory or voluntary, it did use hard data to show the need for action (Anderson, ch. 10; Stevens, pp. 183–187). In 1934, President Franklin Roosevelt created the Committee on Economic Security to consider the whole question of social insurance. NHI did not last long on the agenda. The Committee's Executive Director, Edwin E. Witte, wrote:

> When in 1934 the Committee on Economic Security announced that it was studying health insurance, it was at once subjected to

---

* Both Burrow's books and the Harris articles contain detailed histories and analyses of the AMA's involvement in legislative battles over NHI, the Burrow book detailing them through the 1950s and the Harris articles covering the Medicare struggles.

misrepresentation and vilification. In the original social security
bill there was one line to the effect that the Social Security Board
should study the problem and make a report thereon to Congress.
That little line was responsible for so many telegrams to the members of Congress that the entire social security program seemed
endangered until the Ways and Means Committee unanimously
struck it out of the bill.[*] (Anderson, p. 108)

The President wanted the basic Social Security Act, one of the
cornerstones of the New Deal. It was passed with no reference to
NHI.

The next major legislative foray was made by Senator Robert
F. Wagner, Sr., of New York State, whose landmark Wagner Act
of 1938 had established the right to collective bargaining for all
nonpublic employees in the United States. In 1939, he introduced
S. 1620 "to provide for the general welfare by enabling the several states to make more adequate provision for public health,
prevention and control of disease, maternal and child health services, construction and maintenance of needed hospitals and health
centers, care of the sick, disability insurance, and training of personnel" (Sigerist, pp. 189–190). The bill proposed to subsidize
state public health programs (this later became federal policy
through a series of acts), the construction of hospitals (enacted
in 1946 as the Hill-Burton Act), and state programs for medical
care for the poor (eventually enacted in part in 1960 as the
Kerr/Mills Medical Assistance for the Aged, then expanded as
Title 19 of the Social Security Act—Medicaid—in 1965). The bill
also offered cash sickness benefits (a standard feature of the
European/Japanese approach to NHI that has never made headway in the United States) and a program of federal subsidies to
those states enacting comprehensive health insurance programs
(Sigerist, pp. 190–191; Harris, July 2, 1966, pp. 31–32). The bill
died in committee, after being vigorously attacked by the AMA
(Harris, July 2, 1966, pp. 38–40).

Senator Wagner tried again in 1943, this time in concert with
Senator Murray and Congressman Dingell. Their S. 1161 "advocated a national (i.e., federal) compulsory system of health
insurance, financed from payroll taxes and providing comprehensive health and medical benefits through entitlement to specified
medical service (service benefits) . . ." (Stevens, p. 272). This
was the first major legislative proposal for a federal rather than

* The principal opposition came from the American Medical Association (Burrow, p. 193).

state-based system. Once again, the AMA responded with vigor (Harris, July 2, 1966, pp. 40–42). The bill was reintroduced in several successive Congresses, as S. 1606 in 1945 and S. 1320 in 1947 (Anderson, pp. 112–113). That year, Senator Robert Taft, Sr., also introduced a proposal (S. 545) for federal subsidies to the states to pay for medical care for the poor (Stevens, p. 273).

In 1949, the newly reelected President, Harry Truman, having Democratic majorities in both houses of Congress, decided to make NHI a major goal of his administration. He proposed a national, compulsory system, to be paid for by a combination of social security and general taxation, based upon the following principles, which he had originally enunciated in 1945:

> Everyone should have ready access to all necessary medical, hospital, and related services. . . . A system of required prepayment would not only spread the costs of medical care, it would also prevent much serious disease. . . . Such a system of prepayment should cover medical, hospital, nursing, and laboratory services. It should cover dental care—[as far as] resources of the system permit . . . the nation-wide system must be highly decentralized in administration. . . . Subject to national standards, methods and rates of paying doctors and hospitals should be adjusted locally. . . . People should remain free to choose their own physicians and hospitals. . . . Likewise physicians should remain free to accept or reject patients. . . . Our voluntary hospitals and our city, county, and state general hospitals, in the same way, must be free to participate in the system to whatever extent they wish . . . what I am recommending is not socialized medicine. Socialized medicine means that all doctors work as employees of government. . . . No such system is here proposed. . . . (Truman, pp. 629–630)

The AMA mounted a furious attack on the plan, based primarily on the thesis that it was indeed "socialized medicine" (Harris, July 2, 1966, pp. 40–62). Using a major public relations firm and a war chest of over $2,000,000, the AMA, with allies from the drug and insurance industries (Stevens, pp. 273–274), was successful that year and in succeeding years through 1952, when, with the election of a Republican government, it was able to breathe easily (Burrow, pp. 361, 385).

A number of factors contributed to the success of the AMA and other opponents of NHI. The nation's economy was relatively prosperous following World War II, particularly with "rearmament" underway, beginning in 1948. A Republican majority controlled both houses of Congress during 1946–1948. Voluntary health insurance, given a major stimulus by wartime wage-stabilization policies which had allowed more expansion of fringe benefits than of wages, was providing increasing numbers of employed workers with at least partial coverage of their medical bills (Stevens, p. 271). The AMA did engineer a remarkable, if not entirely straightforward, public relations campaign. (It is unfortunate that they have never chosen to put the same kind of effort and money into campaigns against cigarette-smoking, alcohol abuse, or overeating.)

Finally, the Cold War was a decisive influence. Although President Truman was a moderate opponent of the most virulent forms of McCarthyite anti-Communism at home, he is frequently considered to have been one of the coldest of Cold Warriors abroad (Freeland). In a climate of domestic and foreign anti-Communism, it was difficult for Truman to win support at home for a program consistently attacked as "Communist," or at least "socialist," but in any case "red" (Harris, July 2, 1966, p. 50). Thus, in 1951, on the recommendation of Oscar Ewing, the Federal Security Administrator, the Truman administration withdrew its support for NHI and began the campaign that led to the passage of Medicare, limited health insurance for the aged, in 1965 (Harris, July 2, 1966, pp. 58–60; Stevens, p. 274).

Medicare and Medicaid

The campaign for what is now called Medicare* was long and arduous (Stevens, pp. 432–443; Harris, July 9, 16, 23, 1966). The AMA, ever-vigilant, in 1952 opposed and defeated a proposal to expand the Old Age and Survivors Insurance Program of the Social Security Act. Part of that proposal would have provided pensions to persons under 65 who were permanently and totally disabled. The AMA opposed it because the Social Security Administration would have had the authority to hire physicians to determine whether applicants were indeed permanently and totally disabled (Anderson, p. 133). The AMA apparently saw this provision as the tip of the iceberg. With Medicare, the threat was evident; the AMA fought hard, but in the end lost. (Or did they? In fact, physicians have done rather well financially under

---

* Before the passage of Title 18 of the Social Security Act in 1965, "Medicare" referred to a medical care program for dependents of armed forces personnel (Somers and Somers, p. 528).

Medicare. They will probably do well financially under NHI too, as they have done in Canada [Le Clair, p. 69].) In any case, Medicare and its companion Medicaid did indeed represent a step on the road to NHI. The major operational aspects of both programs are described in Chapter 9.*

Both programs, of course, had their historical antecedents. In almost every country in which the central government has undertaken some responsibility for providing or supervising the provision of health insurance on a national scale, the plan started by taking care of only part of the population. This part was ordinarily segregated by income. This is the basic principle of Medicaid, although Medicaid cannot strictly be considered an *insurance* program since the beneficiaries make no direct contributions at all. The concept first appeared in the United States in the earliest AALL proposals, although they were aimed at the working poor, whereas Medicaid covers the nonworking poor. Medicaid-like proposals appeared in Senator Wagner's prewar bill and Senator Taft's postwar bills. Segregation of an eligible population by age, was, however, a new twist, going back only to 1950.

Although they were passed together, Medicare and Medicaid are in principle quite different measures, aside from the different population groups at which they were aimed. Medicare is a uniform federal program, based in the Social Security Administration, financed primarily by social security taxes, available to all persons 65 and over regardless of income (persons ineligible for Social Security may buy into the program). It has copayment and deductible features, offers a limited range of benefits and separate plans for in-hospital and out-of-hospital services, uses fiscal intermediaries (insurance companies) to make payments to providers, and pays hospitals on a cost-reimbursement basis and individual providers on an "usual and customary fee" basis. Medicaid is 50 different state programs, under the general supervision of the Medical Services Administration of HEW's "W" unit, the Social and Rehabilitation Service, but in fact run by 50 different state agencies. It embodies the means-test principle, has, in theory, unlimited benefits, but in reality limited ones because of chronic money shortages, is financed from general taxation, rarely provides for coinsurance, may or may not use fiscal inter-

---

* The provisions of both Medicare and Medicaid as they stood in the mid-70s are presented in detail by Wilson and Neuhauser in their descriptive outline of the United States health care delivery system (1974, pp. 126–146).

mediaries, pays hospitals on a cost-reimbursement basis and individual providers on a fee-schedule.

The experience with Medicare and Medicaid has been mixed (Stevens, chs. 19, 20; Davis, 1975b, pp. 41–55; Lander, pp. 4–35). Some persons, in both the 65-and-over age group and in the medically indigent group, have undoubtedly benefited. However, both programs lack stringent cost-controls and are thought to have contributed significantly to the acceleration in the rise of health care costs experienced since 1965 (Lander, pp. 20–25; Davis, 1973; Finance Committee, chs. 2, 3). Medicaid, in particular, has suffered from uneven implementation (since it comprises 50 different state programs) and is especially sensitive to expenditure-cutting when states find themselves short of funds (Lander, p. 28; Stevens, pp. 479–482; *New York Times,* Sept. 30, 1971; *Health PAC,* April, 1973; *New York Times,* Dec. 27, 1975). Medicare too, although intended as a uniform program, has suffered from some unevenness in implementation, benefitting higher-income and white people and lower-income and nonwhite people differentially (Davis, 1975b).

Since serious attempts to create some kind of *national* health insurance program had been under way since 1912, there was no reason to expect that they would stop with the passage of Medicaid and Medicare. Thus, after a short respite, the struggle started anew (Falk).

National Health Insurance in the 1970s

More legislative proposals for NHI than we have room to describe have been made since the late 1960s. The original group, made in the 1969–71 period, have been widely discussed (Falk; Bills; Burns; New York Academy of Medicine; Eilers; Eilers and Moyerman). Since that time, the major proposals have been summarized periodically by the Ways and Means Committee of the House of Representatives, as in a 1974 publication (Committee on Ways and Means). The American Hospital Association (AHA), the Committee for National Health Insurance (CNHI, Washington, D.C.), and other major interest groups publish summaries of the details of current NHI legislative proposals periodically. A commercial service began publishing a periodical, *Washington Information: National Health Insurance,* in 1974, which keeps current with the various legislative proposals, hearings, and the like.

Rather than reviewing legislative proposals in detail, then, we shall discuss the major issues, the major policy questions, and the major alternative approaches put forward by the principal interest groups. Although these groups have made minor changes in their specific legislative proposals (Consumers' Union) from Congress to Congress, their basic postures have remained the same, with two exceptions: Senator Edward Kennedy's temporary wavering in regard to organized labor's main plan in 1974 (Davis, 1975b, pp. 105-109), and the major alteration in the AMA's position in 1975 (H. R. 6222).* It is interesting to note that the basic arguments concerning NHI have changed little since midcentury (McKittrick; Boas; Falk; Schwartz).

There are also proposals for a national health *service* advanced by such groups as the Medical Committee for Human Rights (Bodenheimer et al.; Bodenheimer; Kotelchuk and Levy; Jonas, 1974b; Lander, pp. 58-61) and the Committee for a National Health Service (CNHS) (1976). Congressman Ronald Dellums had announced his intention to introduce a bill based on the concept (1974), but by the spring of 1976 had not done so. Draft legislation to create a "community-controlled" National Community Health Service was put forward by the Institute of Policy Studies (1976). The Committee for a National Health Service had developed a somewhat different approach. Although based on the concept of "community control," it emphasized national coordination of policy in quality control, health sciences education, occupational safety and health, use of drugs, health rights, and finance and planning (1976). A national health service would bypass the insurance mechanism entirely, providing services directly to patients itself. It could do this in one of two ways: by owning and operating all health care facilities and employing all health workers itself, or by contracting with institutional and individual providers to supply health services and reimbursing them on a basis other than payment-for-item-of-service. Financing would be either from general taxation or through a special, progressive health care tax. Since by the spring of 1976 a formal legislative proposal of this type had not yet reached the floor of Congress, we shall not discuss it at length.

* An excellent review of the situation in the mid-1970s, covering all of the major legislative proposals with the exception of the changed AMA approach, is contained in a book by Karen Davis (1975b). A good deal of the material in this section comes from her book, especially Chapters 4 and 5.

Issues in National Health Insurance

Benefits. Decisions must be made as to what services to cover. By the mid-70s, it had been generally accepted that there should be unlimited (or almost unlimited) provision for basic hospital in-patient and out-patient services, physician services, laboratory and X-ray services, and prescription drugs. Services generally considered more optional are certain kinds of psychiatric care, eyeglasses and hearing aids, medical appliances, dental care, home health care, ambulance services, and nursing home care. Questions of principle may be involved in at least some of the limitations, but essentially they are determined by considerations of commercial interest, cost, and available supply of services.

Coverage. By 1975, most proposals accepted that all U.S. residents would have health insurance made available to them by one means or another, with special provisions to be made for resident and nonresident aliens in certain cases. Still disputed, however, was whether such coverage should be "voluntary" or "compulsory." (Those terms could be applied to both beneficiaries and payors other than beneficiaries.) Those who feel that coverage should not be compulsory for beneficiaries—such as the American Hospital Association, the Health Insurance Association of America, and the American Medical Association—usually refer to "principles of freedom of choice." Those who support the principle of complusion for beneficiaries—such as the Committee for National Health Insurance (a UAW-AFL-CIO coalition)—usually point out that the people most likely to "opt out" are the healthiest members of the population. Thus the financial support of low-volume users would be lost and the system would be loaded with high-volume users. The general association of sickness and low income (Kane et al., p. 6; National Center for Health Statistics, Nov. 1975, pp. 5-8) only increases the financial strains on the noncompulsory system. In systems that are to be financially supported at least in part by direct employer-employee contributions, noncompulsion for employers, advocated only by the Health Insurance Association of America (presumably to enable commercial insurance companies to maintain a significant amount of private business), would only exacerbate the problems that would be created by noncompulsion for employees. In no plan does beneficiary compulsion mean that beneficiaries must *use* the service; it simply means that they must pay their share of the cost. Once having paid that share, all persons would remain free to pay for care privately if they so chose.

Number of plans. Most of the recent major proposals for NHI have advocated multiple plans, usually three, covering different segments of the population and financed in different ways. In the approach advocated by the AMA and the HIAA, Medicare, with a broadened benefit package financed through social security taxes, would be retained for those 65 and over. A second plan, with separate employer-employee financing, would be created for employed workers and their families, and a third program, supported by general taxation, would be developed to cover all other persons. The AHA would abolish Medicare and have two plans, one for employed workers and their families and one for everyone else. The CNHI favors one plan to cover all persons. Financing for the total plan would come from a combination of general taxation and employer/employee contributions under Social Security. The AMA, AHA, and HIAA approaches, which would use general taxation revenues only to pay for health insurance for the poor (in certain cases with state as well as federal taxes), require a separation of the plan for the poor, even if the benefits would theoretically be the same. By the same token, continuation of Social Security tax financing for health insurance for persons 65 and older requires the maintenance of Medicare. A national health service would cover all persons under one care delivery system, and would be financed primarily by taxation rather than by premiums and/or employer/employee contributions.

Multiple plans do present potentially serious problems, however. Since the aged and the poor tend to be sicker than employed workers, undue financial strains could be placed on those plans. If they were then to require increasing tax subsidies, there could be a move to cut benefits, as happened under Medicaid (Lander, p. 28), or to increase deductibles and co-insurance as happened under Medicare, for those persons who happen to need more, not less, care. A separate plan for the poor does require means-testing, with all of the moral and administrative problems that entails. Even more administrative problems are created by those people who change job or financial status. All of this means paperwork, delays, frustration, and high cost. Japan presents a classic example of the difficulties that can arise from a multiple-plan approach to national health insurance (Jonas, 1975a).

Cost-sharing. A critical and sometimes emotionally charged issue is "cost-sharing," wherein the user of services pays some of the cost directly out-of-pocket. Payment can take the form of a "deductible," an amount that the user must pay during a given time period before the insurance plan begins to pay, or of "co-insurance," an amount representing part of the cost that the user must pay for each service. The arguments on this issue have raged hot and heavy over the years (Davis, 1975b, pp. 59-67). Proponents of user copayments usually cite two arguments in their favor, not always at the same time. First, they say they are needed to hold down the amount of tax funds and employer-employee contributions necessary to finance NHI. Second, they say that copayments are required to control utilization of services, on the theory that patients will "overutilize" and "abuse" entirely free services.

This theory of patient abuse of services free at the time of service has a long history. It is based on the supposition that health services are like any other commodity of service; people will use all that they can get their hands on. However, there is little, if any, evidence in support of this point, and logic argues against it, since health services are associated with sickness, an unpleasant event, rather than with health. Furthermore, though a frequent user of health services may not be "sick" in the eyes of the average provider, he may actually be presenting with an illness characterized by the need to seek care, in the basic sense of the word, frequently. In addition, there is a great deal of concern that copayments can easily constitute a serious barrier to the utilization of needed services (as need is defined by providers, not patients) (Roemer et al.).

Those who worry about patient abuse of services also assume that patients make most or all decisions regarding utilization. It is obvious from the nature of the U.S. health care system, however, that after a patient first chooses to seek health services, decisions concerning further utilization, particularly of expensive services like hospitalization and diagnostic testing, are not made by the patient but rather by providers, usually physicians (Worthington).

Major advocates of copayments have been concerned that an NHI plan without significant copayments would result in so much overutilization, particularly of ambulatory services, that the delivery system would be "wrecked" (Newhouse et al.) Research has been done in the field and in the literature to support their premises (Newhouse et al., 1974; Brian and Gibbens, 1974), but the work has been criticized on methodological and theoretical grounds (Jonas, 1977; Myers; Greenlick; Kasten; Roemer et al.; Hopkins et al., Parts 1 and 2). Furthermore, experience in other countries that have introduced NHI programs providing care free at the time of service indicates that the "swamping" effect proponents of copayments predict does not occur (Jonas, 1977).

Reimbursement. Modes of reimbursement for both institutional and individual providers were discussed in Chapter 9. For institutions, under NHI, there are only two feasible methods. One is by rates that are negotiated for a specific time period in the future, based on audited costs occurring during a specific time period in the past, with the institution claiming reimbursement at the agreed-to rates for each item of service rendered. The other is by a negotiated budget for a given time period in the future, based once again on past experience, which a hospital receives regardless of costs incurred.

These are both referred to as "prospective reimbursement" methods, but they differ in nature. The former is a common method used by Blue Cross to reimburse hospitals, often called cost reimbursement. It means that hospitals get paid for rendering services, which can be considered as an inducement to hospitals to provide services. There are no particular incentives to hospitals to control costs, except for the indirect one of state insurance commission limitations on health insurance carrier rate increases, which limit the amount of money available. The global budget method (already in use nationally, of course, in virtually all government hospitals in federal, state, and local jurisdictions), takes hospital income out of a direct relationship to volume of care, and provides direct incentives for cost controls, that is, if provisions are made for allowing hospitals to keep at least some of any savings achieved for program enrichment. If all savings must be returned to the fiscal agent, as commonly occurs in government hospital operations, the only incentive is to spend one's whole budget, for fear of losing funds the next year. On the other hand, with negotiated budgets, rather than with negotiated rates, methods for guaranteeing maintenance of effort and quality become especially important. In general, provider-oriented groups like negotiated rates, whereas patient-oriented groups like negotiated budgets.

Individual provider reimbursement can be by salary, capitation, or fee-for-service, as was discussed in Chapter 9. Although the vast majority of health workers in the United States are salaried, the mode of reimbursement is critical for the controllers of medical practice, the physicians. All major existing approaches to NHI assume that the predominant fee-for-service mode of physician payment will continue in some form. The AMA and HIAA advocate continuing the Medicare mode of reimbursing physicians on the "usual and customary fee" basis. The AHA encourages capitation; otherwise it would have a Medicaid-type fee schedule. CNHI allows for salary, capitation, or fee-for-service, but discourages the last through something called the "pool system." Under the CNHI approach, money for NHI would be allotted annually to defined geographical regions, each region's budget related to both its fiscal experience and its projected health care needs. Thus a fixed pool of money would be provided for each region, to which all providers, institutional and individual, would have claim—except that fee-for-service practitioners would have the last claim, after the institutions and those individual providers choosing to get paid on a salary or capitation basis. A fee schedule would be established, but physicians could get paid only for as long as the money lasted. This system does put a lid on potential earnings and is in a sense a backwards approach to a salaried service. A pool system has been in use in Germany for many years, and is used in this country in Foundations for Medical Care (see Chapter 6).

Under a national health service, individual providers would most likely be paid by salary or capitation, while most institutions would operate on a global budget basis, whether owned by the service or not. It should be noted that any reimbursement method for either institutions or individuals is subject to abuse. Such abuse can best be controlled through motivation, not coercion.

Role of the private insurance companies. As discussed in Chapter 9, in the United States there are two types of insurance companies: the commercial, for-profit type and the Blue Cross/Blue Shield type that are not-for-profit, at least in the sense that retained earnings are distributed neither to shareholders nor policyholders. By the mid-1970s, the Blues had not yet actively entered the NHI proposal competition. However, the commercial insurance companies certainly had; they are one of the four major interest groups that we have been discussing.

The most critical struggle in the development of NHI in the United States centers on the role of the private insurance companies (Jonas, 1974a, 1975b). The United States is the only country in the world in which commercial insurance companies play a significant role in the health care delivery system. They make large profits, which would be increased by any increase in the volume of premiums handled, since most profits come from investment of premiums, not from an excess of premiums over benefits paid.

Furthermore, increasing control by commercial insurance companies over the fiscal administration of the health care delivery system could eventually lead to these companies taking over the whole system to operate it directly for profit. The possibility of such an eventuality should not be taken lightly; the development of Health Maintenance Organizations by commercial insurance companies may well be part of the same strategy (Salmon). The major insurance companies are the largest corporations in the United States in terms of assets and are inextricably linked to the major banks and manufacturing companies by financial dealings and interlocking boards of directors (Navarro). Thus, an NHI plan that provides a major role for the commercial insurance companies could pave the way for a corporate takeover of the United States health care delivery system (Jonas, 1974a,b; 1975b).

In various ways, the approaches of the AMA, the AHA, and, as one would expect, the HIAA, all put the private insurance companies in a prominent position. For most beneficiaries, insurance policies meeting federal/state standards would be purchased from private insurance companies, either by employers for employed workers, or by state or federal government for nonworking persons, with Medicare being retained for persons 65 and older in the AMA and HIAA plans. No proposals distinguish between the for-profit and the not-for-profit insurance companies. Thus the Blues would presumably remain in business, although the competition would be rough. In most of these approaches, regulation would basically be by state governments, with the federal government having a rather limited role.

In the CNHI approach, the private insurance companies would be eliminated entirely, as they would be in any national health service plan. The concept of involving private insurance companies in NHI is historically newer in the United States than not involving them; it arose only as private companies began to become a significant factor in health insurance after World War II. The first legislative proposals for NHI based on private insurance companies did not appear until the late 1940s (Davenport).

The CNHI approach finds its historical forebear in the Wagner-Murray-Dingell bills of the 1940s. The insurance system would be operated entirely by the federal government. The private insurance companies would not be fiscal intermediaries as they are for Medicare, and, in certain states, for Medicaid (Davis, 1975b, p. 73).

This would take the United States in the direction of operating the financing system for health care delivery as a public utility, as is done in all other capitalist countries. Direct federal operation of the insurance system would probably result in lower administrative costs (Davis, 1975b pp. 73-74; Vogel and Blair; *Washington Report*, Nov. 1975), could bring a return investment to the plan if premiums were to be invested (presumably in low-risk situations), would deal with some of the problems inherent in the provider identification of the insurance companies (Law), and would, of course, block the potential corporate takeover of American medical practice.

Administration. Those who advocate multiple plans and buying approved insurance policies from private companies usually favor vesting major responsibility for the administration of the plans with the insurance companies themselves. In this approach, advocated by the AMA and the HIAA, the primary responsibility for regulating the insurance companies would lie with state insurance departments, operating under federal guidelines.

The AHA, which proposes two plans, has a different approach to administration. Insurance policies covering all beneficiaries would be purchased from private companies, but primary administrative responsibilities for the health care delivery system would be vested in a series of "Health Care Corporations" (HCCs). An HCC "is a non-profit private or governmental corporation which (1) is organized for the purpose of furnishing (through its own facilities and personnel or through other providers) non-profit or for-profit comprehensive and coordinated personal health services to persons registered with the corporation . . . and engaging in educational, research, and other activities related or incidental to the furnishing of personal health service . . ." (H.R.1, Sec. 241). They would be regulated by new state agencies, to be called State Health Commissions, in which would be vested "the exclusive authority on behalf of the State to establish and maintain appropriate standards and requirements for all hospitals, nursing facilities, and other institutional health care facilities in the State and to provide for the licensing of such facilities . . ." (Sec. 231).

The HCC concept is intriguing and innovative in that it would vest primary administrative authority neither in the hands of the private insurance industry nor in the hands of government, except insofar as HCCs were governmental corporations within the provisions of the Act. Depending upon how the HCCs were set up, they could lead to control of the system by the AHA's major constituency, the voluntary hospitals, which already have boards of directors used to dealing with health care delivery matters. With appropriate, enforced regulations, they could also lead to broad consumer involvement in health care delivery system operations, in cooperative relationships with providers.

The CNHI approach would vest administrative control in a full-time Health Security Board to be located in the USDHEW. It would exercise its authority through a regional/local administrative system, which is only vaguely defined. State governments would have only a tangential role (S. 3, Part G). The Medical Committee for Human Rights approach to a national health service would place administrative control in a hierarchy of elected boards at the various levels of governmental jurisdiction (Bodenheimer et al.; Institute for Policy Studies). The Committee for a National Health Service would have a similar pattern, with more emphasis on policy coordination at the national level through a series of National Commissions responsible for broad policy areas like quality control and occupational health (1976).

There are several matters of concern in administration. How is the separation of responsibility and authority for the provision of patient-care services to be avoided? Is the system to be turned over to the private insurance industry, in the light of both their past record of performance (Law) and the potential threat of corporate takeover? What role should be assigned to the states? State insurance commissions have an uneven record in dealing with problems of health insurance. Would vesting primary administrative authority in the states lead to 50 different health insurance programs, rather than *national* health insurance, despite federal supervision and "guidelines," as happened under Medicaid (Stevens pp. 477–479; Lander, pp. 28-29)? Would federal control lead to a high degree of centralization, as a trade-off for uniformity of benefits, coverage, financing, and regulations, with resultant bureaucratic strangulation? In any of the systems, how is balanced representation of consumers (tax and premium payers) and providers to be achieved? In striving for such balance, would it be useful to introduce insurance companies, at least some of which would have as their first goal making profits? These are questions which must obviously be considered with care in designing or evaluating any NHI plan.

Effect on health care delivery. Certain NHI plans have more potential than others for changing the basic functioning of the health care delivery system. The key question which must be considered here is how much of what is wrong with the U.S. health care delivery system (as has been discussed by so many observers—see Chapter 1) stems from the way it is financed and paid for, and how much stems from basic organizational and structural problems. Just how important are the matters of the predominant mode of physician organization, fee-for-service private practice, or the predominant mode of hospital organization, the voluntary system, or the predominant role of government in health care delivery, the provision of categorical services with a strong welfare tradition at the state and local levels?

At one end stands the AMA proposal. Their 1975 Bill devotes one paragraph to the matter:

Prohibition Against Any Federal Interference SEC. 41. Nothing in this title shall be construed to authorize any Federal officer or employee to exercise any supervision or control over the practice of medicine or the manner in which medical services are provided, or over the practice of dentistry or the manner in which dental services are provided, or over the selection, tenure, or compensation of any officer or employee or any institution, agency, or person providing health services; or to exercise any supervision or control over the administration or operation of any such institution, agency, or person. (H.R. 6222, Sec. 41)

The HIAA's approach to the maintenance of the medical practice system is similar to the AMA's; however, it does propose—primarily through grant and loan mechanisms—measures "to increase the supply and improve the distribution of health care personnel" (S. 1438, Title II) and "to encourage comprehensive ambulatory health care centers" (S. 1438, Title III), as well as "Provisions to Strengthen Health Planning" (S. 1438, Title IV). The proposed funding levels are very low, but the programs do have some potential for change, particularly if a comprehensive program for ambulatory care were to be implemented.

The AHA's Health Care Corporation concept could lead to vast change (H. R.1, Title II, Part D). Having a single entity responsible for at least all health care payments in a single area is an entirely new approach for the United States. (The AHA proposal provides for, but does not require, such a system. State Health Commissions would be allowed to certify two or more HCCs for

any one area.) (H.R.1, Sec. 236 (b) (3) (B) (iii).) HCCs could
conceivably develop into *the* administrative agencies for all health
services at the local level, even with the maintenance of private
practice and private insurance. These agencies could have a significant degree of autonomy and could provide for a significant
degree of consumer participation in the operation of health care
services, depending upon how the regulations were written.

The CNHI approach to reorganization would be indirect, like
that of the HIAA. Planning, ambulatory care, and health personnel resources would be strengthened and improved, with funding
at much higher levels than provided for by the HIAA proposals.
The formation of Health Maintenance Organizations would be
strongly encouraged as an organizational cornerstone of the
health care delivery system. The CNHI funding mechanisms,
which put private, fee-for-service practice in an unfavorable
position when it comes to reimbursement, could have far-reaching effects on the health care delivery system.

Only a national health service would begin with reform of
health care delivery and then design a financing mechanism to fit
the desired structure, rather than vice versa. Those who see
health care delivery system change as the primary goal will probably advocate this approach.

Quality control. The various plans also differ in the extent to
which they stress quality control. The AMA and HIAA proposals
treat quality control rather briefly, apparently being content to
go along with existing systems (S. 1438, Sec. 2008 (c) (1) (A) ;
H.R. 6222, Sec. 45 (b) (3)). The AHA plan *could* significantly
reorient the quality evaluation and control system through the
powers granted to the State Health Commissions (H.R. 1, Sec.
236 (a) (19)), and to the Health Care Corporations (H.R. 1,
Sec. 244).

Of the insurance programs, CNHI clearly has the most comprehensive approach to quality evaluation and control. A Commission on the Quality of Health Care would be established and
given a very comprehensive list of powers and responsibilities
(S. 3, Title III). It would be required to advise and assist the
Health Security Board in meeting its assigned objective "to
require the highest practicable quality of care that is attainable
in substantially all parts of the United States" (S. 3, Title I, Part
H). There would be national standards for all institutional and
individual providers. All providers licensed after the initiation of
the program would be required to meet national licensure stand-

ards. A somewhat similar, even more comprehensive approach to quality control is envisioned by the CNHS plan (1976, p. 2).

Consumer participation. A similar spectrum of approaches emerges on the issue of consumer participation (Kindig and Sidel, pp. 15-22, 38-43). The AMA and HIAA consign a rather minor role to consumers. The AHA plan has a large *potential* role for the consumer, again with the SHC/HCC structure. CNHI emphasizes consumer participation, encouraging consumer groups to sponsor Health Maintenance Organizations, which are viewed as the most favored mode of delivering health care services (Kennedy, p. 3). On the other hand, the Dellums/MCHR approach would place control of the entire system clearly in the hands of consumers of service (Lander, p. 58), as would the Committee for a National Health Service program (1976).

Cost. One way to look at the cost of NHI is to determine how much the plan itself would cost. Obviously, plans that cover more services will cost more in terms of dollars spent through the plan than those that cover fewer services. On this basis, an evaluation carried out during the Nixon Administration in 1974 (USDHEW) showed that the then current administration NHI proposal would be rather "economical" compared to the "extravagant" CNHI approach. However, a more useful approach is to examine the effect various plans would have on total expenditures for health services.

Under NHI, *total* expenditures could go up, go down, or remain the same. The magnitude of the outlay made through the plan does not necessarily indicate what effect it would have on total expenditures. It must be remembered that ultimately all dollars spent for health services come from the pockets of the consumers of care, whether as direct payments, as taxes, as insurance premiums, or as parts of the payments for goods and services sold by companies that pay taxes and insurance premiums. A plan that funnels a majority of the total expenditure for health service through itself looks very expensive on paper. Yet it might conceivably lead to a reduction of total expenditures if it were able to increase the use of ambulatory services, particularly for prevention, decrease hospitalization rates (the most expensive service), better regulate the incomes of physicians and dentists, and generally address itself to improving the efficiency of the delivery system. Conversely, a plan with no regulatory mechanisms for physician reimbursement and little control over physician use of the delivery system's resources, particularly hospitals, could ultimately be expensive, though it is cheap on paper. This view is supported by data from the Congressional Budget Office.

The three trade associations—the AMA, the AHA, and the HIAA—treat their own particular interests well when it comes to costs. The AMA uses the "usual and customary or reasonable charges" approach to physician reimbursement, but is slightly stricter with hospitals, requiring some kind of prospective reimbursement method (H.R. 6222, Secs. 32 (3) and (4)). The HIAA is just about as liberal as the AMA with physicians and hospitals (S. 1438, Secs. 2002 (e) (1) (A) and (C) and 2008). The HIAA plan has unique provisions for protecting insurance companies against insolvency (S. 1438, Sec. 2016). The AHA would have a fee schedule for physicians (H.R.1, Sec. 246). They would also make sure that "the financial requirements of hospitals and other health care institutions shall be prescribed by regulations," that is, not in any NHI law itself, but in the administrative regulations written to implement it (McMahon, p. 17). This provision would take good care of the hospitals, particularly in areas in which they feel they have trouble with reimbursement formulae now: education, renovation, major construction, maintaining an "adequate" cash flow, receiving a "reasonable" surplus, and the like.

The CNHI approach would attempt to meet the cost problem head on through stringent quality control measures, annual budgeting rather than reimbursement by item of service for hospitals, making fee-for-service the least favored mechanism for paying doctors, and the like. Fee-for-service private practice presumably has an inflationary effect by allowing physicians a great deal of influence over both their own income levels and total volume of service provided.

When calculating the cost of NHI, then, we must consider not only the number of dollars that would flow through the plan but also the effect the plan, when in full operation, will have on the total expenditure for health services.

Catastrophic health insurance. "Catastrophic health insurance" must be considered an interim step on the road to NHI. We have pointed out that most other countries have commenced NHI by covering part of the expenses of the elderly and of the nonworking poor. "Catastrophic" would extend coverage to all Americans for very high expenditures for health care: it would be "major medical" insurance for all. The principal supporters of the catastrophic approach in the Congress have been Senators Long and

Ribicoff. Their bill in the 94th Congress (S. 2470) had three parts. The first would provide Medicare benefits to persons who incurred medical costs of $2,000 or were hospitalized for 60 days. It would be financed through the Social Security System. The second part would federalize Medicaid, providing for uniform eligibility standards and benefits; extend the coverage to the working as well as the nonworking poor; and transfer its administration from the Social and Rehabilitation Service to the Social Security Administration. The third part would provide a "certification" program for private health insurers' policies. The federal government would set minimum standards, and after three years Medicare intermediaries would have to offer "certified" policies to the general public.

The supporters of this approach point out that it would provide protection against bankrupting illness for all, extend uniform benefits to all of the nation's poor, and set guidelines for private insurers. It would not, however, deal with rising costs, maldistribution of personnel and facilities, delivery system reform, or quality control. The Committee for National Health Insurance was particularly sharp in its critique, saying that catastrophic insurance would:

1. Distract Congress and the public from the serious study of a comprehensive national health insurance program for several years.
2. Exacerbate the current inflation of health-care costs by adding to incentives for very expensive care.
3. Invite less scrupulous providers to *raise prices* especially for the seriously ill and dying, on the excuse that the family or individual would thereby become eligible for catastrophic benefits.
4. Create incentives for longer hospitalization—there would be enormous family pressure to keep the patient hospitalized until the trigger point for catastrophic [coverage] is reached.
5. Weaken efforts to institute quality controls (even any controls written into the bill could not be instituted until after the 60th day of hospitalization).
6. Because of high deductibles proposed and over-whelming emphasis on major illness, further distort the allocation of national health care resources—turning them increasingly toward hospitalization or other institutional treatment and away from prevention, health maintenance, home health care, and other neglected aspects of the system.

7. Strengthen the hands of the insurance companies vis-à-vis national health insurance . . .

9. Further skew manpower away from rural and small town areas by increasing the funds available to pay lucrative specialties in the urban areas . . .

12. Increase the fragmentation and complexities of the financing system. (*Health Security News*, p. 1)

Finally, catastrophic insurance would markedly enhance the position of the private insurance companies, almost guaranteeing that they would take over in any successor comprehensive NHI program.

Insurance against Sickness or for Health?

Because of the huge amounts of money and power involved, the stakes in the outcome of the struggle over the design of an NHI system are higher than in any other major conflict in health care delivery in the United States. The corporate sector, as represented by the commercial insurance industry, is a principal contender in the struggle, since the health care delivery system is one of the few remaining major sectors of the economy offering significant new opportunities for profit-making. The providers, both individual and institutional, as well as the consumers, have major interests in the design of an NHI system. The providers are concerned about their continuing existence in modes acceptable to them; usually, they want little or no change. Consumers want "better" and "cheaper" health services, but often find it difficult to translate those vague desires into feasible, practical proposals.

Among these contending forces and complex issues, we often lose sight of the central question: what is the relationship between national health insurance and health? For the consumer, health service is a means to the end of gaining and maintaining health. Providers are concerned both with the health of the population and with protection of their interests. (Although some providers appear to be more interested in the latter than the former, particularly in the proprietary sectors, most, in their heart of hearts, will put a healthy population first.) The commercial insurance industry, on the other hand, exists primarily to make profits for its shareholders or policy holders and thus that consideration must come first.

In any case, there is little relationship between health and NHI as it is currently being discussed in the United States. In Chapter

2 it was pointed out that for the most part, medical care is not responsible for the improvement in the general health level of the population that has occurred in the past 200 years. Most of the major measurable advances have resulted from improved nutrition, pure water supply and sanitary sewage disposal, environmental sanitation, and communicable disease control; outside of the health field, improved housing, education, and workplace safety have been important factors. One of the major advances involving medical care directly is the use of antibiotics, the proper application of which require medical diagnosis. Another, demonstrated by the reduction in maternal mortality, is the application of asepsis and improved technique to obstetrics.

NHI deals primarily with the financing of medical care, and could secondarily affect the organization of services, depending upon which plan is chosen. Therefore, it would have a limited relationship to measureable health levels in the population, since medical care deals not with health in the population, but sickness in individuals. Curing sickness is extremely important, of course, and should be done as well as possible. Skilled surgery, for example, is of vital importance to persons with acute appendicitis, severe gall-bladder disease, or a subdural hematoma. Any NHI plan must ensure excellence in medical care; however, ensuring health in the population requires other measures. Therefore, even supporters of a national health service responsive to consumers cannot be considered to be dealing with anything more than sickness unless the system is specifically designed to emphasize prevention.

Leon White put it very well:

> The situation reminds me of the old story of the drunk who lost his quarter. The drunk was searching around near a lamppost when a passerby noticed him and asked what he was doing. "Looking for a quarter I lost," replied the drunk. "Where did you lose it?" asked the passerby. "Further down the road," answered the drunk. "Then why are you looking here?" asked the passerby. "Because the light's better," replied the drunk. There is no doubt that the light shines brightest around the health-care system, but is better health to be found there? Maybe we should begin to look elsewhere, if we are really interested in discovering ways to improve health. (White, p. 773)

The ten major killers in the United States are, in order, heart disease, cancer, stroke, accidents, influenza and pneumonia, diabetes mellitus, cirrhosis of the liver, certain problems in early infancy, and bronchitis, emphysema, and asthma (National Center for Health Statistics, June 27, 1974, Table 8). Respiratory system cancer is the fourth leading single cause of death. The ten leading hospital discharge diagnoses are, in order: complications of pregnancy, childbirth, and the puerperium; malignant neoplasms; ischemic heart disease, including myocardial infarction; mental illness; diseases of the urinary system; fractures; tonsillar hypertrophy; other heart and hypertensive disease; infectious disease; and other neoplasms (National Center for Health Statistics, June 10, 1975, Table 1).

A number of these causes of mortality and morbidity, although not all of them, are associated with cigarette smoking, carcinogens in the environment, dysnutrition, alcohol abuse, lack of exercise, unsafe motor vehicles, and unsafe workplaces and iatrogenesis (Report of the Advisory Committee to the Surgeon General; Surgeon General; National Conference on Preventive Medicine,* Report of Task Force III, Sections II and VI, and Volume 6; Susser; Winkelstein; Ross; Terris, 1972, 1975; Meade; Breslow; White; *New York Times*, January 26-30, 1976). NHI can obviously deal with only certain of the major causes of morbidity and mortality. If it has an effective quality control system, it can deal with iatrogenesis. Good medical care per se has been shown to reduce infant mortality (Kessner et al., p. 1). Good medical care can control hypertension and apparently the incidence of complications in diabetes mellitus. Screening procedures, which involve medical care, may be effective measures in the control of hypertension, diabetes, certain cancers, and certain other diseases and conditions (National Conference on Preventive Medicine, Task Force 3 Report and Bibliography). Good all-around health care can certainly make old age more comfortable. Example-setting by health care providers in all personal habits, especially smoking, drinking, diet, and physical fitness might have a positive effect.

Medical care can influence the major environmental risk factors only to the extent that it can affect individual decision-making on a one-to-one basis. It is unlikely that individual per-

*Since this chapter was written, the major task force reports of the National Conference on Prevention (1975) were published in several volumes under the general title *Preventive Medicine, U.S.A.*, by Prodist, in New York (1976).

suasion will do much to lower cigarette and alcohol consumption, or to increase the use of automobile seat-belts. It might have some effect on diet and on getting people to exercise. Individual persuasion is virtually unrelated to making motor vehicles and workplaces safer.

Milton Terris has brought to our attention that alcohol consumption—and cirrhosis of the liver—have been markedly reduced in Great Britain by raising taxes on alcoholic beverages and limiting, but not eliminating, their availability (1975). The same measures could be taken in the United States, for alcohol as well as cigarettes. Taxes, federal and state, could be raised, equalized, and collected at the point of production so that bootlegging from low-tax to high-tax states would prove unprofitable. All advertising of both products could be prohibited, on the assumption that advertising must stimulate sales, since manufacturers would not otherwise bother to advertise. One could go further, setting up a rationing system with increasing cost for increasing consumption, for example, but the simpler measures would probably accomplish the objective.

Controls could be placed on food production and advertising so as to improve the nutritional content of the food which Americans eat. Incentives for weight control, at least, could be conceivably built into the premium structure of an NHI program. It is probably impossible to approach exercise by any other means than individual persuasion. Compulsory seat-belt laws are reported to have reduced traffic-accident fatalities in European countries, as have heavy penalties for drunken driving. A wide variety of other less drastic control measures are available (Baker and Haddon). A simple reduction of the speed limit, when it was enforced, was associated with a drop in motor vehicle accident mortality (Winkelstein). A variety of control measures are available to reduce the levels of environmental carcinogens and to make workplaces safer (National Conference on Preventive Medicine, Volume 6, Part 2).

Some claim that community health service measures that aim at controlling personal habits infringe on individual freedom (Meenan). However, few personal habits affecting health can now be considered entirely personal matters. The public cigarette smoker is polluting others' air. The drunk driver may well kill the innocent. Anyone who increases his risk of a morbid event requiring health care service is increasing the total cost of health care services, which must be borne by the population as a whole.

Some proposed control measures are opposed on the grounds that they may harm important industries and put many people out of work. For example, it is said that lowered cigarette consumption would impoverish many farmers, put tobacco companies out of business and their employees out of work, reduce the incomes of advertising agencies, and harm the newspaper and magazine industries. This is all true. It means that the American people are subsidizing tobacco farmers, the cigarette industry, advertising agencies, and the major newspapers and magazines with millions if not billions of dollars spent on health services that would not be needed if people did not smoke cigarettes. Worse, the subsidy is also made in the form of unnecessary suffering during life and needless premature death. Let tobacco farmers grow food, and provide subsidies as necessary. Let the tobacco companies diversify, with government assistance if necessary, as many of them are already doing. And let the advertising and publishing industries adjust to a changed financial environment, just as the television industry did after cigarette advertising was banned.

It is preventive measures of this kind—rather than utilization controls or even health care delivery system reform—that will best effect cost control: by raising health levels, they will reduce the need for sickness services. Much of the debate over NHI in the United States deals with how to rearrange the existing pieces of the system. Even those who advocate improving hospital environments for both staff and patient and making doctors different kinds of people are still talking about doctors and hospitals—that is, about sickness, not health.

Clearly, the delivery of personal health services is important; reform of the United States health care delivery system is essential; and the design of an NHI program will have a critical impact on the future shape of that system. Still, even a superb NHI system, one guaranteeing access for all persons to high quality health care humanely delivered, with due emphasis on personal preventive measures, will not solve our health problems as long as cigarette smoking and alcohol drinking are unabated, automobile drivers are unbelted, overeaters are sated, the dangers of environmental hazards are underrated, and unsafe workplaces are unregulated. Terris has put it succinctly: ". . . it is a serious error—unfortunately a common one—to consider a national health care program as synonymous with a national health program. The health of a population is determined only in part by the health care system. . . . Prevention should be made the keystone of the national health program . . ." (1972).

References

Anderson, O. W. *The Uneasy Equilibrium: Private and Public Financing of Health Services in the United States, 1875–1965.* New Haven, Conn.: College and University Press, 1968.

Baker, S. P., and Haddon, W. "Reducing Injuries and Their Results: The Scientific Approach." *Health and Society, 52,* 377, 1974.

Bills, S. S. "National Health Insurance: The Battle Takes Shape." *Hospitals, J.A.H.A.,* April 16, 1975, p. 126.

Boas, F. P. "Why Do We Need National Health Insurance?" Society for Ethical Culture, 1945. Reprinted in Committee on Medical Care Teaching of the Association of Teachers of Preventive Medicine, *Readings in Medical Care,* p. 655. Chapel Hill: University of North Carolina Press, 1958.

Bodenheimer, T. "The Hoax of National Health Insurance." *American Journal of Public Health, 62,* 1324, 1972.

Bodenheimer, T. et al., eds. *Billions for Band-Aids, An Analysis of the U.S. Health Care System and of Proposals for Its Reform.* San Francisco, Calif.: San Francisco Bay Area Chapter, Medical Committee for Human Rights, 1972.

Breslow, L. "A Quantitative Approach to the World Health Organization Definition of Health: Physical, Mental and Social Well-Being." *International Journal of Epidemiology, 1,* 347, 1972.

Brian, E. "Medi-Cal Criticisms in Perspective." *Medical Care, 13,* 360, 1975.

Brian, E. W., and Gibbens, S. F. "California's Medi-Cal Copayment Experiment." *Medical Care, 12,* Supplement, December, 1974.

Burns, E. M. "Health Insurance: Not If, or When, But What Kind?" *American Journal of Public Health, 61,* 2164, 1971.

Burrow, J. G. *AMA: Voice of American Medicine.* Baltimore, Md.: Johns Hopkins Press, 1963.

Committee for a National Health Service. *Summary of a Bill to Create a National Health Service.* Box 2125, New York, N.Y., 10001, 1976.

Committee on the Costs of Medical Care. *Medical Care for the American People.* Chicago, Ill.: University of Chicago Press, 1932. Reprinted, Washington, D.C.: USDHEW, 1970.

Committee on Ways and Means, House of Representatives. *National Health Insurance Resource Book*. Washington, D.C.: Government Printing Office, 1974.

Congressional Budget Office. *Estimates of Minimal Costs of Health Services*. Washington, D.C.: U.S. Congress, 1976.

Consumers' Union. "National Health Insurance: Which Way to Go?" February, 1975, p. 118.

Davenport, R. W. "Health Insurance is Next." *Fortune*, March, 1950, p. 63. Reprinted in Committee on Medical Care Teaching of the Association of Teachers of Preventive Medicine, *Readings in Medical Care*, p. 640. Chapel Hill: University of North Carolina Press, 1958.

Davis, K. "Hospital Costs and the Medicare Program." *Social Security Bulletin, 36*, 18, 1973.

Davis, K. "Equal Treatment and Unequal Benefits: The Medicare Program." *Health and Society, 53*, 449, 1975 (a).

Davis, K. *National Health Insurance: Benefits, Costs, and Consequences*. Washington, D.C.: The Brookings Institution, 1975 (b).

Dellums, R. "Health Rights and Community Health Services." *Congressional Record*, October 17, 1974.

Douglas-Wilson, I., and McLachlan, G. *Health Service Prospects: An International Survey*. Boston: Little, Brown, 1973.

Eilers, R. D. "National Health Insurance: What Kind and How Much." Parts 1 and 2. *New England Journal of Medicine, 284*, 881, 945, 1971.

Eilers, R. D., and Moyerman, S. S. *National Health Insurance: Proceedings of the Conference on National Health Insurance*. Homewood, Ill.: R. D. Irwin, 1971.

Falk, I. S. "Medical Care in the USA—1932–1972. Problems, Proposals and Programs *from the* Committee on the Costs of Medical Care *to the* Committee for National Health Insurance." *Health and Society, 51*, 1, 1973.

Finance Committee, United States Senate. *Medicare and Medicaid: Problems, Issues and Alternatives*. Washington, D.C., February 9, 1970.

Freeland, R. M. *The Truman Doctrine and the Origins of McCarthyism*. New York: Knopf, 1975.

Fry, J., and Farndale, W. A. J., eds. *International Medical Care*. Oxford, England: MTP, 1972.

Greenlick, M. R. "California's Medi-Cal Copayment Experiment." *Medical Care, 12*, 1054, 1974.

Harris, R. "Annals of Legislation: Medicare." *The New Yorker*, July 2, July 9, July 16, July 23, 1966.

Health-PAC. "Medicaid: The Fading of a Dream." *Bulletin*, April, 1973, p. 13.

Health Security News. "Catastrophic Still a Threat." October–November, 1974, p. 1.

Hopkins, C. E. et al. "Cost-Sharing and Prior Authorization Effects on Medicaid Services in California: Part I: The Beneficiaries' Reactions." *Medical Care, 13,* 582, 1975.

———. "Cost-Sharing and Prior Authorization Effects on Medicaid Services in California: Part II: The Providers' Reactions." *Medical Care, 13,* 643, 1975.

H. R. 1. "The National Health Care Services Reorganization and Financing Act." House of Representatives, Washington, D.C., 1975.

H. R. 6222. "Comprehensive Health Care Insurance Act of 1975." House of Representatives, Washington, D.C., 1975.

Institute for Policy Studies. *Model Legislation for a National Community Health Service.* Washington, D.C.: Community Health Alternatives Project, 1976.

Jonas, S. "Issues in National Health Insurance in the United States of America." *The Lancet,* July 20, 1974, p. 413. (a)

Jonas, S. "Review Article: Billions for Band-Aids." *International Journal of Health Services, 4,* 723, 1974. (b)

Jonas, S. "Japan Strains under Complex Health System." *Hospitals, J.A.H.A.,* September 1, 1975. (a)

Jonas, S. "The Economy and Health Care Policy: The Corporatization of American Medical Practice." Presented at the Annual Meeting of the American Public Health Association, November, 1975, Chicago, Illinois. (b)

Jonas, S. "Copayment and National Health Insurance in the United States: A Critique of Work by Newhouse, Phelps and Schwartz." *International Journal of Health Services, 7* (2), 1977.

Kane, R. L. et al., eds. *The Health Gap: Medical Services and the Poor.* New York: Springer Publishing Co., 1976.

Kasten, J. "California's Medi-Cal Copayment Experiment." *Medical Care, 12,* 1958, 1974.

Kennedy, E. M. "A Complete Plan of Health Care for All Americans." *Congressional Record,* January 15, 1975.

Kessner, D. M. et al. *Infant Death: An Analysis by Maternal Risk and Health Care.* Washington, D.C.: Institute of Medicine, 1973.

Kindig, D. A., and Sidel, V. W. "Impact of National Health Insurance Plans on the Consumer." Ch. 1 in Eilers, R. D., and Moyerman, S. S., *National Health Insurance.* Homewood, Ill.: Richard D. Irwin, 1971.

Kotelchuk, R., and Levy, H. "MCHR: An Organization in Search of an Identity." *Health/PAC Bulletin,* March/April, 1975, p. 1.

Lander, L. "National Health Insurance: He Who Pays the Piper Lets the Piper Call the Tune." New York: Health/PAC, 1975.

Law, S. A. *Blue Cross: What Went Wrong?* New Haven, Conn.: Yale
     University Press, 1974.
Le Clair, M. "The Canadian Health Care System." Ch. 1 in Andreopou-
     los, S., ed., *National Health Insurance: Can We Learn From
     Canada?* New York: John Wiley, 1975.
Lynch, M. J., and Raphael, S. S. *Medicine and the State.* Springfield,
     Ill.: Charles C Thomas, 1963.
McKittrick, L. S. "Medical Care for the American People: Is Compul-
     sory Health Insurance the Solution? *New England Journal of
     Medicine, 240,* 998, 1949. Reprinted in Committee on Medical Care
     Teaching of the Association of Teachers of Preventive Medicine,
     Readings in Medical Care, p. 647. Chapel Hill: University of
     North Carolina Press, 1958.
McMahon, J. A. *Statement of the American Hospital Association on
     National Health Insurance before the Health Subcommittee of the
     House Committee on Ways and Means, November 10, 1975.* Wash-
     ington, D.C.: American Hospital Association.
Meade, T. W. "Our Lives and Hard Times." *The Lancet,* November 29,
     1975, p. 1953.
Meenan, R. F. "Improving the Public's Health—Some Further Reflec-
     tions." *New England Journal of Medicine, 294,* 45, 1976.
Myers, B. A. "California's Medi-Cal Copayment Experiment." *Medical
     Care, 12,* 1051, 1974.
National Center for Health Statistics. "Provisional Statistics: Annual
     Summary for the United States, 1973." *Monthly Vital Statistics
     Report.* Vol. 22, June 27, 1974.
————. "Utilization of Short-Stay Hospitals, by Diagnosis: United
     States, 1973." *Monthly Vital Statistics Report.* Vol. 24, June 10,
     1975.
————. "Selected Vital and Health Statistics in Poverty and Nonpov-
     erty Areas of 19 Large Cities, United States, 1969–71." *Vital and
     Health Statistics,* Series 21, No. 26, November, 1975.
National Conference on Preventive Medicine. *Report.* Bethesda, Md.:
     Fogarty International Center, May, 1975.
Navarro, V. "The Political Economy of Medical Care." *International
     Journal of Health Services, 5,* 65, 1975.
Newhouse, J. P. et al. "Policy Options and the Impact of National
     Health Insurance." *New England Journal of Medicine, 290,* 1345,
     1974.
New York Academy of Medicine. "Toward a National Health Pro-
     gram." The 1971 Health Conference. *Bulletin of the New York
     Academy of Medicine, 48,* January, 1972.
New York Times. "Cuts in Medicaid Put into Effect." September 30,
     1971.
————. "Fund-Short States Cut Services." December 27, 1975.

————. "The Problem of Incompetent Doctors." Series of five articles, January 26–30, 1976.

Report of the Advisory Committee to the Surgeon General of the Public Health Service. *Smoking and Health.* Washington, D.C.: USDHEW, 1964.

Roemer, M. I. et al. "Copayments for Ambulatory Care: Penny-Wise and Pound-Foolish." *Medical Care, 13,* 457, 1975.

Ross, R. S. "The Case for Prevention of Coronary Heart Disease." *Circulation, 51,* May, 1975.

Salmon, J. W. "The Health Maintenance Organization Strategy: A Corporate Takeover of Health Services Delivery." *International Journal of Health Services, 5,* 609, 1975.

S. 1438. "Natural Healthcare Act of 1975." U.S. Senate, 94th Congress, 1st Session.

S. 3 "The Health Security Act." U.S. Senate, Washington, D.C., 1975.

Schwartz, H. *The Case for American Medicine: A Realistic Look at Our Health Care System.* New York: David McKay, 1972.

Sigerist, H. E. *On the Sociology of Medicine.* Edited by M. I. Roemer. New York: MD Publications, 1960.

Somers, H. M., and Somers, A. R. *Doctors, Patients, and Health Insurance.* Washington, D.C.: The Brookings Institution, 1961.

Stevens, R. *American Medicine and the Public Interest.* New Haven, Conn.: Yale University Press, 1971.

Surgeon General of the United States. *The Health Consequences of Smoking.* Washington, D.C.: USDHEW, 1967. (See also subsequent reports, 1968–1974.)

Susser, M., chairman. "Prevention and Health Maintenance Revisited." *Bulletin of the New York Academy of Medicine,* 2nd Series, *51,* 5–258, 1975.

Terris, M. "The Need for a National Health Program." *Bulletin of the New York Academy of Medicine,* 2nd Series, *48,* 24, 1972.

Terris, M. "Breaking the Barriers to Prevention: Legislative Approaches." *Bulletin of the New York Academy of Medicine,* 2nd Series, *51* 242, 1975.

Truman, H. S. *Message from the President of the United States, Transmitting His Request for Legislation for Adoption of a National Health Program.* 79th Congress, 1st Session. Washington, D.C.: Government Printing Office, 1945. Reprinted in: Committee on Medical Care Teaching of the Association of Teachers of Preventive Medicine, *Readings in Medical Care,* p. 629. Chapel Hill: University of North Carolina Press, 1958.

USDHEW. *Estimated Health Expenditures under Selected National Health Insurance Bills.* A Report to the Congress, 1974.

Vogel, R. J., and Blair, R. D. *Health Insurance Administrative Costs.* Washington, D.C.: USDHEW, 1975.

Washington Report on Medicine and Health. "Social Security Adminis-
    tration Officials." November 3, 1975.
White, L. S. "How to Improve the Public's Health." *New England Jour-
    nal of Medicine, 293,* 773, 1975.
Wilson, F. A., and Neuhauser, D. *Health Services in the United States.*
    Cambridge, Mass.: Ballinger, 1974.
Winkelstein, W. "Contemporary Perspectives on Prevention." *Bulletin
    of the New York Academy of Medicine,* 2nd Series, *51,* 27, 1975.
Worthington, N. L. "Expenditures for Hospital Care and Physicians'
    Services: Factors Affecting Annual Changes." *Social Security
    Bulletin,* November, 1975. p. 3.

Appendix I

Sources of Data

Introduction

This guide to the principal sources of health and health services data for the United States has two parts. Part A contains descriptions of the major data sources: who publishes them, how frequently they are published as of 1976, from whom they may be ordered, and what categories of data they contain. All of the tables in the text that derive from sources listed here (that is, all tables from recurring sources), are keyed to Part A—for example, source notes to text tables taken from the *Statistical Abstract of the United States* include the phrase "(See Appendix I, A1)" at the end of the relevant bibliographical information.

Part B lists categories of data and indicates in which publications they can be found. Most of the data sources are obviously the same as those described in Part A; they are simply looked at from a different perspective. Each source listed in Part B that appears in Part A is keyed to Part A so that the reader may locate it with ease.

Using this appendix and the keys in those text tables that derive from recurring sources, the reader can keep the book—or at least the tables—up-to-date. He must determine for himself whether the text has become out-of-date in light of new data.

A. Major Sources of Data

1. *Statistical Abstract of the United States*
   Published annually by the Bureau of the Census, Social and Economic Statistics Administration, U.S. Department of Commerce, Washington, D.C.* The *Statistical Abstract* reproduces a vast selection of tables containing informa-

---

* Almost all U.S. government publications are to be purchased from the Government Printing Office (GPO), Washington, D.C., 20402, rather than directly from the agency producing them.

tion from many different government agencies. They are accumulated under the following headings: Population; Vital Statistics, Health and Nutrition; Immigration and Naturalization; Education; Law Enforcement, Federal Courts, and Prisons; Geography and Environment; Public Lands, Parks, Recreation and Travel; Federal Government Finances and Employment; State and Local Government Finances and Employment; Social Insurance and Welfare Services; National Defense and Veterans Affairs; Labor Force, Employment, and Earnings; Income, Expenditure, and Wealth; Prices; Elections; Banking, Finance and Insurance; Business Enterprise; Communications; Energy; Science; Transportation—Land; Transportation—Air and Water; Agriculture; Forests and Forest Products; Fisheries; Mining and Mineral Products; Construction and Housing; Manufacturers Distribution and Services; Foreign Commerce and Aid; and Comparative International Statistics.

2. *U.S. Census of Population*
The Bureau of the Census is part of the Social and Economic Statistics Administration of the U.S. Department of Commerce, Washington, D.C., 20233. The Constitution requires that a census be taken every 10 years, at the beginning of each decade. The original purpose was to apportion seats in the House of Representatives and thus in the Electoral College. In modern times, in addition to the simple counts, a great deal of demographic data is collected by the Census Bureau. Hardcover compendia of decennial national census data are published periodically. Also available are special analyses for a wide variety of geographical subdivisions of the country. Many reports on the decennial censuses are published by the Census Bureau, but a good place to begin is in Section 1 of the *Statistical Abstract*.

3. *Current Population Reports*
In addition to reports from the decennial censuses, the Census Bureau publishes eight series of reports on a continuing basis. These include estimates, projections, sample counts, and special studies of selected segments of the population. The eight series each have a "P" number. They

are: P-20, Population Characteristics; P-23, Special
Studies; P-25, Population Estimates and Projections; P-26,
Federal-State Cooperative Program for Population Estimates; P-27, Farm Population; P-28, Special Censuses;
P-60, Consumer Income; P-65, Consumer Buying Indicators. Information on the content of each series is of course
available from the Census Bureau. Subscriptions are not
available for individual series but must be taken for the
whole set. However, single copies of reports from all series
except P-28 may be ordered from the GPO.

4. *Monthy Vital Statistics Report*
   This report, which is published by the National Center for
   Health Statistics of the Health Resources Administration
   of the USDHEW, 5600 Fishers Lane, Rockville, Md., 20852,
   has several sections. *Provisional Statistics*, published
   monthly, contains the most recent data for the traditional
   "Vital Statistics"—deaths, births, marriages, and divorces.
   There are also a series of "Supplements," containing a
   variety of data, which appear on a semiregular basis. They
   include data from the *Health Interview Survey;* the *Hospi-*
   tal Discharge Survey (which contains data in the following
   categories: Utilization of Short-Stay Hospitals—Nonmedical Statistics; Utilization of Short-Stay Hospitals, by
   Diagnosis; and Surgery in Short-Stay Hospitals); the
   National Ambulatory Medical Care Survey; and *Final*
   Statistics for each year for deaths, births, marriages, and
   divorces. (See Chapter 3 for a further description of these
   data sources.) This publication may be ordered by annual
   subscription; one subscription covers all of the regular reports and the supplements.

5. *Vital Statistics of the United States*
   This is the annual report of the National Center for Health
   Statistics (NCHS) concerning vital statistics. The address
   of the NCHS is given above.

6. *Vital and Health Statistics*
   This periodic publication of the NCHS appears at irregular intervals. There are 12 series, not numbered consecutively, most of which report data from ongoing studies and
   surveys that the NCHS carries out. In recent years, some

reporting of data—from, for example, the *Hospital Discharge Survey* and the *National Ambulatory Medical Care Survey*—has been shifted to *Monthly Vital Statistics Report*. Periodically, the NCHS publishes a useful guide, *Current Listing and Topical Index to the Vital and Health Statistics Series*. The 12 series in *Vital and Health Statistics* are as follows:

Series 1. "Programs and Collection Procedures."

Series 2. "Data Evaluation and Methods Research."

Series 3. "Analytical Studies." Primarily of mortality, they stress international comparisons.

Series 4. "Documents and Committee Reports."

Series 10. "Data from the Health Interview Survey." These contain patient-perspective health, illness, and health services utilization data.

Series 11. "Data from the Health Examination Survey."

Series 12. "Data from the Health Records Survey." Reports data from two studies of nursing homes carried out in the 1960s.

Series 13. "Data from the Hospital Discharge Survey." Three categories: by diagnosis, nonmedical statistics, and surgical operations. The HDS now appears in *Monthly Vital Statistics Report*.

Series 14. "Data on Health Resources: Manpower and Facilities." Reports dealing with optometry, ophthalmology, and podiatry. Health resources data now appear principally in *Health Resources Statistics*, a biennial publication of the NCHS.

Series 20. "Data on Mortality." Reports of time-trends analyses for the United States.

Series 21. "Data on Natality, Marriage, and Divorce."

Series 22. "Data from the National Natality and Mortality Surveys." This series differs from the one above in that special studies are reported.

7. *Morbidity and Mortality Weekly Report*

This is a regular publication of the Center for Disease Control (CDC) of the USDHEW, and is available on an annual subscription basis from the CDC, Atlanta, Georgia, 30333. It is concerned primarily with the communicable diseases for which reporting is required by law. Most of the diseases covered are no longer of much importance in the United States, and for many of them the reporting rates are poor. Nevertheless, it provides an important perspective. Each week, case reports of specific outbreaks of communicable diseases are reported; there are also occasional international notes, status reports on communicable disease control programs, and statements of official United States Public Health Service positions on various issues in communicable disease control.

8. *Health Resources Statistics*
   Health Resources Statistics is a formerly annual, now biennial publication of the National Center for Health Statistics. It has three major parts, on manpower, inpatient facilities, and outpatient and nonpatient health services. It is a voluminous work, reporting numbers, distribution, and some facilities and services utilization data. It is the major source of census data on health manpower and facilities in the United States, although the American Hospital Association and American Medical Association do, of course, report data on hospitals and physicians respectively.

9. *Health, United States*
   The first edition of this work was published in 1976 under the title *Health, United States, 1975*. It is not known how frequently it will appear. It is a combined effort of the National Center for Health Statistics and the National Center for Health Services Research and is available from the NCHS. It has four parts: Part A covers "Financial Aspects of the Nation's Health Care"; Part B condenses material from *Health Resources Statistics*; Part C covers "Health Status"; Part D reports on "Use of Health Services." If it continues to appear on a regular basis, it will be a boon to students and researchers on health care delivery because it provides "one-stop shopping" for most important health and health care data.

10. "Guide Issue," *Hospitals, Journal of the American Hospital Association*
    This publication of the American Hospital Association, 840 North Lake Shore Drive, Chicago, Ill., 60611, appears on August 1 of each year. It has two parts. The first, part of the regular journal, contains a listing of almost every hos-

pital in the United States by location, and basic data on size, type, ownership, and facilities, as well as a great deal of information on the AHA and the hospital supply industry. The second part, *Hospital Statistics,* was included through 1972 with part one, but now must be purchased separately. *Hospital Statistics* contains a great deal of summary utilization and financial data on United States hospitals, by many different cross-tabulations. Some of the data are presented historically. The "Guide Issue" and *Hospital Statistics* together contain the most detailed available data on hospitals in the United States.

11. "Hospital Indicators," *Hospitals, J.A.H.A.*
    Appearing in alternate issues of the biweekly journal of the American Hospital Association, "Hospital Indicators" reports up-to-date summary data on utilization, personnel, and finances and also has periodic special studies of particular aspects of hospital operations.

12. *Social Security Bulletin*
    The *Bulletin* is a monthly publication of the Social Security Administration, USDHEW, 1875 Connecticut Ave., N.W., Washington, D.C., 20009. In the winter and/or spring of each year, it publishes two important articles: "National Health Expenditures" for the most recent fiscal year, and "Private Health Insurance" for the fiscal year preceding the most recent one. These articles contain the basic financial data for the health care delivery system. The former also presents summary data going back to 1929. The data include total amount, where the money comes from and where it goes. Monthly, there are summary data on expenditures under SSA programs, as well as Consumer Price Index data.

13. "Datagrams" of the Association of
    American Medical Colleges
    The "Datagrams" were formerly separate publications, but in recent years have appeared monthly in the *Journal of Medical Education.* The AAMC is located at 1 DuPont Circle, Washington, D.C., 20036. Together with the annual issue of the *Journal of the American Medical Association* on medical education (usually the last issue of the year),

"Datagrams" provide the principal source of data on medical education in the United States: schools, faculty, curricula, admissions, students, and the like.

14. Center for Health Services Research and Development of the American Medical Association

The Center, which is located in AMA national headquarters, 535 North Dearborn St., Chicago, Ill., 60610, produces a wide variety of very useful data on physician manpower from its own files. Two annual or biennial publications containing these data, as well as secondary source material, are *Profile of Medical Practice* and *Socioeconomic Issues of Health*. Other major professional organizations are good sources of data on their own members.

B. Categories of Data: Sources
1. Population Data

a. *Statistical Abstract of the United States,* Section 1 (A1)
b. *U.S. Census of Population* (A2)
c. *Current Population Reports* (A3)
d. State and local governments. Some state and local governments, and/or state and local independent planning agencies use detailed Census Bureau data on their local areas which the Bureau does not routinely publish, to produce very detailed compendia of local and/or state census data. Local inquiries must be made to determine if such information is available for a particular area.
e. Utility companies. In many parts of the country, utility companies publish, on a regular, periodic basis, estimates of population changes since the most recent census, and often add other information, particularly concerning economic growth. Local inquiries should be made.

2. Vital Statistics

a. *Monthly Vital Statistics Report* (A4)
b. *Vital Statistics of the United States* (A5)
c. *Vital and Health Statistics* (A6). Summary vital statistics data appear from time to time in Series 3, 20, 21, and 22.
d. Life Tables. These indicators, which are based on mortality data, are published independently, and periodically, by the National Center for Health Statistics.
e. *Statistical Abstract of the United States* (A1). Selected

vital statistics appear annually in Section 2, "Vital Statistics, Health and Nutrition," in about 30 tables.

f. Health Departments. Some state and local health departments publish compendia of vital statistics for their jurisdictions.

g. *Current Population Reports* (A3). Fertility data, which are regarded technically as vital statistics, are collected by the Bureau of the Census and published in Current Population Reports, Series P-20.

3. Morbidity

a. *Vital and Health Statistics* (A6). A wide variety of morbidity data from many different sources is published periodically in Series 10, 11, 12, and 13.

b. *Monthly Vital Statistics Report* (A4). Although they are not technically vital statistics, a variety of morbidity data, some of which also appear, or have appeared, in *Vital and Health Statistics,* are published on an irregular basis. They include data from the *Health Interview Survey,* the *National Ambulatory Medical Care Survey,* and the *Hospital Discharge Survey.*

c. *Morbidity and Mortality Weekly Report* (A7)

d. *Statistical Abstract of the United States* (A1). Selected morbidity statistics appear annually in Section 2, "Vital Statistics, Health and Nutrition," in about 10 tables.

e. Health Departments. State and local health departments sometimes publish morbidity surveys for their jurisdictions.

4. Utilization of Health Services

a. *Vital and Health Statistics* (A6). Series 10 presents patient-perspective data from the *Health Interview Survey.* Provider-perspective data are provided from the *National Ambulatory Medical Care Survey* (Series 2) and the *Hospital Discharge Survey* (Series 13).

b. *Monthly Vital Statistics Report* (A4). Provider-perspective ambulatory service data are provided from the *National Ambulatory Medical Care Survey.* Provider-perspective hospital utilization data are provided from the *Hospital Discharge Survey.*

c. "Guide Issue," *Hospitals, J.A.H.A.* (A10)

d. "Hospital Indicators" (A11)

e. *Health, United States* (A9). Part D contains patient- and provider-perspective utilization data.

f. American Medical Association (A14). *Profile of Medical Practice* and *Socioeconomic Issues in Health* present provider-perspective utilization data.

5. Institutions

a. *Statistical Abstract of the United States* (A1). Basic data on health care institutions is contained in Section 2.

b. *Vital and Health Statistics* (A6). Data on institutions appear in Series 12, 13, and 14.

c. *Health Resources Statistics* (A8). Parts II and III.

d. *Health, United States* (A9). Part B.

e. "Guide Issue," *Hospitals, J.A.H.A.* (A10)

f. "Hospital Indicators" (A11)

g. "Datagrams" (A13)

6. Health Manpower

a. *Statistical Abstract of the United States* (A1)

b. *Vital and Health Statistics* (A6). Series 14.

c. *Health Resources Statistics* (A8). Part I.

d. *Health, United States* (A9). Part B.

e. *Center for Health Services Research and Development of the AMA* (A14)

7. Financing

a. *Statistical Abstract of the United States* (A1). Section 2.

b. *Health, United States* (A9). Part A.

c. "Guide Issue," *Hospitals, J.A.H.A.* (A10). Certain financial data concerning hospitals appear.

d. "Hospital Indicators" (A11). Certain financial data concerning hospitals appear.

e. *Social Security Bulletin* (A12)

f. "Datagrams" (A13). Certain financial data concerning medical schools appear.

g. Center for Health Services Research and Development of the AMA (A14). Certain financial data concerning physicans appear.

Appendix II

Additional Topics

Dentistry

An excellent introduction to and overview of the dental health care system in the U. S. is provided by *Oral Health, Dentistry, and the American Public: The Need for an Improved Oral Care Delivery System,* edited by William E. Brown (Norman, Okla.: University of Oklahoma Press, 1974). It presents, with commentaries, six papers prepared at the behest of the Dental Health Research and Education Advisory Committee, National Institutes of Health. The papers are extensively referenced. Two additional papers typifying the organized approach to problems of dental health services are:

Hirsch, G. B., and Killingworth, W. R. "A New Framework for Projecting Dental Manpower Requirements." *Inquiry, 12,* 126, 1975.

Wan, W. T. H., and Yates, A. S. "Prediction of Dental Utilization: A Multivariate Approach." *Inquiry, 12,* 143, 1975.

Nursing Homes

The nursing home industry is one which is periodically wracked with scandal and revelations of shockingly poor care, as we pointed out in Chapter 7. Among the works which deal with such problems are:

Moreland Act Commission. *Regulating Nursing Home Care: The Paper Tigers.* Albany, N.Y., October, 1975.

Subcommittee on Long-Term Care. *Nursing Home Care in the United States: Failure in Public Policy.* Washington, D.C.: Special Committee on Aging, U.S. Senate, November, 1974.

Temporary State Commission on Living Costs and the Economy. *Report on Nursing Homes and Health Related Facilities in New York State.* Albany, N.Y., April, 1975.

Thomas, W. C. *Nursing Homes and Public Policy: Drift and Decision in New York State.* Ithaca, N.Y.: Cornell University Press, 1969.

There is also an academic literature dealing with nursing homes. Among the more important papers are:

Earle, P. W. "The Nursing Home Industry. Parts 1 and 2." *Hospitals, J.A.H.A.*, Feb. 16, 1970, p. 45; March 1, 1970, p. 60.

Frank, K. D. "Government Support of Nursing-Home Care." *New England Journal of Medicine, 287*, 538, 1972.

Kane, R. L. et al. "Is Good Nursing-Home Care Feasible?" *Journal of the American Medical Association, 235*, 516, 1976.

Schwarz, A. et al. "Evaluating Quality of Care in Nursing Homes." *Journal of the American College of Nursing Home Administration, 1*, 9, 1973.

Shulman, D., and Galanter, R. "Reorganizing the Nursing Home Industry: A Proposal." *Health and Society, 54*, 129, 1976.

Solon, J. A. "Medical Care: Its Social and Organizational Aspects: Nursing Homes and Medical Care." *New England Journal of Medicine, 269*, 1067, 1973.

Willard, H.N. "Improving Hospital-Nursing Home Relationships." *Hospitals, J.A.H.A.*, July 16, 1975, p. 57.

Occupational Safety and Health

This is an immense field with an extensive literature. The Occupational Safety and Health Administration of the Department of Labor in Washington, D.C., and the National Institute of Occupational Safety and Health of the National Institutes of Health in Bethesda, Md. are the two principal federal agencies involved in the field. They both maintain lists of current publications. A useful bibliography was published in 1975:

Carnow, B. W. et al. "A Bookshelf on Occupational Health and Safety." *American Journal of Public Health, 65*, 503, 1975.

Among the many books on the subject are:

Bond, R. G. et al. *Environmental Health and Safety in Health Care Facilities.* New York: Macmillan, 1973.

Brodeur, P. *Expendable Americans: The Incredible Story of How Tens of Thousands of Americans—Men and Women—Die Each Year of Preventable Industrial Disease.* New York: Viking Press, 1966.

Commoner, B. *Science and Survival.* New York: Viking Press, 1966.

Page, J. A., and O'Brien, M. W. *Bitter Wages.* New York: Grossman Publishers, 1972.

Scott, R. *Muscle and Blood.* New York: E. P. Dutton, 1974.

Stellman, J. M., and Daum. S. M. *Work Is Dangerous to Your Health: A Handbook of Health Hazards in the Work-Place and What You Can Do About Them.* New York: Vintage Books, 1971.

Work in America: Report of a Special Task Force to the Secretary of Health, Education and Welfare. Foreword by Eliot Richardson. Cambridge, Mass.: MIT Press, 1972.

Pharmaceutical Industry

The production and marketing of drugs forms one of the most important sectors of the health care industry. After all, the right to prescribe prescription drugs is one of the most important powers separating physicians and other health professionals. An important series of papers was published by the *International Journal of Health Services,* Vol. 4, No. 1, pp. 59–204. The authors include Paul Stolley; David Rabin and Patricia Bush; P. E. Sartwell; Henry Simmons; O. L. Wade and Linda Beeley; Benjamin Hodes; Leonard Schifrin; Charlotte Muller; T. Donald Rucher; Sheila West; Jerrold Schneider; Paul Liebman; and D. A. Knapp and D. E. Knapp.

Other papers of interest include:

Business Week. "The Drug Industry's Clouded Future." November 23, 1974.
Doherty, N. "Excess Profits in the Drug Industry and Their Effect on Consumer Expenditures." *Inquiry, 10,* 19, 1973.
Fuchs, V. R. "Drugs: The Key to Modern Medicine." Ch. 5 in V. R. Fuchs, *Who Shall Live?* New York: Basic Books, 1974.
Goddard, J. L. "The Medical Business." *Scientific American,* September, 1973, p. 161.
Murray, M. J. 'The Pharmaceutical Industry: A Study in Corporate Power." *International Journal of Health Services, 4,* 625, 1974.

Prison Health Services

At any one time, there are about 200,000 persons in state and federal prisons, plus an unknown additional number in local government prisons, juvenile detention facilities, and the like. While in prison, the only health services which persons receive will be from prison health services. Among the useful works on this topic are the following:

Alexander, S. "The Captive Patient: The Treatment of Health Problems in American Prisons." *Clearinghouse Review,* May, 1972, p. 163.
American Medical News. "Medical Care behind Bars—a Horror Story." March 11, 1974, p. 13.
Bach-y-Rita, G. "The Prisoner as an Experimental Subject." *Journal of the American Medical Association, 229,* July 11, 1974.

Goldsmith, S. "The Status of Prison Health Care: A Review of the Literature." *Public Health Reports, 89,* 569, 1974.
Health-PAC Bulletin. "Prison Health." No. 53, September, 1973.
Jails and Prisons Task Force, Program Development Board. *Standards for the Health Services in Correctional Institutions.* Washington, D.C.: American Public Health Association, 1976.
Prout, C. "Massachusetts Department of Public Health; Prison Health Services." *New England Journal of Medicine, 290,* April 11, 1974.
Steinwald, C. et al. *Medical Care in U.S. Jails.* Chicago, Ill.: American Medical Association, 1973.
Turin, E. et al. "Hospital Operates Health Program at Jail." *Hospitals,* July 16, 1975.

Rural Health Care

Health services for Americans living in rural areas have always presented serious problems. A classic in the field is *Rural Medicine* by F. D. Mott, one of the monograph series published for the Committee on Medicine and the Changing Order of The New York Academy of Medicine by The Commonwealth Fund in 1946. This was followed shortly by *Rural Health and Medical Care* by F. D. Mott and M. I. Roemer (New York: McGraw-Hill, 1948).

Among the useful papers published in the 1970s are:

Borhani, N. O., and Kraus, J. F. "Use of Health Services in a Rural Community." *Health Services Reports, 88,* 275, 1973.
Falk, L. A. "The Potential Role of the Medical School in Rural Health Care Delivery." In Nolan, R. L., and Schwartz, J. L., *Rural and Appalachian Health,* pp. 79–95. Springfield, Ill.: Charles C Thomas, 1973.
Fenderson, D. A. "Health Manpower Development and Rural Services." *Journal of the American Medical Association, 225,* 1627, 1973.
Kane, R. L., and Moeller, D. "Rural Service Elements Foil Coordination." *Hospitals, J.A.H.A.,* Oct. 1, 1974, p. 79.
Navarro, V. "The Political and Economic Determinants of Health in Rural America." *Inquiry, 13,* 3, 1976.
Waller, J. A. "Urban-Oriented Methods: Failure to Solve Rural Emergency Care Problems." *Journal of the American Medical Association, 226,* 1441, 1973.

School Health Care

School health services are available to the vast majority of the 60 million schoolchildren in the United States. Among the basic works on school health are:

Eisner, V., and Callan, L. *Dimensions of School Health.* Springfield, Ill.: Charles C Thomas, 1974.

Knotts, G. R., and McGovern, J., eds. *School Health Problems*. Spring-
    field, Ill.: Charles C Thomas, 1975.
Smolensky, J., and Bonvechio, R. *Principles of School Health*. Boston,
    Mass.: Heath & Co,. 1966.
The Journal of School Health is the major academic publication in the
    field.

University Health Services

In 1976, there were about 9 million persons enrolled in institutions of higher education in the United States. An unknown, but
significant proportion of them received all or part of their health
care from services provided by these institutions. The major
source for articles on university health services is the *Journal of
the American College Health Association*. Several useful papers
from the mid-70s are listed.

Burke, W. "Attitudes and the Utilization of Health Services." *Journal
    of the American College Health Association, 22*, April, 1973.
Du Bois, D. "Measuring the Effects and Qualities of College Health
    Programs." *Journal of the American College Health Association,
    21*, April, 1973.
Nichols, D. "Some Recent Data on Community College Health Service
    Programs." *Journal of the American College Health Association,
    22*, October, 1973.
Raymond, R. "The Yale Health Plan." *Yale Alumni Magazine*, March,
    1976, p. 26.
Woody, R. "College Health Services: Demise or Rebirth?" *Journal of
    School Health, 43*, September, 1973.